Soft Tissue Sarcomas: Treatment and Management

Soft Tissue Sarcomas: Treatment and Management

Editors

Shinji Miwa
Po-Kuei Wu
Hiroyuki Tsuchiya

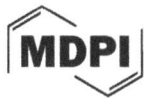

Basel • Beijing • Wuhan • Barcelona • Belgrade • Novi Sad • Cluj • Manchester

Editors

Shinji Miwa
Kanazawa University
Kanazawa
Japan

Po-Kuei Wu
National Yang Ming Chiao
Tung University
Taipei
Taiwan

Hiroyuki Tsuchiya
Kanazawa University
Kanazawa
Japan

Editorial Office
MDPI
St. Alban-Anlage 66
4052 Basel, Switzerland

This is a reprint of articles from the Topic published online in the open access journals *Biology* (ISSN 2079-7737), *Cancers* (ISSN 2072-6694), *Current Oncology* (ISSN 1718-7729), *International Journal of Environmental Research and Public Health* (ISSN 1660-4601), and *Onco* (ISSN 2673-7523) (available at: https://www.mdpi.com/topics/STS).

For citation purposes, cite each article independently as indicated on the article page online and as indicated below:

Lastname, A.A.; Lastname, B.B. Article Title. *Journal Name* **Year**, *Volume Number*, Page Range.

ISBN 978-3-7258-0603-4 (Hbk)
ISBN 978-3-7258-0604-1 (PDF)
doi.org/10.3390/books978-3-7258-0604-1

© 2024 by the authors. Articles in this book are Open Access and distributed under the Creative Commons Attribution (CC BY) license. The book as a whole is distributed by MDPI under the terms and conditions of the Creative Commons Attribution-NonCommercial-NoDerivs (CC BY-NC-ND) license.

Contents

Shinji Miwa, Po-Kuei Wu and Hiroyuki Tsuchiya
Soft Tissue Sarcomas: Treatment and Management
Reprinted from: *Cancers* **2024**, *16*, 1042, doi:10.3390/cancers16051042 1

Yoshinori Imura, Satoshi Takenaka, Hidetatsu Outani, Takaaki Nakai, Naohiro Yasuda, Sho Nakai, et al.
Impact of Surgery and Chemotherapy on Metastatic Extrauterine Leiomyosarcoma
Reprinted from: *Curr. Oncol.* **2022**, *29*, 2301–2311, doi:10.3390/curroncol29040187 6

Saya Tamura, Takuma Hayashi, Tomoyuki Ichimura, Nobuo Yaegashi, Kaoru Abiko and Ikuo Konishi
Characteristic of Uterine Rhabdomyosarcoma by Algorithm of Potential Biomarkers for Uterine Mesenchymal Tumor
Reprinted from: *Curr. Oncol.* **2022**, *29*, 2350–2363, doi:10.3390/curroncol29040190 17

Sebastián Cruz-Morande, Javier Dotor and Mikel San-Julian
P144 a Transforming Growth Factor Beta Inhibitor Peptide, Generates Antifibrogenic Effects in a Radiotherapy Induced Fibrosis Model
Reprinted from: *Curr. Oncol.* **2022**, *29*, 2650–2661, doi:10.3390/curroncol29040217 31

Yeon-Jin Kim, Jai-Min Ryu, Se-Kyung Lee, Byung-Joo Chae, Seok-Won Kim, Seok-Jin Nam, et al.
Primary Angiosarcoma of the Breast: A Single-Center Retrospective Study in Korea
Reprinted from: *Curr. Oncol.* **2022**, *29*, 3272–3281, doi:10.3390/curroncol29050267 43

Na Cao, Hongtao Liang, Ruoyu Zhang, Yanhua Li and Hui Cao
A New Nonlinear Photothermal Iterative Theory for Port-Wine Stain Detection
Reprinted from: *Int. J. Environ. Res. Public Health* **2022**, *19*, 5637, doi:10.3390/ijerph19095637 . . . 52

Ankit Mangla, Gino Cioffi, Jill S. Barnholtz-Sloan and Richard T. Lee
Treatment Outcomes for Primary Hepatic Angiosarcoma: National Cancer Database Analysis 2004–2014
Reprinted from: *Curr. Oncol.* **2022**, *29*, 3637–3646, doi:10.3390/curroncol29050292 64

Manabu Hoshi, Naoto Oebisu, Tadashi Iwai, Yoshitaka Ban and Hiroaki Nakamura
Does Systemic Chemotherapy Influence Skeletal Growth of Young Osteosarcoma Patients as a Treatment-Related Late Adverse Effect?
Reprinted from: *Curr. Oncol.* **2022**, *29*, 4081–4089, doi:10.3390/curroncol29060325 74

Megan Delisle, Bader Alshamsan, Kalki Nagaratnam, Denise Smith, Ying Wang and Amirrtha Srikanthan
Metastasectomy in Leiomyosarcoma: A Systematic Review and Pooled Survival Analysis
Reprinted from: *Cancers* **2022**, *14*, 3055, doi:10.3390/cancers14133055 83

Haidong Zhang, Tianxiang Jiang, Mingchun Mu, Zhou Zhao, Xiaonan Yin, Zhaolun Cai, et al.
Radiotherapy in the Management of Gastrointestinal Stromal Tumors: A Systematic Review
Reprinted from: *Cancers* **2022**, *14*, 3169, doi:10.3390/cancers14133169 105

Xiang Fang, Yan Xiong, Fang Yuan, Senlin Lei, Dechao Yuan, Yi Luo, et al.
Preoperative Planning Using Three-Dimensional Multimodality Imaging for Soft Tissue Sarcoma of the Axilla: A Pilot Study
Reprinted from: *Cancers* **2022**, *14*, 3185, doi:10.3390/cancers14133185 122

Zhengxiao Ouyang, Sally Trent, Catherine McCarthy, Thomas Cosker, Duncan Whitwell, Harriet Branford-White and Christopher Leonard Maxime Hardwicke Gibbons
Nomogram Predicting the Risk of Postoperative Major Wound Complication in Soft Tissue Sarcoma of the Trunk and Extremities after Preoperative Radiotherapy
Reprinted from: *Cancers* **2022**, *14*, 4096, doi:10.3390/cancers14174096 . . . . **134**

Abdulhameed Alfagih, Abdulaziz AlJassim, Bader Alshamsan, Nasser Alqahtani and Timothy Asmis
Gastrointestinal Stromal Tumors: 10-Year Experience in Cancer Center—The Ottawa Hospital (TOH)
Reprinted from: *Curr. Oncol.* **2022**, *29*, 7148–7157, doi:10.3390/curroncol29100562 . . . . **145**

Viktor Grünwald, Daniel Pink, Gerlinde Egerer, Enrico Schalk, Marinela Augustin, Christoph K. W. Deinzer, et al.
Trabectedin for Patients with Advanced Soft Tissue Sarcoma: A Non-Interventional, Prospective, Multicenter, Phase IV Trial
Reprinted from: *Cancers* **2022**, *14*, 5234, doi:10.3390/cancers14215234 . . . . **155**

Jintao Guo, Qichao Ge, Fan Yang, Sheng Wang, Nan Ge, Xiang Liu, et al.
Small Gastric Stromal Tumors: An Underestimated Risk
Reprinted from: *Cancers* **2022**, *14*, 6008, doi:10.3390/cancers14236008 . . . . **170**

Andrea York Tiang Teo, Vivian Yujing Lim and Valerie Shiwen Yang
MicroRNAs in the Pathogenesis, Prognostication and Prediction of Treatment Resistance in Soft Tissue Sarcomas
Reprinted from: *Cancers* **2023**, *15*, 577, doi:10.3390/cancers15030577 . . . . **181**

Silvia Hofer, Leopold Hentschel, Stephan Richter, Veronika Blum, Michael Kramer, Bernd Kasper, et al.
Electronic Patient Reported Outcome (ePRO) Measures in Patients with Soft Tissue Sarcoma (STS) Receiving Palliative Treatment
Reprinted from: *Cancers* **2023**, *15*, 1233, doi:10.3390/cancers15041233 . . . . **203**

Mina Fazel, Armelle Dufresne, Hélène Vanacker, Waisse Waissi, Jean-Yves Blay and Mehdi Brahmi
Immunotherapy for Soft Tissue Sarcomas: Anti-PD1/PDL1 and Beyond
Reprinted from: *Cancers* **2023**, *15*, 1643, doi:10.3390/cancers15061643 . . . . **211**

Munehisa Kito, Keisuke Ae, Masanori Okamoto, Makoto Endo, Kunihiro Ikuta, Akihiko Takeuchi, et al.
Clinical Outcome of Low-Grade Myofibroblastic Sarcoma in Japan: A Multicenter Study from the Japanese Musculoskeletal Oncology Group
Reprinted from: *Cancers* **2023**, *15*, 2314, doi:10.3390/cancers15082314 . . . . **225**

Katharina Seidensaal, Matthias Dostal, Andreas Kudak, Cornelia Jaekel, Eva Meixner, Jakob Liermann, et al.
Preoperative Dose-Escalated Intensity-Modulated Radiotherapy (IMRT) and Intraoperative Radiation Therapy (IORT) in Patients with Retroperitoneal Soft-Tissue Sarcoma: Final Results of a Clinical Phase I/II Trial
Reprinted from: *Cancers* **2023**, *15*, 2747, doi:10.3390/cancers15102747 . . . . **237**

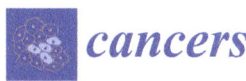

Editorial

Soft Tissue Sarcomas: Treatment and Management

Shinji Miwa [1,*], Po-Kuei Wu [2,3,4] and Hiroyuki Tsuchiya [1]

1. Department of Orthopedic Surgery, Graduate School of Medical Sciences, Kanazawa University, Kanazawa 920-8640, Japan; tsuchi@med.kanazawa-u.ac.jp
2. Department of Orthopedics and Joint Reconstruction, Taipei Veterans General Hospital, Taipei 112, Taiwan; drwuvgh@gmail.com
3. Orthopedic Department of Medicine, National Yang Ming Chiao Tung University, Taipei 112, Taiwan
4. Therapeutical and Research Center of Musculoskeletal Tumor, Taipei Veterans General Hospital, Taipei 112, Taiwan
* Correspondence: smiwa001@yahoo.co.jp

1. Introduction

Due to the rarity and heterogeneity of soft tissue sarcoma (STS), investigating new treatments for this condition has been challenging. Although intensive chemotherapy and the establishment of surgical procedures have improved the outcome of patients with STS, there are ongoing issues such as limited anticancer agents, a high incidence of postoperative complications, and an unsatisfactory curative rate for recurrent/metastatic STS. To improve the clinical outcomes of patients with STS, there is a need for further investigations into molecular biology, the microenvironment, anticancer agents, and the management of STS. Thus, this Special Issue collates various high-quality original/review articles on basic and clinical research into STS.

2. An Overview of Published Articles

This Special Issue comprises both original and review articles focusing on systemic treatment and complications in STS management. Grünwald et al. conducted a prospective phase 4 study assessing the use of trabectedin in 128 patients with STS [contribution 1]. The progression-free survival rates at 3 and 6 months were 61% and 45%, respectively. Of the study participants, 1 patient had a complete response, 14 had a partial response, and the objective response rate was 12%. Common grade 3/4 adverse events included leukopenia (27%), thrombocytopenia (16%), neutropenia (13%), and increased alanine aminotransferase (11%). Two patients died as a result of sepsis and pneumonia, and these were deemed to be treatment-related adverse events. Hoshi et al. investigated the influence of systemic chemotherapy on skeletal growth in 20 patients (aged ≤18 years) with osteosarcoma [contribution 2]. According to their findings, systemic chemotherapy did not inhibit skeletal growth in young patients with osteosarcoma. Fazel et al. summarized the state of the art of immunotherapy in STS in their review article [contribution 3]. Recent clinical studies on immune checkpoint inhibitors suggest that the efficacy of this treatment was limited, necessitating further studies on combination therapies, innovative adoptive therapies, and biomarkers. To assess global health-related quality of life during treatment with pazopanib or physician-preferred chemotherapy over a 9-week period, a prospective, randomized, controlled, multicenter study (PazoQoL) was designed [contribution 4]. Although the study was discontinued due to the pandemic, continuous electronic patient-reported outcomes enabled early detection of the onset of deterioration and initiation of countermeasures. The Time Trade-off demonstrated that the prolongation of life and the side effect profile of continued therapy failed to meet patients' expectations.

This Special Issue also includes three articles on gastrointestinal stromal tumors (GISTs). Management of small gastrointestinal stromal tumors (GISTs), which are less than

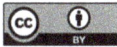

2 cm in size, remains controversial. Guo et al. reported a high overall mutation rate (96%) and high mutation rate of oncogenic BRAF-V600E in small GISTs [contribution 5]. Although previous studies showed a significantly lower mutation rate of small GISTs compared with large tumors [1–3], these results indicate that genetic alterations are common in early GIST generation. Alfagih et al. presented pathological data, management strategies, and clinical outcomes of 248 patients diagnosed with GISTs in a single cancer center [contribution 6]. At diagnosis, 206 patients (83%) had a localized tumor. A total of 213 patients (86%) underwent curative surgical resection, while 49 patients (20%) underwent adjuvant imatinib. The 5-year overall survival rates of patients with low-, intermediate-, high-risk, and advanced tumors were 100%, 94%, 91%, 88%, and 65%, respectively. Univariate analysis revealed that the location of the tumor, Eastern Cooperative Oncology Group performance status, secondary malignancy, size, and mitosis were predictors for overall survival. GISTs are believed to be resistant to radiation therapy [4]. On the other hand, objective responses to radiation therapy have been described in case reports and cases series [5,6]. To assess the role of radiation therapy in GISTs, Zhang et al. conducted a systematic review of radiation therapy for the treatment of GISTs [contribution 7]. In the review, bone was the site most commonly treated with radiation therapy. In the review, radiation therapy showed objective response in some patients with advanced or metastatic GISTs, although no survival benefit was observed. The symptom palliation rate was 79%, and radiation therapy was generally well tolerated. Further studies on radiation therapy for GISTs are needed to identify the indication of radiation therapy for GIST.

Although radiation therapy is thought to be an effective treatment option in patients with high-grade sarcoma, positive margin, or unresectable sarcomas, this type of therapy increases wound complications. Seidensaal et al. conducted a prospective, one-armed, single-center phase 1/2 study on preoperative dose-escalated intensity-modulated radiotherapy (IMRT) and intraoperative radiation therapy (IORT) in patients with retroperitoneal STS [contribution 8]. In their study, 37 patients underwent preoperative IMRT of 45–50 Gy with a simultaneous integrated boost of 50–56 Gy, surgery, and IORT. Twenty-seven participants underwent IORT, thirty-five patients underwent tumor resection, and the surgical margin was positive in twenty-eight patients (80%) and negative in seven patients (20%). The 5-year overall survival rate was 60%. The authors described that stratification by grading and histology should be considered for future studies. Radiation-induced fibrosis, a severe side effect of radiation therapy, is induced by TGF-β1, Smad2/3 phosphorylation, and profibrotic target genes [7,8]. Cruz-Morande et al. reported that P144, a TGF-β1 peptide inhibitor, reduced radiation-induced fibrosis and significantly reduced Smad2/3 phosphorylation [contribution 9]. Further studies on the optimal dosage and timing of P144 administration in model of radiation-induced fibrosis are required. Preoperative radiation therapy increases the risk of postoperative wound complication in the treatment of STS. Ouyang et al. conducted a retrospective study using the Oxford University Hospital database [contribution 10], which included 126 patients with STS who underwent preoperative radiation therapy. In multivariate analysis, age, tumor size, and metastasis were identified as independent risk factors for major wound complication. They also used a nomogram, a useful tool that enables clinicians to assess the risk of major wound complication by graphical calculation of each predictor, and it showed a good predictive value for major wound complications in this study.

This Special Issue also includes several studies on the management of metastatic leiomyosarcomas. Delisle et al. conducted a systematic review and pooled analysis to investigate survival in patients who underwent metastasectomy for leiomyosarcoma and to compare their outcomes based on the site of metastasis [contribution 11]. The median survival rates were 73 months for lung metastasectomy, 35 months for liver metastasectomy, 14 months for spine metastasectomy, and 14 months for brain metastasectomy. Two studies comparing outcomes between patients revealed that metastasectomy was associated with significantly better survival rates. Although these studies were nonrandomized, these data suggest that metastasectomy offers numerous clinical benefits. Imura et al. investigated the clinical features, outcomes, and prognostic factors of metastatic extrauterine leiomyosarcoma [contribution 12]. Sixty-one patients with metastatic extrauterine leiomyosarcoma were included in the retrospective study. The five-year overall survival of the study patients was 38%. Univariate analysis showed that primary tumor size (>10 cm), initial metastatic sites >1, synchronous metastasis, and no metastasectomy were significantly associated with poor overall survival. In multivariate analysis, primary tumor size was identified as an independent prognostic factor for poor overall survival. Among 24 patients who underwent metastasectomy, the interval from the initial diagnosis to development of metastasis ($\leq$6 months) was significantly associated with poor overall survival. In 37 patients without metastasectomy, chemotherapy was significantly associated with better overall survival. This study suggested that metastasectomy and chemotherapy could improve overall survival in patients with metastatic extrauterine leiomyosarcoma.

Due to the rarity of angiosarcoma of the breast, the optimal treatment method remains unclear. Kim et al. reported clinicopathological features, treatment, and oncological outcomes of primary angiosarcomas of the breast [contribution 13]. In their study, 15 patients with primary angiosarcoma of the breast underwent surgical tumor resection. The mean age of the patients was 33 years and mean tumor size was 7.7 cm. The histological grades were low-grade in three cases, intermediate-grade in five cases, high-grade in six cases, and unidentified-grade in one case. The 5-year disease-free and overall survival rates were 24% and 37%, respectively. Histological grade was significantly associated with overall survival ($p = 0.024$). Because the roles of chemotherapy and radiotherapy remain unclear, surgical resection with appropriate surgical margin is thought to be the best approach to treating angiosarcoma of the breast. Mangla et al. investigated the risk of mortality and prognostic factors for primary hepatic angiosarcoma using the National Cancer Database (NCDB) [contribution 14]. In their study, 346 patients with primary hepatic angiosarcoma were included. The mean age of the patients was 63 years. One-third of the patients (36%) underwent chemotherapy, while 15% underwent surgical tumor resection. The survival rates in patients with surgical tumor resection and those without surgical resection were 8 and 2 months, respectively ($p < 0.001$). Patients who underwent chemotherapy had significantly better survival than patients without chemotherapy (5 months vs. 1 month, $p < 0.001$), although no long-term survival benefit was observed.

Kito et al. conducted a retrospective multicenter study that explored the clinical features and prognosis of low-grade myofibroblastic sarcoma [contribution 15]. The study included 24 patients with low-grade myofibroblastic sarcoma; of these, 22 patients underwent surgical tumor resection and 2 patients underwent radiation therapy. The status of the surgical margin was R0 in 14 cases, R1 in 7 cases, and R2 in 1 case. The local recurrence-free survival was 91% at 2 years and 75% at 5 years. The two patients who underwent radiation therapy showed one complete response and one partial response. This study suggests that tumor resection with appropriate surgical margin is considered to be the standard treatment, and radiation therapy is an alternative treatment option in unresectable low-grade myofibroblastic sarcoma.

MicroRNAs (miRNAs), short non-coding RNA molecules, target and modulate various dysregulated genes and/or signaling pathways in cancer cells. miRNAs are believed have utility in the diagnosis, prognosis prediction, and treatment of STS. In their review article, Teo et al. provided an updated discussion of roles and potential use of miRNAs in management of STS [contribution 16].

A computer-generated 3D tumor model can reveal tumor and adjacent neurovascular structures. Fang et al. reported that using a computer-generated 3D tumor model of axillary STS reduced intraoperative blood loss, operative time, and hospital stay [contribution 17]. This technique can be expected to improve operative planning in patients with STS adjacent to important organs.

Cao et al. developed a theoretical model for thermal nonlinear photoacoustic detection related to port-wine stain samples [contribution 18].

Tamura et al. reported a case of pleomorphic rhabdomyosarcoma during the follow-up of a uterine leiomyoma [contribution 19].

In summary, this Special Issue presents a collection of articles that discuss the latest basic and clinical studies on STS. Although there are limited treatment options for patients with STS, recent studies have demonstrated promising therapeutic targets, anticancer agents, and combinations of these treatments. We hope the articles presented in this Special Issue will help improve the management of STS. We greatly appreciate the contributions of the authors of the articles published in this Special Issue.

Conflicts of Interest: The authors declare no conflicts of interest.

List of Contributions

1. Grunwald, V.; Pink, D.; Egerer, G.; Schalk, E.; Augustin, M.; Deinzer CK, W.; Kob, V.; Reichert, D.; Kebenko, M.; Brandl, S.; et al. Trabectedin for Patients with Advanced Soft Tissue Sarcoma: A Non-Interventional, Prospective, Multicenter, Phase IV Trial. *Cancers* **2022**, *14*, 5234.
2. Hoshi, M.; Oebisu, N.; Iwai, T.; Ban, Y.; Nakamura, H. Does Systemic Chemotherapy Influence Skeletal Growth of Young Osteosarcoma Patients as a Treatment-Related Late Adverse Effect? *Curr. Oncol.* **2022**, *29*, 4081–4089.
3. Fazel, M.; Dufresne, A.; Vanacker, H.; Waissi, W.; Blay, J.Y.; Brahmi, M. Immunotherapy for Soft Tissue Sarcomas: Anti-PD1/PDL1 and Beyond. *Cancers* **2023**, *15*, 1643.
4. Hofer, S.; Hentschel, L.; Richter, S.; Blum, V.; Kramer, M.; Kasper, B.; Riese, C.; Schuler, M.K. Electronic Patient Reported Outcome (ePRO) Measures in Patients with Soft Tissue Sarcoma (STS) Receiving Palliative Treatment. *Cancers* **2023**, *15*, 1233.
5. Guo, J.; Ge, Q.; Yang, F.; Wang, S.; Ge, N.; Liu, X.; Shi, J.; Fusaroli, P.; Liu, Y.; Sun, S. Small Gastric Stromal Tumors: An Underestimated Risk. *Cancers* **2022**, *14*, 6008.
6. Alfagih, A.; AlJassim, A.; Alshamsan, B.; Alqahtani, N.; Asmis, T. Gastrointestinal Stromal Tumors: 10-Year Experience in Cancer Center-The Ottawa Hospital (TOH). *Curr. Oncol.* **2022**, *29*, 7148–7157.
7. Zhang, H.; Jiang, T.; Mu, M.; Zhao, Z.; Yin, X.; Cai, Z.; Zhang, B.; Yin, Y. Radiotherapy in the Management of Gastrointestinal Stromal Tumors: A Systematic Review. *Cancers* **2022**, *14*, 3169.
8. Seidensaal, K.; Dostal, M.; Kudak, A.; Jaekel, C.; Meixner, E.; Liermann, J.; Weykamp, F.; Hoegen, P.; Mechtersheimer, G.; Willis, F.; et al Preoperative Dose-Escalated Intensity-Modulated Radiotherapy (IMRT) and Intraoperative Radiation Therapy (IORT) in Patients with Retroperitoneal Soft-Tissue Sarcoma: Final Results of a Clinical Phase I/II Trial. *Cancers* **2023**, *15*, 2747.
9. Cruz-Morande, S.; Dotor, J.; San-Julian, M. P144 a Transforming Growth Factor Beta Inhibitor Peptide, Generates Antifibrogenic Effects in a Radiotherapy Induced Fibrosis Model. *Curr. Oncol.* **2022**, *29*, 2650–2661.
10. Ouyang, Z.; Trent, S.; McCarthy, C.; Cosker, T.; Whitwell, D.; Branford-White, H.; Gibbons, C. Nomogram Predicting the Risk of Postoperative Major Wound Complication in Soft Tissue Sarcoma of the Trunk and Extremities after Preoperative Radiotherapy. *Cancers* **2022**, *14*, 4096.
11. Delisle, M.; Alshamsan, B.; Nagaratnam, K.; Smith, D.; Wang, Y.; Srikanthan, A. Metastasectomy in Leiomyosarcoma: A Systematic Review and Pooled Survival Analysis. *Cancers* **2022**, *14*, 3055.
12. Imura, Y.; Takenaka, S.; Outani, H.; Nakai, T.; Yasuda, N.; Nakai, S.; Wakamatsu, T.; Tamiya, H.; Okada, S. Impact of Surgery and Chemotherapy on Metastatic Extrauterine Leiomyosarcoma. *Curr. Oncol.* **2022**, *29*, 2301–2311.
13. Kim, Y. J.; Ryu, J. M.; Lee, S. K.; Chae, B. J.; Kim, S. W.; Nam, S.J.; Yu, J. H.; Lee, J. E. Primary Angiosarcoma of the Breast: A Single-Center Retrospective Study in Korea. *Curr. Oncol.* **2022**, *29*, 3272–3281.
14. Mangla, A.; Cioffi, G.; Barnholtz-Sloan, J. S.; Lee, R. T. Treatment Outcomes for Primary Hepatic Angiosarcoma: National Cancer Database Analysis 2004–2014. *Curr. Oncol.* **2022**, *29*, 3637–3646.
15. Kito, M.; Ae, K.; Okamoto, M.; Endo, M.; Ikuta, K.; Takeuchi, A.; Yasuda, N.; Yasuda, T.; Imura, Y.; Morii, T.; et al. Clinical Outcome of Low-Grade Myofibroblastic Sarcoma in Japan: A Multicenter Study from the Japanese Musculoskeletal Oncology Group. *Cancers* **2023**, *15*, 2314.
16. Teo, A.Y.T.; Lim, V.Y.; Yang, V.S. MicroRNAs in the Pathogenesis, Prognostication and Prediction of Treatment Resistance in Soft Tissue Sarcomas. *Cancers* **2023**, *15*, 577.

17. Fang, X.; Xiong, Y.; Yuan, F.; Lei, S.; Yuan, D.; Luo, Y.; Zhou, Y.; Min, L.; Zhang, W.; Tu, C.; et al. Preoperative Planning Using Three-Dimensional Multimodality Imaging for Soft Tissue Sarcoma of the Axilla: A Pilot Study. *Cancers* **2022**, *14*, 3185.
18. Cao, N.; Liang, H.; Zhang, R.; Li, Y.; Cao, H. A New Nonlinear Photothermal Iterative Theory for Port-Wine Stain Detection. *Int. J. Environ. Res. Public Health* **2022**, *19*, 5637.
19. Tamura, S.; Hayashi, T.; Ichimura, T.; Yaegashi, N.; Abiko, K.; Konishi, I. Characteristic of Uterine Rhabdomyosarcoma by Algorithm of Potential Biomarkers for Uterine Mesenchymal Tumor. *Curr. Oncol.* **2022**, *29*, 2350–2363.

References

1. Rossi, S.; Gasparotto, D.; Toffolatti, L.; Pastrello, C.; Gallina, G.; Marzotto, A.; Sartor, C.; Barbareschi, M.; Cantaloni, C.; Messerini, L.; et al. Molecular and clinicopathologic characterization of gastrointestinal stromal tumors (GISTs) of small size. *Am. J. Surg. Pathol.* **2010**, *34*, 1480–1491. [CrossRef] [PubMed]
2. Agaimy, A.; Wunsch, P.H.; Hofstaedter, F.; Blaszyk, H.; Rummele, P.; Gaumann, A.; Dietmaier, W.; Hartmann, A. Minute gastric sclerosing stromal tumors (GIST tumorlets) are common in adults and frequently show c-KIT mutations. *Am. J. Surg. Pathol.* **2007**, *31*, 113–120. [CrossRef] [PubMed]
3. Soreide, K. Cancer biology of small gastrointestinal stromal tumors (<2 cm): What is the risk of malignancy? *Eur. J. Surg. Oncol.* **2017**, *43*, 1344–1349. [PubMed]
4. Ahmed, K.A.; Caudell, J.J.; El-Haddad, G.; Berglund, A.E.; Welsh, E.A.; Yue, B.; Hoffe, S.E.; Naghavi, A.O.; Abuodeh, Y.A.; Frakes, J.M.; et al. Radiosensitivity Differences Between Liver Metastases Based on Primary Histology Suggest Implications for Clinical Outcomes After Stereotactic Body Radiation Therapy. *Int. J. Radiat. Oncol. Biol. Phys.* **2016**, *95*, 1399–1404. [CrossRef] [PubMed]
5. Lolli, C.; Pantaleo, M.A.; Nannini, M.; Saponara, M.; Pallotti, M.C.; Scioscio, V.D.; Barbieri, E.; Mandrioli, A.; Biasco, G. Successful radiotherapy for local control of progressively increasing metastasis of gastrointestinal stromal tumor. *Rare Tumors* **2011**, *3*, e49. [CrossRef] [PubMed]
6. Cuaron, J.J.; Goodman, K.A.; Lee, N.; Wu, A.J. External beam radiation therapy for locally advanced and metastatic gastrointestinal stromal tumors. *Radiat. Oncol.* **2013**, *8*, 274. [CrossRef] [PubMed]
7. Randall, K.; Coggle, J.E. Expression of transforming growth factor-beta 1 in mouse skin during the acute phase of radiation damage. *Int. J. Radiat. Biol.* **1995**, *68*, 301–309. [CrossRef] [PubMed]
8. Randall, K.; Coggle, J.E. Long-term expression of transforming growth factor TGF beta 1 in mouse skin after localized beta-irradiation. *Int. J. Radiat. Biol.* **1996**, *70*, 351–360. [CrossRef] [PubMed]

Disclaimer/Publisher's Note: The statements, opinions and data contained in all publications are solely those of the individual author(s) and contributor(s) and not of MDPI and/or the editor(s). MDPI and/or the editor(s) disclaim responsibility for any injury to people or property resulting from any ideas, methods, instructions or products referred to in the content.

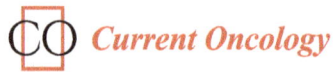

Article

Impact of Surgery and Chemotherapy on Metastatic Extrauterine Leiomyosarcoma

Yoshinori Imura [1,*], Satoshi Takenaka [2], Hidetatsu Outani [1], Takaaki Nakai [1], Naohiro Yasuda [1], Sho Nakai [2], Toru Wakamatsu [2], Hironari Tamiya [2] and Seiji Okada [1]

[1] Department of Orthopaedic Surgery, Osaka University Graduate School of Medicine, 2-2 Yamadaoka Suita, Osaka 565-0871, Japan; h-otani@ort.med.osaka-u.ac.jp (H.O.); taknakai000m@gmail.com (T.N.); o9o5o5442o4@gmail.com (N.Y.); seokada@ort.med.osaka-u.ac.jp (S.O.)

[2] Department of Musculoskeletal Oncology Service, Osaka International Cancer Institute, 3-1-69 Otemae, Osaka 541-8567, Japan; s.takenaka.0816@gmail.com (S.T.); s.nakai.0925@gmail.com (S.N.); evolutionhhh49@yahoo.co.jp (T.W.); tamiyahironari@yahoo.co.jp (H.T.)

* Correspondence: y.imura@ort.med.osaka-u.ac.jp; Tel.: +81-6-6879-3552

Abstract: Background: Few studies have described the characteristics and prognostic factors of patients with metastatic extrauterine leiomyosarcoma (euLMS). Therefore, we retrospectively investigated the clinicopathological features, clinical outcomes, and prognostic factors of patients with euLMS. Methods: We recruited 61 patients with metastatic euLMS treated from 2006 to 2020 and collected and statistically analyzed information on patient-, tumor-, and treatment-related factors. The median follow-up period was 21.1 months. Results: Sixty-one patients with euLMS and a median age of 59 years were included. Furthermore, their five-year overall survival (OS) rate was 38.3%. Univariate analysis revealed that primary tumor size >10 cm, synchronous metastasis, initial metastatic sites >1, and no metastasectomy with curative intent were significantly associated with poor OS rate. Multivariate analysis identified primary tumor size >10 cm as an independent prognostic factor for poor OS. Among 24 patients who received metastasectomy with curative intent, the interval from the initial diagnosis to development of metastasis ≤6 months was significantly correlated with unfavorable OS. Among 37 patients who did not receive metastasectomy, chemotherapy after metastasis development was significantly related to better OS. Conclusions: Complete metastasectomy should be considered for metastatic euLMS treatment. Moreover, chemotherapy could prolong survival in patients with metastasis who are ineligible for metastasectomy.

Keywords: metastatic extrauterine leiomyosarcoma; overall survival; metastasectomy; chemotherapy

Citation: Imura, Y.; Takenaka, S.; Outani, H.; Nakai, T.; Yasuda, N.; Nakai, S.; Wakamatsu, T.; Tamiya, H.; Okada, S. Impact of Surgery and Chemotherapy on Metastatic Extrauterine Leiomyosarcoma. *Curr. Oncol.* **2022**, *29*, 2301–2311. https://doi.org/10.3390/curroncol29040187

Received: 27 February 2022
Accepted: 23 March 2022
Published: 26 March 2022

Publisher's Note: MDPI stays neutral with regard to jurisdictional claims in published maps and institutional affiliations.

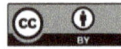

Copyright: © 2022 by the authors. Licensee MDPI, Basel, Switzerland. This article is an open access article distributed under the terms and conditions of the Creative Commons Attribution (CC BY) license (https://creativecommons.org/licenses/by/4.0/).

1. Introduction

Leiomyosarcoma (LMS) represents a heterogeneous subset of soft tissue sarcomas (STSs). Additionally, LMS is a malignant mesenchymal tumor originating from smooth muscle tissues and accounts for 5–10% of all newly diagnosed STSs [1–4]. LMS is commonly diagnosed in the fifth and sixth decades of life, and it can appear at almost all anatomic sites, such as the uterus, retroperitoneum, extremities, and blood vessels.

Surgical resection is the cornerstone treatment for patients with localized LMS, independent of the origin site. The standard surgical procedure involves a complete excision with wide negative margins, offering the best chance of cure. Performing a complete surgical resection at the initial presentation is the most important prognostic factor for survival. Despite this optimal local treatment, the rate of metastatic relapse is approximately 40% [4–6]. Furthermore, metastasis can be present at diagnosis or arise during treatment and follow-up. Prognosis is poor in the metastatic setting, with overall survival (OS) ranging from 10 to more than 30 months [4–10].

Two primary categories can be distinguished, uterine LMS (uLMS) and extrauterine LMS (euLMS) [11]. uLMS is the most common subtype of uterine sarcoma, likely accounting for the single largest site-specific LMS group [12]. First, gene expression profiling studies suggest a small difference between uLMS and euLMS [13]. Second, several studies suggest that uLMS differs in sensitivity to chemotherapy compared with other STS subtypes [14]. Finally, factors influencing the prognosis for patients with metastatic euLMS are not well described, and limited data regarding responses to systemic therapy are available.

This retrospective study investigates the clinicopathological features, clinical course, treatment outcomes, and prognostic factors in patients with metastatic euLMS treated at our institutions.

2. Materials and Methods

We designed a two-institutional retrospective study conducted in Osaka University Hospital and Osaka International Cancer Institute. We collected clinical and pathologic information for patients with metastatic euLMS treated at our institutions between January 2006 and December 2020. Patients' eligibility criteria included metastatic euLMS diagnosis, pathologically confirmed by a musculoskeletal tumor pathologist at each institution. The Institutional Review Board approved this study.

Sixty-one patients with metastatic euLMS treated at our hospitals were included in this study. The median follow-up period was 21.1 months (range, 1.8–158.8 months). Information on patient-related factors (age and sex), tumor-related factors (site of primary lesions; tumor size, depth, and histological grade; metachronous or synchronous metastasis; duration from the date of initial diagnosis to that of metastasis development; and the number of initial metastatic sites and lesions), treatment-related factors (surgery of the primary tumor and metastatic lesions and chemotherapy and radiotherapy status), local and distant relapse, follow-up period, and oncological outcome at final follow-up were anonymously collected from patients' medical charts. Synchronous metastasis was defined as that presenting simultaneously as the primary tumor diagnosis. In contrast, metachronous metastasis was defined as that developing after completion of the initial curative treatment. Unfortunately, we could not obtain data on tumor grade in three patients who received their first surgeries at other hospitals.

Objective responses to chemotherapy were determined by Response Evaluation Criteria in Solid Tumors, v.1.1 (RECIST v.1.1). ORR (objective response rate) was defined as the proportion of confirmed complete response (CR) or partial response (PR) to the best response. However, DCR (disease control rate) was defined as the percentage of confirmed CR, PR, or stable disease (SD) to the best response. We calculated the OS rate from the date of metastasis diagnosis to death from any cause or the last follow-up visit. Furthermore, progression-free survival (PFS) was defined as the duration from the date of chemotherapy initiation to that of radiographic progressive disease (PD), discontinuation due to adverse events, death from any cause, or the last follow-up visit. In addition, we calculated the OS rate and PFS using the Kaplan–Meier method and evaluated the impact of prognostic factors using the log-rank test in a univariate analysis. We conducted multivariate analysis using the Cox proportional-hazards model, with variables chosen using a forward conditional stepwise approach. Hazard ratios (HR) were listed with their 95% confidence intervals (CIs). Differences were considered significant when p-values were <0.05. EZR software (Saitama Medical Center, Jichi Medical University, Saitama, Japan), a graphical user interface for R (The R Foundation for Statistical Computing, Vienna, Austria), was used for statistical analyses.

3. Results

3.1. Patient-, Tumor-, and Treatment-Related Characteristics

Patient-, tumor-, and treatment-related characteristics of the 61 cases are presented in Table 1. The 25 male (41%) and 36 female (59%) patients had a median age of 59 years (range, 25–85 years) at metastatic disease diagnosis. Thirty-four patients (55.7%) were ≤60 years, and 27 patients (44.3%) were >60 years.

Table 1. Patient-, tumor-, and treatment-related characteristics and univariate analysis of prognostic factors for OS in 61 patients with metastatic euLMS. OS, overall survival; euLMS, extrauterine leiomyosarcoma; N.A., not available.

Factors		N (%)	Median OS (Months)	p Value
Age	≤60	34 (55.7)	38.8	0.175
	>60	27 (44.3)	23.3	
Sex	Male	25 (41)	23.3	0.112
	Female	36 (59)	55.9	
Primary site	Extremity	22 (36.1)	29.9	0.502
	Trunk	9 (14.8)	83	
	Retroperitoneum	17 (27.9)	30.4	
	Others	13 (21.3)	28.2	
Size	≤10 cm	37 (60.7)	55.9	<0.001
	>10 cm	24 (39.3)	17.1	
Depth	Superficial	10 (16.4)	N.A.	0.093
	Deep	51 (83.6)	29.9	
Grade	2	25 (43.1)	41.3	0.244
	3	33 (56.9)	23.3	
	N.A.	3	-	-
Presenting status	Metachronous	41 (67.2)	38.8	0.021
	Synchronous	20 (32.8)	24.7	
Number of initial metastatic sites	1	48 (78.7)	41.3	0.034
	>1	13 (21.3)	23.4	
Resection of primary tumor	Yes	53 (86.9)	32.2	0.071
	No	8 (13.1)	24.7	
Metastasectomy with curative intent	Yes	24 (39.3)	88.3	<0.001
	No	37 (60.7)	23.3	
Chemotherapy	Yes	48 (78.7)	32.2	0.917
	No	13 (21.3)	23.3	
Radiotherapy	Yes	24 (39.3)	30.7	0.91
	No	37 (60.7)	29.9	

Sites of primary lesions were the extremities in 22 (36.1%), trunk in 9 (14.8%), the retroperitoneum in 17 (27.9%), and others in 13 (21.3%) patients. The tumor size was ≤10 cm in the greatest dimension in 37 patients (60.7%) and >10 cm in 24 patients (39.3%), with a median size of 8 cm (range, 2.3–24 cm). The tumor depth was categorized as either superficial or deep in the investing fascia. Ten patients (16.4%) had superficial tumors, and fifty-one (83.6%) had deep tumors. Furthermore, we determined the histological grade using the Fédération Nationale des Centers de Lutte Contre le Cancer (FNCLCC) grading system [15]. Twenty-five patients (43.1%) had FNCLCC Grade 2 tumors, and thirty-three (56.9%) had FNCLCC Grade 3 tumors. In addition, 41 patients (67.2%) had metachronous metastases and 20 (32.8%) developed synchronous metastases. For patients with metachronous metastases, the median interval between initial diagnosis and metastatic relapse was 14.7 months (range, 2.1–108.2 months). For example, 48 patients (78.7%) had a single initial metastatic site, and 13 (21.3%) had multiple initial metastatic sites. The most common sites of initial metastases were the lungs (38 patients, 62.3%), followed by the liver (10 patients, 16.4%), muscle (10 patients, 16.4%), lymph nodes (7 patients, 11.5%), and bones (6 patients, 9.8%). Twenty patients (32.8%) had a single metastatic lesion, and 41 patients (67.2%) had multiple metastatic lesions at metastasis diagnosis.

Additionally, fifty-three patients (86.9%) underwent surgery on the primary tumor, and the remaining eight (13.1%) could not undergo surgery of the primary tumor due to metastases at the first visit and inoperative local conditions for surgical treatment. Among

41 patients with metachronous metastases who underwent surgical resection of their primary tumors, ten (24.4%) received neoadjuvant or adjuvant (or both) chemotherapy. In addition, nine patients underwent doxorubicin plus ifosfamide regimens. Thirty patients (49.2%) underwent metastasectomy irrespective of the anatomical site of the metastases. In addition, twenty-four patients (39.3%) underwent complete resection of metastatic lesions, defined as metastasectomy with curative intent. The most common initial metastatic sites where metastasectomy with curative intent was performed were lungs (13 patients), followed by the liver (4 patients), muscle (4 patients), lymph nodes (2 patients), and skin (1 patient).

Chemotherapy and radiotherapy for metastatic lesions were given to 48 (78.7%) and 24 (39.3%) patients, respectively. Various chemotherapy regimens, including doxorubicin, doxorubicin plus ifosfamide, gemcitabine plus docetaxel, pazopanib, trabectedin, and eribulin, were administered. Furthermore, the median number of chemotherapy regimens for patients with metastatic euLMS was 2 (range, 1–5). Of the patients evaluable for response, data for best response, ORR, DCR, and median PFS are described in Table 2.

Table 2. Best response, ORR, DCR, and PFS of chemotherapy regimens. CR, complete response; PR, partial response; SD, stable disease; PD, progressive disease; ORR, objective response rate; DCR, disease control rate; PFS, progression-free survival; DXR, doxorubicin; IFM, ifosfamide; GEM, gemcitabine; DOC, docetaxel; PAZ, pazopanib; TRB, trabectedin; ERB, eribulin.

Regimen	N	Best Response				ORR (%)	DCR (%)	Median PFS (Months)
		CR	PR	SD	PD			
DXR	9	0	1	6	2	11.1	77.7	4.9
DXR + IFM	18	1	4	8	5	27.8	72.2	6.1
GEM + DOC	22	0	7	8	7	31.8	68.2	4.5
PAZ	24	0	1	14	9	4.2	62.5	3.5
TRB	9	0	0	4	5	0	44.4	2.1
ERB	14	0	1	8	5	7.1	64.3	3.5

3.2. Survival and Outcomes

At the final follow-up, 12 patients (19.7%) had no evidence of the disease; however, 15 (24.6%) were alive with the disease, and 34 (55.7%) died of the disease. The five-year OS rate of all patients with metastatic euLMS was 38.3%, with a median OS period of 30.7 months (range, 1.8–158.8 months). Furthermore, among 53 patients who underwent surgery of the primary tumor, local recurrence developed in 11 (20.8%). Finally, surgical removal of the local recurrent tumor was performed in five patients.

3.3. Prognostic Factor Analyses

For all 61 patients with metastatic euLMS, primary tumor size ($p < 0.001$), presenting status at initial diagnosis ($p = 0.021$), number of initial metastatic sites ($p = 0.034$), and metastasectomy with curative intent ($p < 0.001$) were significant prognostic factors for OS in univariate analyses (Table 1; Figure 1a–d). However, multivariate analysis revealed that primary tumor size >10 cm (HR 2.48; 95% CI 1.137–5.411; $p = 0.023$) was a significant prognostic factor for unfavorable OS in all patients (Table 3).

Of the 24 patients who underwent metastasectomy with curative intent, 23 (95.8%) presented with metachronous metastatic disease. Furthermore, all patients undergoing metastasectomy with curative intent had undergone surgical resection of the primary tumor before metastasectomy. Therefore, they had one or two metastatic lesions at a single initial metastatic site. Fourteen patients (58.3%) received systemic chemotherapy before and/or after metastasectomy. By univariate analysis, the interval from the initial diagnosis to metastasis development ≤ 6 months ($p = 0.03$) was a significantly poor prognostic factor for OS (Table 4; Figure 2).

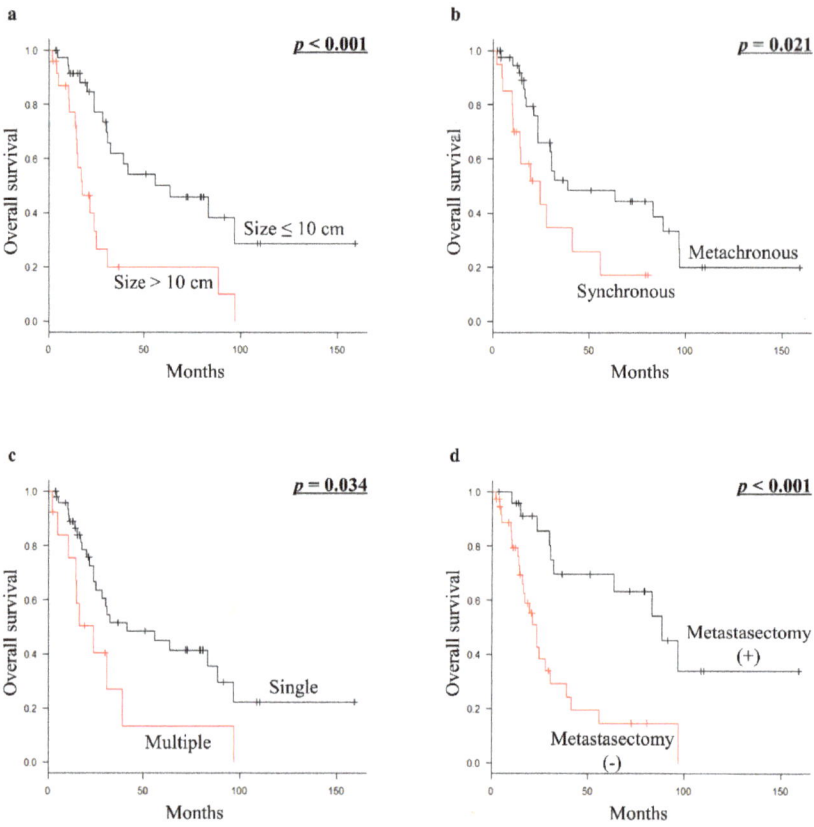

Figure 1. Kaplan–Meier survival curves in all 61 patients with metastatic euLMS: (**a**) OS according to tumor size (≤10 cm vs. >10 cm). (**b**) OS according to presenting status (metachronous vs. synchronous). (**c**) OS according to the number of initial metastatic sites (single vs. multiple). (**d**) OS according to metastasectomy with curative intent (presence vs. absence of metastasectomy with curative intent). euLMS, extrauterine leiomyosarcoma; OS, overall survival.

Table 3. Multivariate analysis of prognostic factors for OS in 61 patients with metastatic euLMS. OS, overall survival; euLMS, extrauterine leiomyosarcoma; HR, hazard ratio; CI, confidence interval.

Factors	Multivariate Analysis		
	HR	95% CI	*p* Value
Size >10 cm	2.48 / 1	1.137–5.411	0.023
Synchronous metastasis	1.756 / 1	0.701–4.4	0.23
Initial metastatic sites > 1	1.039 / 1	0.385–2.803	0.94
No metastasectomy	2.236 / 1	0.773–6.471	0.138

Table 4. Patient-, tumor-, and treatment-related characteristics and univariate analysis of prognostic factors for OS in 24 patients with metastatic euLMS who underwent metastasectomy with curative intent. OS, overall survival; euLMS, extrauterine leiomyosarcoma; N.A., not available.

Factors		N (%)	Median OS (Months)	p Value
Age	≤60	13 (54.2)	96.8	0.208
	>60	11 (45.8)	88.3	
Sex	Male	9 (37.5)	32.2	0.211
	Female	15 (62.5)	96.8	
Primary site	Extremity	10 (41.7)	32.2	0.513
	Trunk	6 (25)	96.8	
	Retroperitoneum	6 (25)	76.05	
	Others	2 (8.3)	30.7	
Size	≤10 cm	19 (79.2)	96.8	0.101
	>10 cm	5 (20.8)	88.3	
Depth	Superficial	7 (29.2)	N.A.	0.289
	Deep	17 (70.8)	83	
Grade	2	10 (45.5)	88.3	0.289
	3	12 (54.5)	83	
	N.A.	2	-	-
Interval from initial diagnosis to metastasis	≤6 months	6 (25)	31.1	0.03
	>6 months	18 (75)	96.8	
Number of initial metastatic lesions	1	18 (75)	88.3	0.888
	2	6 (25)	N.A.	
Chemotherapy prior to or after metastasectomy	Yes	14 (58.3)	83	0.351
	No	10 (41.7)	88.3	
Radiotherapy	Yes	10 (41.7)	83	0.387
	No	14 (58.3)	N.A.	

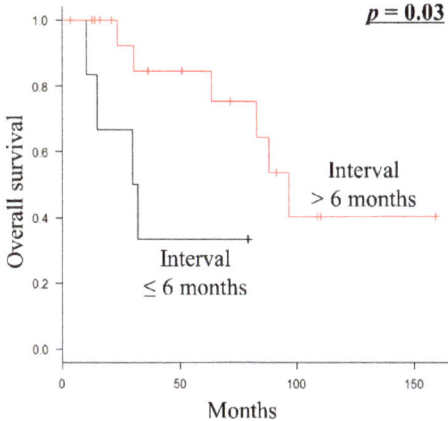

Figure 2. Kaplan–Meier survival curve of OS according to the interval from the initial diagnosis to metastasis (≤6 months vs. >6 months) in 24 patients with metastatic euLMS who underwent metastasectomy with curative intent. OS, overall survival; euLMS, extrauterine leiomyosarcoma.

Palliative chemotherapy ($p < 0.001$) was significantly associated with a better prognosis for OS in 37 patients who were ineligible for metastasectomy with curative intent (Table 5; Figure 3a). Furthermore, among 30 patients who received palliative chemotherapy, the most common first-line chemotherapy regimens were doxorubicin plus ifosfamide (10 patients), followed by gemcitabine plus docetaxel (8 patients), doxorubicin (7 patients), pazopanib (2 patients), eribulin (2 patients), and trabectedin (1 patient). In addition, the prognosis of 24 patients who had non-PD (PR or SD) during first-line palliative chemotherapy ($p = 0.031$) was significantly better than that of 6 patients who had PD (Figure 3b).

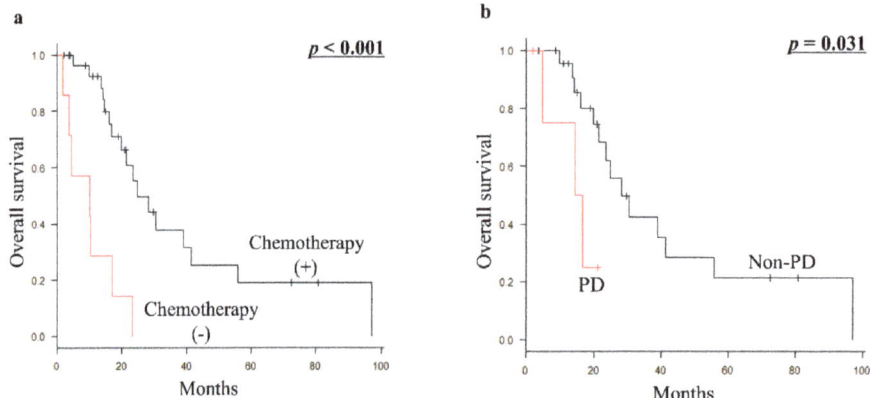

Figure 3. (**a**) Kaplan–Meier survival curve of OS according to palliative chemotherapy (presence vs. absence of chemotherapy) in 37 patients with metastatic euLMS who were ineligible for metastasectomy with curative intent. (**b**) Kaplan–Meier survival curve of OS according to the response of first-line chemotherapy from developing metastasis (non-PD vs. PD) in 30 patients with metastatic euLMS who were ineligible for metastasectomy with curative intent and received palliative chemotherapy. OS, overall survival; euLMS, extrauterine leiomyosarcoma; PD, progressive disease.

Table 5. Patient-, tumor-, and treatment-related characteristics and univariate analysis of prognostic factors for OS in 37 patients with metastatic euLMS who were ineligible for metastasectomy with curative intent. OS, overall survival; euLMS, extrauterine leiomyosarcoma; N.A., not available.

Factors		N (%)	Median OS (Months)	p Value
Age	≤60	21 (56.8)	24.7	0.152
	>60	16 (43.2)	17.1	
Sex	Male	16 (43.2)	19.8	0.205
	Female	21 (56.8)	30.4	
Primary site	Extremity	12 (32.4)	19.8	0.202
	Trunk	3 (8.1)	16.1	
	Retroperitoneum	11 (29.7)	24.7	
	Others	11 (29.7)	28.2	
Size	≤10 cm	18 (48.6)	28.2	0.087
	>10 cm	19 (51.4)	17.1	
Depth	Superficial	3 (8.1)	16.1	0.696
	Deep	34 (91.9)	23.3	

Table 5. Cont.

Factors		N (%)	Median OS (Months)	p Value
Grade	2	15 (41.7)	24.7	0.349
	3	21 (58.3)	16.1	
	N.A.	1	-	-
Presenting status	Metachronous	18 (48.6)	23.3	0.477
	Synchronous	19 (51.4)	19.8	
Number of initial metastatic sites	1	24 (64.9)	23.3	0.702
	>1	13 (35.1)	23.4	
Resection of primary tumor	Yes	29 (78.4)	21.3	0.704
	No	8 (21.6)	24.7	
Chemotherapy	Yes	30 (81.1)	24.7	<0.001
	No	7 (18.9)	10.2	
Radiotherapy	Yes	14 (37.8)	24.7	0.989
	No	23 (62.2)	21.3	

The median OS periods for patients with metastatic euLMS diagnosed from 2006 to 2013 and those diagnosed from 2014 to 2020 were 36.8 and 29.9 months, respectively. There was no significant difference between the two groups ($p = 0.742$).

4. Discussion

A single-center, retrospective review of 353 patients with primary euLMS identified size and grade as distinct factors influencing disease-specific survival [16]. However, there are relatively little data published regarding factors influencing survival in patients with metastatic euLMS. In our study, the median OS from the diagnosis of metastatic disease was 30.7 months, which is higher than the data reported by others [4–10]. Furthermore, univariate analyses of our cohort showed that primary tumor size, presenting status at initial diagnosis, number of initial metastatic sites, and metastasectomy with curative intent were associated with significant differences in OS. We identified primary tumor size >10 cm as an independent risk factor for decreased OS in the metastatic euLMS population. The histological tumor grade was not significantly associated with survival in univariate analysis, suggesting that tumor grade did not affect OS after metastasis development.

Surgical resection of primary tumors is considered the primary local treatment for patients with LMS and localized disease, prolonging their survival [17]. However, treating metastatic LMS remains a challenge, as a curative treatment for metastatic disease is rare. The appropriate treatment for patients with metastatic euLMS remains unknown. In our cohort, surgical resection of primary tumors was performed in 86.9% of all patients with metastatic euLMS but did not significantly prolong their survival. Patients with metastatic LMS of any site should be evaluated to determine whether the resection of metastases may be appropriate. Additionally, favorable five-year survival rates of 38%–52% following pulmonary metastasectomy for LMS have been reported [18–20]. In this study, the five-year OS rate of patients with metastatic euLMS who received metastasectomy with curative intent was 69.5%. They had received surgical resection of primary tumors before metastasectomy, and most of them had metachronous metastatic disease. These results suggest that primary and metastatic lesions should be actively treated to obtain maximum survival time.

Additionally, resection should be considered for patients with a relatively long disease-free interval and an isolated disease site amenable to complete resection, with an acceptably low risk of morbidity. However, in our study, all patients undergoing metastasectomy with curative intent had one or two metastatic lesions at a single initial metastatic site. The extended disease-free interval following resection of a primary tumor to the occurrence of pulmonary metastases has also been demonstrated by several authors to be a positive predictor of survival. The best results are seen with a disease-free interval of 12 months or longer [21]. In this study, the interval from the initial diagnosis to development of metastasis ≤6 months but not 12 months was significantly associated with unfavorable OS among patients who received metastasectomy with curative intent. However, this finding could be the result of the patient selection process. Therefore, establishing the benefit of metastasectomy would require further randomized clinical trials.

Different STS subtypes have recognized variable patterns of chemosensitivity, and LMS shows moderate sensitivity to chemotherapy. Doxorubicin-based chemotherapy is commonly used to treat patients with metastatic STS, alone or with ifosfamide [22]. Combining gemcitabine plus docetaxel, unlike other STSs, seems to be effective in LMS as first- and second-line treatments in patients who have previously received doxorubicin-based therapy. Furthermore, in the phase III multicenter trial, gemcitabine and docetaxel vs. doxorubicin as a first-line treatment in previously untreated advanced unresectable or metastatic soft tissue sarcoma (GeDDiS) did not observe differences in response rate and PFS from first-line gemcitabine plus docetaxel treatment compared with single-agent doxorubicin, with both regimens demonstrating activity in LMS [23]. Therefore, regimens to consider for first-line therapy include doxorubicin-based therapies and gemcitabine plus docetaxel. In this study, the main reasons for avoiding doxorubicin-based regimens were advanced age and cardiac dysfunction.

Several regimens have shown activity in LMS as second-line treatment or later. Since 2012, three anticancer drugs, pazopanib, trabectedin, and eribulin, have been approved in Japan for the second-line or later treatment of patients with advanced STS of any histologic subtype, including LMS. In the randomized phase III study (the PALETTE trial) in 372 patients with advanced non-adipocytic STS, pazopanib improved PFS compared with placebo in STS. However, there was no difference in OS, and ORR was observed in only 4% of patients [24]. Subgroup analysis by histologic subtype and predictive analysis for histology subtype using Cox models showed pazopanib to be effective for LMS in terms of PFS [24,25]. The phase III trial of trabectedin demonstrated trabectedin superiority over dacarbazine in PFS, but not in ORR or OS [26]. Several studies, including data from 431 patients with LMS of any origin treated in a trabectedin-expanded access program, demonstrated an ORR of 7.5% in patients with LMS compared with 5.9% among patients with all-type STS [27]. In the phase III trial of eribulin for L-sarcomas, eribulin demonstrated superior OS benefit than dacarbazine, but this was not the case for PFS or response rate [28]. Subgroup analysis by histologic subtype of the data for OS showed the effect of eribulin on LMS to be similar to that of dacarbazine [29].

In our cohort, palliative chemotherapy for patients with metastatic euLMS ineligible for metastasectomy proved to be of significant prognostic value for better OS. This suggests that palliative chemotherapy may help prolong the survival of these patients. Patients with PR or SD to first-line chemotherapy had significantly better OS than patients whose tumors showed PD regardless of the type of chemotherapy used. It is hoped that biomarkers of response that will help to optimize treatment choices for patients with LMS may be identified.

We believe that our study shows the efficacy of surgery and chemotherapy in patients with metastatic euLMS. There are several limitations to this study. First, the results of this study must be interpreted with caution due to its retrospective design and limited sample size. Second, we could not obtain precise histological grading information in three patients who received surgical resection of the primary tumor in other hospitals. Third, there was possible selection bias concerning receipt of surgery and chemotherapy because frail patients with limited life expectancy are often not offered aggressive multimodality treatment. Fourth, each physician decided the choice of drugs used. During the study period, we could use pazopanib, trabectedin, and eribulin since 2012, 2015, and 2016, respectively.

These limitations should be considered when evaluating the results of this study. Therefore, further investigations, including a prospective randomized study, are needed.

5. Conclusions

The five-year OS rate of patients with metastatic euLMS was 38.3%. Large primary tumor size was significantly associated with poor OS in multivariate analysis. Therefore, complete metastasectomy should be performed for patients with metastatic euLMS whose primary tumors were resected. Moreover, palliative chemotherapy could prolong survival in patients who are ineligible for metastasectomy. A multidisciplinary approach for metastatic euLMS is necessary, and, thus, understanding how to select the best therapies that may benefit patients with advanced euLMS is important.

Author Contributions: Conceptualization, Y.I., S.T., H.O., T.N., N.Y., S.N., T.W., and H.T.; methodology, Y.I. and S.T.; resources, S.T. and S.O.; data curation, Y.I., S.T., H.O., T.N., N.Y., S.N., T.W., and H.T.; writing—original draft preparation, Y.I.; writing—review and editing, S.T., H.O., T.N., N.Y., S.N., T.W., H.T., and S.O.; supervision, S.O.; project administration, Y.I.; funding acquisition, Y.I. All authors have read and agreed to the published version of the manuscript.

Funding: This research was funded by JSPS KAKENHI Grant Number JP19K18481.

Institutional Review Board Statement: The study was conducted according to the guidelines of the Declaration of Helsinki, and was approved by the Osaka University Clinical Research Review Committee (certificate no. 14240-3, date of approval; 1 November 2019) and the Osaka International Cancer Institute Ethics Committee (registration number 1506059008-2, date of approval; 5 June 2015).

Informed Consent Statement: Informed consent was obtained from all subjects involved in the study.

Data Availability Statement: The datasets used in this study are available from the corresponding author on reasonable request.

Acknowledgments: This research was funded by JSPS KAKENHI Grant Number JP19K18481.

Conflicts of Interest: The authors declare no conflict of interest.

References

1. Van Glabbeke, M.; van Oosterom, A.T.; Oosterhuis, J.W.; Mouridsen, H.; Crowther, D.; Somers, R.; Verweij, J.; Santoro, A.; Buesa, J.; Tursz, T. Prognostic factors for the outcome of chemotherapy in advanced soft tissue sarcoma: An analysis of 2185 patients treated with anthracycline-containing first-line regimens—A European Organization for Research and Treatment of Cancer Soft Tissue and Bone Sarcoma Group Study. *J. Clin. Oncol.* **1999**, *17*, 150–157. [PubMed]
2. Blay, J.Y.; van Glabbeke, M.; Verweij, J.; van Oosterom, A.T.; Le Cesne, A.; Oosterhuis, J.W.; Judson, I.; Nielsen, O.S. Advanced soft-tissue sarcoma: A disease that is potentially curable for a subset of patients treated with chemotherapy. *Eur. J. Cancer* **2003**, *39*, 64–69. [CrossRef]
3. Weitz, J.; Antonescu, C.R.; Brennan, M.F. Localized extremity soft tissue sarcoma: Improved knowledge with unchanged survival over time. *J. Clin. Oncol.* **2003**, *21*, 2719–2725. [CrossRef] [PubMed]
4. Coindre, J.M.; Terrier, P.; Guillou, L.; Le Doussal, V.; Collin, F.; Ranchère, D.; Sastre, X.; Vilain, M.O.; Bonichon, F.; N'Guyen Bui, B. Predictive value of grade for metastasis development in the main histologic types of adult soft tissue sarcomas: A study of 1240 patients from the French Federation of Cancer Centers Sarcoma Group. *Cancer* **2001**, *91*, 1914–1926. [CrossRef]
5. Zivanovic, O.; Jacks, L.M.; Iasonos, A.; Leitao, M.M., Jr.; Soslow, R.A.; Veras, E.; Chi, D.S.; Abu-Rustum, N.R.; Barakat, R.R.; Brennan, M.; et al. A nomogram to predict postresection 5-year overall survival for patients with uterine leiomyosarcoma. *Cancer* **2012**, *118*, 660–669. [CrossRef] [PubMed]
6. Svarvar, C.; Böhling, T.; Berlin, O.; Gustafson, P.; Folleràs, G.; Bjerkehagen, B.; Domanski, H.A.; Sundby Hall, K.; Tukiainen, E.; Blomqvist, C.; et al. Clinical course of nonvisceral soft tissue leiomyosarcoma in 225 patients from the Scandinavian Sarcoma Group. *Cancer* **2007**, *109*, 282–291. [CrossRef] [PubMed]
7. Oosten, A.W.; Seynaeve, C.; Schmitz, P.I.; den Bakker, M.A.; Verweij, J.; Sleijfer, S. Outcomes of first-line chemotherapy in patients with advanced or metastatic leiomyosarcoma of uterine and non-uterine origin. *Sarcoma* **2009**, *2009*, 348910. [CrossRef] [PubMed]
8. Shoushtari, A.N.; Landa, J.; Kuk, D.; Sanchez, A.; Lala, B.; Schmidt, N.; Okoli, C.; Chi, P.; Dickson, M.A.; Gounder, M.M.; et al. Overall Survival and response to systemic therapy in metastatic extrauterine leiomyosarcoma. *Sarcoma* **2016**, *2016*, 3547497. [CrossRef]
9. Lamm, W.; Natter, C.; Schur, S.; Köstler, W.J.; Reinthaller, A.; Krainer, M.; Grimm, C.; Horvath, R.; Amann, G.; Funovics, P.; et al. Distinctive outcome in patients with non-uterine and uterine leiomyosarcoma. *BMC Cancer* **2014**, *14*, 981. [CrossRef] [PubMed]

10. Penel, N.; Italiano, A.; Isambert, N.; Bompas, E.; Bousquet, G.; Duffaud, F.; French Sarcoma Group (Groupe Sarcome Français/Groupe d'Etude des Tumeurs Osseuses). Factors affecting the outcome of patients with metastatic leiomyosarcoma treated with doxorubicin-containing chemotherapy. *Ann. Oncol.* **2010**, *21*, 1361–1365. [CrossRef] [PubMed]
11. Yang, J.; Du, X.; Chen, K.; Ylipää, A.; Lazar, A.J.; Trent, J.; Lev, D.; Pollock, R.; Hao, X.; Hunt, K.; et al. Genetic aberrations in soft tissue leiomyosarcoma. *Cancer Lett.* **2009**, *275*, 1–8. [CrossRef] [PubMed]
12. Amant, F.; Coosemans, A.; Debiec-Rychter, M.; Timmerman, D.; Vergote, I. Clinical management of uterine sarcomas. *Lancet Oncol.* **2009**, *10*, 1188–1198. [CrossRef]
13. Skubitz, K.M.; Skubitz, A.P. Differential gene expression in leiomyosarcoma. *Cancer* **2003**, *98*, 1029–1038. [CrossRef] [PubMed]
14. Hensley, M.L.; Blessing, J.A.; Degeest, K.; Abulafia, O.; Rose, P.G.; Homesley, H.D. Fixed-dose rate gemcitabine plus docetaxel as second-line therapy for metastatic uterine leiomyosarcoma: A Gynecologic Oncology Group phase II study. *Gynecol. Oncol.* **2008**, *109*, 323–328. [CrossRef] [PubMed]
15. Trojani, M.; Contesso, G.; Coindre, J.M.; Rouesse, J.; Bui, N.B.; de Mascarel, A.; Goussot, J.F.; David, M.; Bonichon, F.; Lagarde, C. Soft-tissue sarcomas of adults; study of pathological prognostic variables and definition of a histopathological grading system. *Int. J. Cancer* **1984**, *33*, 37–42. [CrossRef]
16. Gladdy, R.A.; Qin, L.X.; Moraco, N.; Agaram, N.P.; Brennan, M.F.; Singer, S. Predictors of survival and recurrence in primary leiomyosarcoma. *Ann. Surg. Oncol.* **2013**, *20*, 1851–1857. [CrossRef] [PubMed]
17. Anaya, D.A.; Lev, D.C.; Pollock, R.E. The role of surgical margin status in retroperitoneal sarcoma. *J. Surg. Oncol.* **2008**, *98*, 607–610. [CrossRef]
18. Blackmon, S.H.; Shah, N.; Roth, J.A.; Correa, A.M.; Vaporciyan, A.A.; Rice, D.C.; Hofstetter, W.; Walsh, G.L.; Benjamin, R.; Pollock, R.; et al. Resection of pulmonary and extrapulmonary sarcomatous metastases is associated with long-term survival. *Ann. Thorac. Surg.* **2009**, *88*, 877–884; discussion 884–885. [CrossRef] [PubMed]
19. Anraku, M.; Yokoi, K.; Nakagawa, K.; Fujisawa, T.; Nakajima, J.; Akiyama, H.; Nishimura, Y.; Kobayashi, K.; Metastatic Lung Tumor Study Group of Japan. Pulmonary metastases from uterine malignancies: Results of surgical resection in 133 patients. *J. Thorac. Cardiovasc. Surg.* **2004**, *127*, 1107–1112. [CrossRef] [PubMed]
20. Burt, B.M.; Ocejo, S.; Mery, C.M.; Dasilva, M.; Bueno, R.; Sugarbaker, D.J.; Jaklitsch, M.T. Repeated and aggressive pulmonary resections for leiomyosarcoma metastases extends survival. *Ann. Thorac. Surg.* **2011**, *92*, 1202–1207. [CrossRef]
21. van Geel, A.N.; Hoekstra, H.J.; van Coevorden, F.; Meyer, S.; Bruggink, E.D.; Blankensteijn, J.D. Repeated resection of recurrent pulmonary metastatic soft tissue sarcoma. *Eur. J. Surg. Oncol. J. Eur. Soc. Surg. Oncol. Br. Assoc. Surg. Oncol.* **1994**, *20*, 436–440.
22. Judson, I.; Verweij, J.; Gelderblom, H.; Hartmann, J.T.; Schöffski, P.; Blay, J.Y.; Kerst, J.M.; Sufliarsky, J.; Whelan, J.; Hohenberger, P.; et al. Doxorubicin alone versus intensified doxorubicin plus ifosfamide for first-line treatment of advanced or metastatic soft-tissue sarcoma: A randomised controlled phase 3 trial. *Lancet Oncol.* **2014**, *15*, 415–423. [CrossRef]
23. Seddon, B.; Strauss, S.J.; Whelan, J.; Leahy, M.; Woll, P.J.; Cowie, F.; Rothermundt, C.; Wood, Z.; Benson, C.; Ali, N.; et al. Gemcitabine and docetaxel versus doxorubicin as first-line treatment in previously untreated advanced unresectable or metastatic soft-tissue sarcomas (GeDDiS): A randomised controlled phase 3 trial. *Lancet Oncol.* **2017**, *18*, 1397–1410. [CrossRef]
24. van der Graaf, W.T.; Blay, J.Y.; Chawla, S.P.; Kim, D.W.; Bui-Nguyen, B.; Casali, P.G.; Schöffski, P.; Aglietta, M.; Staddon, A.P.; Beppu, Y.; et al. Pazopanib for metastatic soft-tissue sarcoma (Palette): A randomised, double-blind, placebo-controlled phase 3 trial. *Lancet* **2012**, *379*, 1879–1886. [CrossRef]
25. Sleijfer, S.; Ray-Coquard, I.; Papai, Z.; Le Cesne, A.; Scurr, M.; Schöffski, P.; Collin, F.; Pandite, L.; Marreaud, S.; De Brauwer, A.; et al. Pazopanib, a multikinase angiogenesis inhibitor, in patients with relapsed or refractory advanced soft tissue sarcoma: A phase II study from the European Organisation for Research and Treatment of Cancer-soft tissue and bone sarcoma group (EORTC study 62043). *J. Clin. Oncol.* **2009**, *27*, 3126–3132. [PubMed]
26. Demetri, G.D.; von Mehren, M.; Jones, R.L.; Hensley, M.L.; Schuetze, S.M.; Staddon, A.; Milhem, M.; Elias, A.; Ganjoo, K.; Tawbi, H.; et al. Efficacy and safety of trabectedin or dacarbazine for metastatic liposarcoma or leiomyosarcoma after failure of conventional chemotherapy: Results of a Phase III randomized multicenter clinical trial. *J. Clin. Oncol.* **2016**, *34*, 786–793. [CrossRef] [PubMed]
27. Samuels, B.L.; Chawla, S.; Patel, S.; von Mehren, M.; Hamm, J.; Kaiser, P.E.; Schuetze, S.; Li, J.; Aymes, A.; Demetri, G.D. Clinical outcomes and safety with trabectedin therapy in patients with advanced soft tissue sarcomas following failure of prior chemotherapy: Results of a worldwide expanded access program study. *Ann. Oncol.* **2013**, *24*, 1703–1709. [CrossRef] [PubMed]
28. Schöffski, P.; Chawla, S.; Maki, R.G.; Italiano, A.; Gelderblom, H.; Choy, E.; Grignani, G.; Camargo, V.; Bauer, S.; Rha, S.Y.; et al. Eribulin versus dacarbazine in previously treated patients with advanced liposarcoma or leiomyosarcoma: A randomised, open-label, multicentre, phase 3 trial. *Lancet* **2016**, *387*, 1629–1637. [CrossRef]
29. Blay, J.Y.; Schöffski, P.; Bauer, S.; Krarup-Hansen, A.; Benson, C.; D'Adamo, D.R.; Jia, Y.; Maki, R.G. Eribulin versus dacarbazine in patients with leiomyosarcoma: Subgroup analysis from a phase 3, open-label, randomised study. *Br. J. Cancer* **2019**, *120*, 1026–1032. [CrossRef]

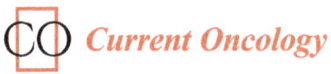

Case Report

Characteristic of Uterine Rhabdomyosarcoma by Algorithm of Potential Biomarkers for Uterine Mesenchymal Tumor

Saya Tamura [1], Takuma Hayashi [2,3,*], Tomoyuki Ichimura [4], Nobuo Yaegashi [5], Kaoru Abiko [1] and Ikuo Konishi [1,6]

[1] National Hospital Organization Kyoto Medical Center, Department of Obstetrics and Gynecology, Kyoto 612-8555, Japan; nho.kmc.rc@hotmail.com (S.T.); hiroyukiaburatani@yahoo.co.jp (K.A.); ikuokonishi08@yahoo.co.jp (I.K.)
[2] Section of Cancer Medicine, National Hospital Organization Kyoto Medical Center, Kyoto 612-8555, Japan
[3] START-Program, Japan Science and Technology Agency (JST), Tokyo 102-8666, Japan
[4] Department of Obstetrics and Gynecology, Osaka City University School of Medicine, Osaka 545-8586, Japan; kenjisano12@yahoo.co.jp
[5] Department of Obstetrics and Gynecology, Tohoku University School of Medicine, Miyagi 980-8575, Japan; nobuoyaegashi@yahoo.co.jp
[6] Department of Obstetrics and Gynecology, Kyoto University School of Medicine, Kyoto 606-8501, Japan
* Correspondence: yoyoyo224@hotmail.com or takumah@shinshu-u.ac.jp; Tel.: +81-263372629

Abstract: Background/Aim: Patients with uterine sarcoma comprise 2–5% of all patients with uterine malignancies; however, the morbidity of uterine sarcoma is low compared with that of other gynecological cancers. For many cases, malignant uterine tumors are diagnosed during follow-up of benign uterine leiomyoma. Of the uterine sarcomas, rhabdomyosarcoma is considered a mixed tumor containing components of epithelial cells and mesenchymal cells. Therefore, the onset of primary uterine rhabdomyosarcoma during follow-up of uterine leiomyoma is extremely rare. Rhabdomyosarcoma is a relatively common malignant tumor in children, but rhabdomyosarcoma in adults is extremely rare, accounting for approximately 3% of all patients with soft tissue sarcoma. Rhabdomyosarcoma in children is highly sensitive to chemotherapy and radiation therapy; however, the response to chemotherapy and radiation therapy in adult rhabdomyosarcoma is low and survival in adult rhabdomyosarcoma with metastatic lesions to other organs is approximately 14 months. We experienced a case of pleomorphic rhabdomyosarcoma during the follow-up of a uterine leiomyoma. Materials and Methods: We examined the oncological properties of uterine rhabdomyosarcoma in adults using molecular pathological techniques on tissue excised from patients with uterine leiomyoma. Result: A differential diagnosis was made for this case by molecular pathology, which included candidate biomarkers for uterine smooth muscle tumors. The oncological nature of uterine rhabdomyosarcoma was found to be similar to the oncological properties of uterine leiomyosarcoma. However, in uterine rhabdomyosarcoma, LMP2/β1i-positive cells were clearly observed. Conclusion: It is expected that establishing a diagnostic and treatment method targeting characteristics of mesenchymal tumor cells will lead to the treatment of malignant tumors with a low risk of recurrence and metastasis.

Keywords: rhabdomyosarcoma; leiomyoma; leiomyosarcoma; mesenchymal tumor

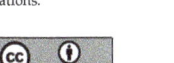

1. Introduction

Uterine mesenchymal tumors are broadly classified into two types: benign and malignant tumors. However, for uterine mesenchymal tumors, cells with various histological types and cell morphologies are mixed. Furthermore, the components contained within the cells also vary. Therefore, surgical pathological diagnosis for uterine mesenchymal tumor is challenging. Uterine sarcoma in gynecologic oncology is a rare disease and, in most cases, it develops in the uterine body. Therefore, sarcomas that occur outside of the uterus, such as the vagina, vulva, and ovaries, are extremely rare. In 2020, the International Classification for Gynecologic Tumors published by the World Health Organization classified uterine sarcoma as cancer of the uterine body [1]. As a result, the histological types of uterine sarcoma are classified as uterine leiomyosarcoma, endometrial stromal sarcoma (low and high grade), and undifferentiated uterine sarcoma [2]. As a somewhat rare uterine sarcoma, the development of uterine adenosarcoma, which is a malignant tumor, may occur.

In clinical practice, histopathologically poor prognostic factors for uterine adenosarcoma include lymphovascular invasion, differentiation into uterine rhabdomyosarcoma, and overgrowth of sarcoma components [3]. Uterine adenosarcoma is a mixed tumor consisting of components of benign glandular epithelial tissue and sarcoma tissue. Uterine adenosarcoma is known to form foliate polyp-like elevated lesions. The incidence of uterine adenosarcoma is only 1/9 of that observed for uterine carcinosarcoma [4]. The age of onset of uterine adenosarcoma is younger compared with that of uterine carcinosarcoma and the results of a clinical study with 100 patients indicated that the distribution by age was 14–89 years, with a median of 58 years [5]. The site of onset of uterine adenosarcoma is the uterine endometrium in 76% of all cases, the cervix endometrium in 6%, and the myometrium layer of the uterus in 4%. Atypical components of the sarcomatous tissue of uterine adenosarcoma are not always pathologically evident. Uterine adenosarcoma is diagnosed as an intimal or cervical polyp and repeated recurrences occur, thus regular examination is required. As a treatment for uterine adenosarcoma, like other uterine sarcomas, surgery by simple abdominal hysterectomy and bilateral adnexectomy is standard practice. However, as a clinical treatment for uterine adenosarcoma, the effectiveness of lymph node dissection and post-operative treatment has not been established. Compared with other uterine sarcomas, uterine adenosarcoma exhibits a better prognosis, and clinical studies have indicated that the five-year survival rate is 79% in pre-operative stage I cases and 48% in cases considered stage III [4].

The pathological findings of uterine adenosarcoma are characterized by spindle-shaped cells displaying significant fission. In many cases of uterine adenosarcoma, the expression of cluster of differentiation (CD) 10, an epithelial cell marker, is diffusely positive, and the expression of alpha smooth muscle actin (αSMA) and desmin, a marker of smooth muscle cells, is negative [6,7]. In addition, in cases of uterine adenosarcoma, the expression of the hormone receptors, estrogen receptor (ER) and progesterone receptor (PgR), may be positive or negative [8,9]. Thus, the expression of these receptors differs depending on the case. Surgical pathology of uterine rhabdomyosarcoma is performed based on the differentiation of uterine adenosarcoma into uterine rhabdomyosarcoma and the molecular pathological characteristics of uterine rhabdomyosarcoma. For uterine rhabdomyosarcoma, immunohistochemical expression of desmin, muscle-specific actin, myogenin, myogenic and differentiation antigen 1 (MyoD1) is observed, and the expression status of these markers can be used as a diagnostic reference for uterine rhabdomyosarcoma [10].

Using surgical pathology, we examined neonatal-sized uterine tumors, pelvic lymph nodes, para-aortic lymph nodes, and left supraclavicular lymph nodes with bulky mass. The onset of uterine leiomyosarcoma and malignant lymphoma was suspected based on a significantly raised abdomen, a large mass on the left subclavian lymph node, ultrasonographic images, computed tomography images, and high lactic acid dehydrogenase (LDH) levels (3631 U/L). However, based on the results, the patient's uterine tumor was diagnosed as a rhabdomyosarcoma originating from the uterus and metastasis to the left supraclavicular lymph node. The frequency of rhabdomyosarcoma at different sites within the female genital tract varies by histological subtype [11]. Pleomorphic rhabdomyosarcoma typically occurs in the corpus. In the lower female genital tract, embryonal rhabdomyosarcoma is most common in the vagina in children and in the cervix and corpus in adolescents and adults, whereas alveolar rhabdomyosarcoma is most common in the vulva. We examined the difference between uterine leiomyosarcoma and uterine rhabdomyosarcoma using molecular pathological techniques. Our results provide a new molecular marker for the diagnosis of gynecologic tumors.

2. Materials and Methods

2.1. Tissue Collection

A total of 101 patients between 32 and 83 years of age and diagnosed as having smooth muscle tumors of the uterus were selected from pathological files. Serial sections were cut from at least two tissue blocks from each patient for hematoxylin and eosin staining and immunostaining. All tissues were used with the approval of the Ethical Committee of Shinshu University after obtaining written consent from each patient. The pathological diagnosis of uterine smooth muscle tumors was performed using established criteria (Hendrickson and Kempson, 1995) with some modification. Briefly, usual leiomyoma (usual LMA) was defined as a tumor showing typical histological features with a mitotic index (MI) (obtained by counting the total number of mitotic figures (MFs) in 10 high-power fields (HPFs)) of <5 MFs per 10 HPFs. Cellular leiomyoma (cellular LMA) was defined as a tumor with significantly increased cellularity (>2000 myoma cells/HPF) and a MI < 5, but without cytologic atypia. Bizarre leiomyoma (BL) was defined as a tumor either with diffuse nuclear atypia and a MI < 2 or with focal nuclear atypia and a MI < 5 without coagulative tumor cell necrosis. A tumor of uncertain malignant potential (UMP) was defined as tumor with no mild atypia and a MI < 10 but with coagulative tumor cell necrosis. Leiomyosarcoma (LMS) was diagnosed in the presence of a MI > 10 with either diffuse cytologic atypia, coagulative tumor cell necrosis, or both. Of the 105 smooth muscle tumors, 52 were diagnosed as LMA, 3 were BL, 2 were intravenous leiomyomatosis, 58 were uterine LMS, 1 was uterine LANT-like tumor, and 2 were uterine rhabdomyosarcoma. Of the 58 LMS, 48 were histologically of the spindle-cell type and 10 were of the epithelioid type. The clinical stage of the LMS patients was stage I in 11 cases, stage II or III in 31 cases, and stage IV in 16 cases. Protein expression studies with cervix epithelium and carcinoma tissues were performed using tissue array (uterus cancer tissues, AccuMax Array, Seoul, Korea). Details about tissue sections are indicated in the manufacturer's information (AccuMax Array).

2.2. Immunohistochemistry (IHC)

IHC staining for caveolin-1, cyclin B, cyclin E1, large multifunctional peptidase 2/β1i (LMP2/β1i), Ki-67, desmin, and myogenin was performed using serial human uterine mesenchymal tumor sections obtained from patients with uterine mesenchymal tumor. A monoclonal antibody against yclin E1 (CCNE1/2460) was purchased from Abcam (Cambridge Biomedical Campus, Cambridge, UK) and a monoclonal antibody against Ki-67 (clone MIB-1) was purchased from Dako Denmark A/S (DK-2600 Glostrup, Denmark). Monoclonal antibodies against desmin (clone RM234) and myogenin (clone MGN185) were purchased from Gene Tex, Inc. (Irvine, CA, USA). The monoclonal antibody against caveolin-1, cyclin B1, LMP2/β1i were purchased from Santa Cruz Biotechnology Inc. (Santa Cruz, CA, USA). IHC was performed using the avidin–biotin complex method as described previously [12–14]. Briefly, one representative 5-mm tissue section was cut from a paraffin-embedded sample of a radical hysterectomy specimen from each patient with a uterine mesenchymal tumor.

The sections were incubated with a biotinylated secondary antibody (Dako, DK-2600 Glostrup, Denmark) followed by the streptavidin complex (Dako). The completed reaction was developed using 3,39-diaminobenzidine and the slides were counterstained with hematoxylin. Normal myometrium portions in the specimens were used as positive controls. The negative controls consisted of tissue sections incubated with normal rabbit IgG instead of primary antibody. Shinshu University approved the experiments according to internal guidelines (approval no. M192). The expression of cyclin E and Ki-67 was indicated by brown 3,3′-diaminobenzidine, tetrahydrochloride (DAB) staining. Normal rabbit or mouse antiserum was used as a negative control for the primary antibody. The entire brown 3,3′-diaminobenzidine, tetrahydrochloride-stained tissue was scanned with a

BZ-X800 digital microscope (Keyence, Osaka, Japan). Black dots indicated the expression of cyclin E and Ki-67.

IHC staining for CD31 and lymphatic vessel endothelial hyaluronan receptor 1 (LYVE-1) was performed on sections from the excised tissue. Briefly, tumor tissue sections were incubated with the appropriate primary antibodies at 4 °C overnight. Rabbit polyclonal antibodies to LYVE-1 (1:200) and a mouse monoclonal antibody to CD31 (1:200) were the primary antibodies. A monoclonal antibody for CD31 (clone JC/70A) was purchased from Gene Tex, Inc. (Irvine, CA, USA). The antibody for LYVE-1 (bs-20353R) was purchased from Bioss Inc. (Boston, MA, USA). Following incubation with an Alexa Fluor® 488-conjugated anti-mouse IgG or Alexa Fluor® 546-conjugated anti-rabbit IgG secondary antibody (1:200; Invitrogen, Waltham, MA, USA), the sections were washed, cover-slipped with mounting medium and 40,6-diamidino-2-phenylindole (DAPI) (Vectashield; Vector Laboratories, Burlingame, CA, USA), and visualized by confocal microscopy (Leica TCS SP8, Wetzlar, Germany) according to the manufacturer's instructions. Normal rabbit or mouse antiserum was used as a negative control for the primary antibody. The experiments with human tissues were conducted at the National Hospital Organization Kyoto Medical Center in accordance with institutional guidelines (approval no. NHO H31-02).

2.3. Ethical Approval and Consent to Participate

This study was reviewed and approved by the Central Ethics Review Board of the National Hospital Organization Headquarters in Japan (Tokyo, Japan) and Shinshu University (Nagano, Japan). Ethical approval was obtained on 17 August 2019, and the code was NHO H31-02. The authors attended educational lectures on medical ethics in 2020 and 2021, which were supervised by the Japanese government. The completion numbers for the authors are AP0000151756, AP0000151757, AP0000151769, and AP000351128. Consent to participate was required as this research was considered clinical research. Subjects signed an informed consent form when they were briefed on the clinical study and agreed with content of the research. The authors attended a seminar on the ethics of experimental research using small animals on 2 July 2020 and 20 July 2021. They became familiar with the importance and ethics of animal experiments (National Hospital Organization Kyoto Medical Center and Shinshu University School of Medicine). The code number for the ethical approval for experiments involving small animals was KMC R02-0702.

3. Results

Case 1. On 31 May 2021, a 58-year old woman arrived at our hospital with a markedly swollen abdomen and swollen left supraclavicular lymph nodes (Supplementary Material S1). Hematological examination before surgical treatment revealed a high LDH value of 3631 U/L and she excreted a blood clot during long-term follow-up of uterine leiomyoma delivery. Therefore, we considered a diagnosis of uterine leiomyosarcoma accompanied by uterine leiomyoma. We performed molecular pathological analysis with multiple index markers for various soft tissue tumors including candidate biomarkers for uterine leiomyosarcoma using the tissues removed during surgical treatment.

Macroscopic findings of the excised tissue are shown below. The resected uterine tumor was markedly hypertrophied, and the findings of the cut surface indicated that the uterine wall was replaced by a white solid phyllodes lesion with necrosis. A part of the uterine tumor exhibited a hard nodule and calcification that appeared to be uterine leiomyoma.

The pathological findings are shown below. Significant necrosis was observed at the tumor site on the uterus and a viable mass remained primarily at the margin and around the blood vessels. Many tumor cells found in a patient's uterine tumor are round-shaped cells or short-spindle-shaped cells with a high nuclear-cytoplasmic ratio (N/C). Furthermore, rhabdoid/rhabdomyoblastic cells, epithelioid cells, cells with bizarre large nuclei, large multi-nucleated cells, and spindle-shaped cells comprised the uterine tumor. Many fission cells were also observed in the tumor. Five factors (caveolin, cyclin B, cyclin

E, LMP2/β1i, Ki-67) were evaluated as markers to differentiate uterine leiomyosarcoma from other mesenchymal tumors [15,16] (Figures 1 and 2).

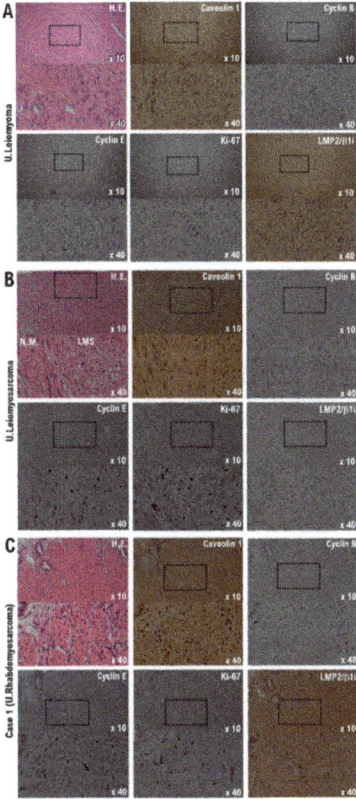

Figure 1. Differential expression of cyclin B, cyclin E, caveolin-1, ki-67, and LMP2/b1i as potential biomarkers in the normal myometrium, uterine leiomyoma, uterine leiomyosarcoma, and the Case 1 uterine tumor. (**A**) The image shows spindle cell leiomyoma. Low-power view (10× field) shows a well-circumscribed tumor nodule in the myometrium composed of broad fascicles of spindle cells. A high-power view (40× field) shows uterine leiomyoma (spindle cell) with bland cytological features, elongated nuclei, and fine nuclear chromatin. Immunohistochemistry of uterine leiomyoma tissue sections was performed using monoclonal antibodies. (**B**) The image shows uterine epithelioid leiomyosarcoma. Low power view (10× field) shows a uterine mass and an irregular interface with the myometrium composed of round to polygonal cells with granular eosinophilic cytoplasm. The presence of significant nuclear atypia and mitoses is evident. High-power view (40× field) shows tumor cells that are round to ovoid. The tumor cells have eosinophilic granular cytoplasm and irregular-shaped nuclei. Immunohistochemistry of the leiomyosarcoma tissue sections was performed using the appropriate monoclonal antibodies. (**C**) Case 1 uterine tumor appears as an admixture of round, polygonal, bizarre, or spindle cells, with marked atypia, with or without giant cells and rhabdomyoblasts. Some tumors invaded the lymphatic vessels. Low-power view (10× field) shows no obvious high-grade nuclear atypia or mitotic cell proliferation, and necrosis is observed. The high-power view (40× field) showing tumor cells with significant pleomorphism, whereas some are multinucleated and rhabdomyoblastic differentiation is evident. Immunohistochemistry with the of normal myometrium, leiomyoma, leiomyosarcoma, and the Case 1 uterine tumor was performed using appropriate monoclonal antibodies.

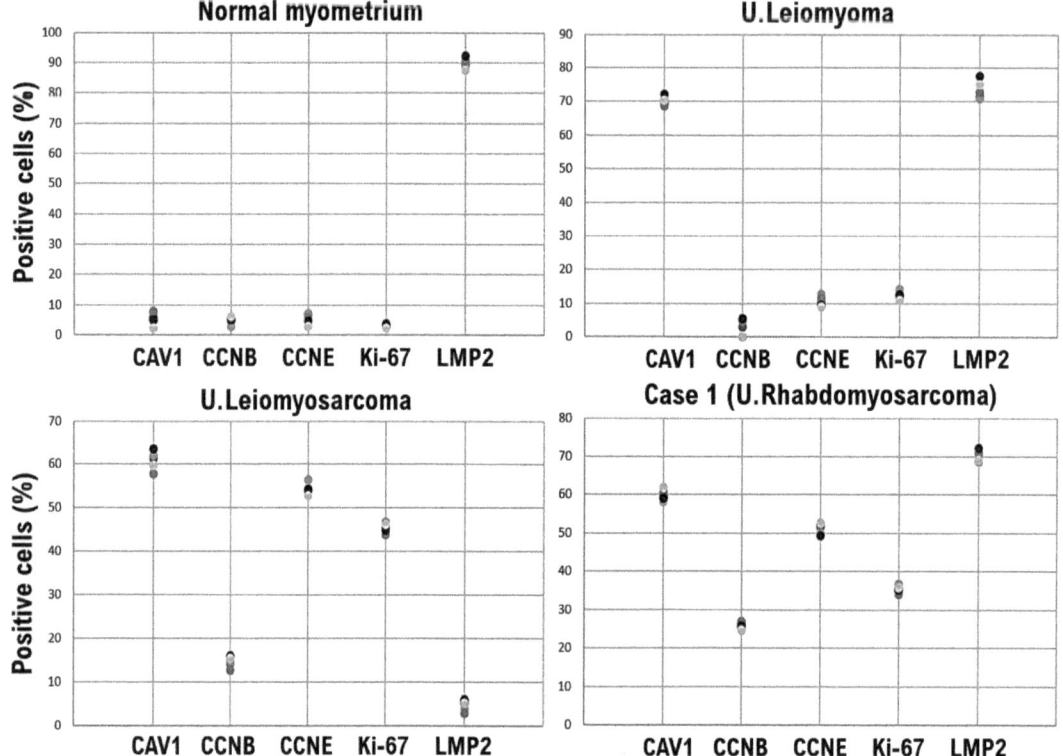

Figure 2. Significance of LMP2/b1i-positive uterine mesenchymal tumor cells in the Case 1 tumor as well as normal myometrium and uterine leiomyoma. Immunohistochemistry of normal myometrium, uterine leiomyoma, uterine leiomyosarcoma, and Case 1 uterine tumor tissues was performed using appropriate monoclonal antibodies. The tissues were randomly selected from normal myometrium, uterine leiomyoma, uterine leiomyosarcoma, and the Case 1 uterine tumor. Under a 40× field of view, the positive rates for five biomarkers were determined in four tissue sites under a microscope (Panthera Shimadzu Co. Ltd., Kyoto, Japan). The positive rates at each site for each tissue are displayed in a scatter plot. CAV1, caveolin-1; CCNB, cyclin B; CCNE, cyclin E; LMP2, LMP2/β1i.

The expression of caveolin, a candidate biomarker for uterine mesenchymal tumors, was confirmed in the uterine leiomyoma and uterine tumor of the patient (Figures 1 and 2). Mild expression of cyclin B, which is considered a biomarker for malignant tumors, was confirmed in the uterine leiomyosarcoma and uterine tumors of the patient (Figures 1 and 2). Strong expression of cyclin E and Ki-67, biomarker candidates for malignant mesenchymal tumors, was also observed in the uterine leiomyosarcoma and uterine tumors (Figures 1 and 2). Previous studies have indicated that the spontaneous onset of uterine leiomyosarcoma is observed in LMP2/β1i-deficient mice, which is one of the subunits of the immunoproteasome [17,18]. In human uterine leiomyosarcoma, the expression of LMP2/β1i is significantly reduced [17–19]. However, similar to normal uterine smooth muscle tissue and uterine leiomyoma, strong expression of LMP2/β1i was observed in the uterine tumor (Figures 1 and 2). These results indicate that the uterine tumor appears to be malignant, as the possibility of a uterine leiomyosarcoma is low (Table 1).

Table 1. Differential expressions of SMA, caveolin-1, cyclin B, cyclin E, LMP2, NT5DC2, CD133, and Ki-67 in human uterine mesenchymal tumors and uterine LANT-like tumor.

Mesenchymal Tumor Types	Age Years	n	Protein Expression *							
			SMA	CAV1	CCNB	CCNE	LMP2	NT5DC2	CD133	Ki-67
Normal	30–80 s	74	+++	-	-	-	+++	-	-	-
Leiomyoma (LMA) (Ordinally leiomyoma) (Cellular leiomyoma)	30–80 s	40 (30) (10)	+++	++	-/+	-/(+)	+++	-/+	-	+/-
			+++	++	-/+	-	+++	-/+		+/-
			++	++	-/+	-/(+)	++	-/+		+/-
STUMP	40–60 s	12	++	++	+	-/+	-/+	-/+	NA	+/+++
Bizarre Leiomyoma	40–50 s	4	++	++	-/+	+	Focal+	+	NA	+
Intravenous LMA	50 s	3	++	++	+	+	-	NA	++	+
Benign metastasizing	50 s	1	++	++	+	++	-	NA	NA	++
Leiomyosarcoma	30–80 s	54	-/+	+	++	+++	-/+	++	++	++/+++
Rhabdomyosarcoma	10 s, 50 s	2	NA	++	-/+	+++	+++	NA	NA	NA
U.LANT#-like tumor	40 s	1	++	+	NA	++	-	NA	NA	-

* Staining score of expression of SMA (smooth muscle actin), CAV1 (caveolin-1), CCNB (cyclin B), CCNE (cyclin E), LMP2 (low molecular protein 2), NT5DC2 (5′-nucleotidase domain containing 2) and Ki-67 from results of IHC experiments. Protein expression *; estimated-protein expressions by immunoblot analysis, immunohistochemistry (IHC) and/or RT-PCR (quantitative-PCR), -/+; partially positive (5% to 10% of cells stained), Focal+; Focal-positive (focal or sporadic staining with less than 5% of cells stained), ++; staining with 5% or more, less than 90% of cells stained, +++; diffuse-positive (homogeneous distribution with more than 90% of cells stained), -; negative (no stained cells). U.LANT-like tumor (uterine leiomyomatoid angiomatous neuroendocrine tumor-like tumor), LMP2 [13,20], cyclin E [13,20], caveolin-1 [13], NT5DC2 [21], CD133 [15], Ki-67 [13,20]. STUMP (smooth muscle tumor of uncertain malignant potential) [21,22]. Cyclin E, LMP2, caveolin-1 are potential biomarker for human uterine mesenchymal tumors. LANT #, leiomyomatoid angiomatous neuroendocrin tumor (LANT) is described as a dimorphic neurosecretory tumor with a leiomyomatous vascular component [23]. NA; no answer.

In histopathological diagnosis, desmin, myoglobin, myogenin, MyoD1, αSMA, and familial hyperinsulinemic hypoglycemia-35 (HHF-35) are used as markers for myogenic tissue. Desmin and HHF-35 are positive in both striated and smooth muscle tissues and are positive in many cases including uterine leiomyoma, rhabdomyosarcoma, uterine leiomyoma, and nodular fasciitis. Myogenin, MyoD1, and myoglobin are markers specific to striated muscle. Myogenin is highly sensitive and specific for rhabdomyosarcoma and is useful for differential diagnosis [24]. The results of immunohistochemical staining indicated strong expression of desmin, a molecular marker of muscle cells, in the uterine tumor and uterine leiomyosarcoma. Desmin expression was not evident in the normal uterine smooth muscle tissue (Figure 3). Strong expression of myogenin, a molecular marker of muscle cells, was observed in the uterine tumor, whereas high expression of myogenin was not observed in the uterine leiomyosarcoma (Figure 3). Given the positive status of myogenin, it was not considered to be a localized ectopic component of other tumors. Mild expression of synaptophysin, a neuroendocrine marker, and cytokeratin AE1/AE3, a marker of epithelial cells, was observed in the uterine tumor (Supplementary Material S2).

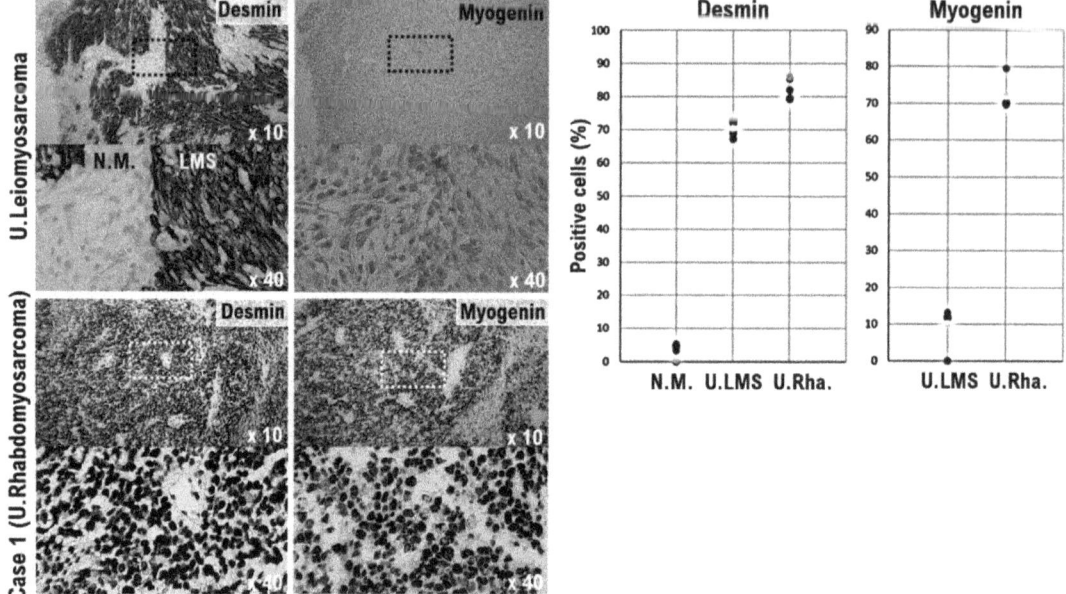

Figure 3. Significance of myogenin-positive uterine mesenchymal tumor cells in the Case 1 tumor. Differential expression of desmin and myogenin as potential biomarkers in normal myometrium, uterine leiomyosarcoma, and the Case 1 uterine tumor. The photograph shows uterine epithelioid leiomyosarcoma and normal myometrium. The low power view (10× field) shows the uterine mass irregular interface with normal myometrium, which is composed of round to polygonal cells with granular eosinophilic cytoplasm. The presence of significant nuclear atypia and mitoses is evident. A high-power view (40× field) shows tumor cells that are round to ovoid. The tumor cells have eosinophilic granular cytoplasm and irregular shaped nuclei. Immunohistochemistry (IHC) with the tissue sections of leiomyosarcoma was performed using the appropriate monoclonal antibodies (left upper panel). Case 1 uterine tumor is an admixture of round, polygonal, bizarre, or spindle cells, with marked atypia, with or without giant cells and rhabdomyoblasts. Some tumors invaded the lymphatic vessels. The low-power view (10× field) shows no obvious high grade nuclear atypia or mitotic cell proliferation. The high-power view (40× field) shows that tumor cells exhibit significant pleomorphism and some show multi-nucleated, rhabdomyoblastic differentiation. IHC with the Case 1 uterine tumor was performed using the appropriate monoclonal antibodies (left lower panel). The five tissue sites were randomly selected from normal myometrium, uterine leiomyosarcoma, and the Case 1 uterine tumor. In a 40× field of view, the positive rates for the two biomarkers were determined in three tissue sites under a microscope (Panthera Shimadzu Co. Ltd., Kyoto, Japan) (right panel). The positive rates at the sites for each tissue are shown in a scatter plot.

Circular cells with a high nuclear cytoplasm ratio (N/C) were found in the biopsy of the tumors of the left supraclavicular lymph node, as well as cells infiltrating the lymph vessels within the patient's uterine tumor (Figure 4). In addition, intravascular infiltration by the uterine tumor cells was observed (Figure 4). Based on this observation, we determined that the tumor of the left supraclavicular lymph node was not a malignant lymphoma, but a lymph node metastasis derived from a malignant mesenchymal tumor originating in the uterus. Lymphatic endothelial cells (CD31 and LYVE1-positive cells), which were not found in the uterine leiomyosarcoma, were observed in the uterine tumor (Figure 4). Although lymphatic metastases are rarely found in uterine leiomyosarcoma, in pleomorphic rhabdomyosarcoma, distant metastases to other organs and lymph node metastases are common [25].

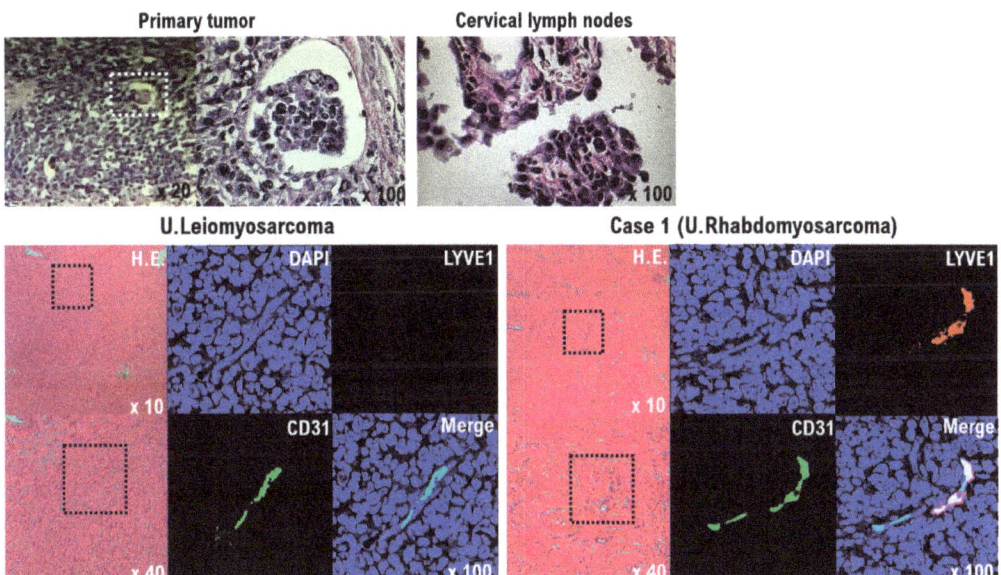

Figure 4. Significance of lymphatic endothelial cells in the primary Case 1 uterine tumor. Tumor cells infiltrating the lymph vessels within the uterine tumor are round cells with a high nuclear cytoplasmic ratio (N/C) (upper left panel). Circular cells with a high nuclear cytoplasm ratio (N/C) were also found in the biopsy from the tumor of the left supraclavicular lymph node (upper right panel). The results indicate that tumor cells from the primary uterine tumor formed metastases in the left supraclavicular lymph node by lymphatic metastasis. H&E staining and immunofluorescence of uterine leiomyosarcoma and the Case 1 uterine tumor with an anti-human CD31 (green) and anti-human LYVE-1 antibody (red) (lower panels). Human vascular endothelial cells and lymphatic endothelial cells were detected as CD31 and LYVE-1 double-positive cells. The tumor cells from the Case 1 uterine tumor appear to differentiate into lymphatic endothelial cell progenitors (lower light panel), but the tumor cells from the uterine leiomyosarcoma do not appear to have differentiated to lymphatic endothelial cell progenitors (lower left panel).

Based on these molecular pathological results, the patient was diagnosed with pleomorphic rhabdomyosarcoma. Pleomorphic rhabdomyosarcoma typically occurs in postmenopausal patients who present with abnormal vaginal bleeding [11]. The characteristics of pleomorphic rhabdomyosarcoma are consistent with the clinical findings.

Hematological examination before surgical treatment showed that the ovarian carcinoma antigen-125 (CA125) value was as high as 82, so it is possible that the giant uterine tumor may be a malignant tumor derived from epithelial cells, such as endometrial or ovarian cancer. No obvious malignant cells were observed in the fallopian tube tissue; however, endometriosis was observed in the tissues of the appendages, including the fallopian tubes. Thus, epithelial cells with nuclear swelling, so-called atypical endometriosis, were observed. Because CA125 is also produced in the peritoneum, thoracic membrane, or uterine/endometrial membrane, it is also elevated in benign and inflammatory diseases, such as benign ovarian cysts, endometriosis, uterine fibroids, inflammation, intestinal obstruction, pancreatitis, and cholecystitis. Therefore, the cause of high CA125 levels in patient serum is considered to be endometriosis.

4. Discussion

Rhabdomyosarcoma is the third most common solid childhood cancer outside of the central nervous system (after Wilms tumor and neuroblastoma). Rhabdomyosarcoma accounts for 3–4% of all childhood cancers. It belongs to a group of tumors known as soft tissue sarcoma and the number of patients with rhabdomyosarcoma is the highest among soft tissue sarcomas. The incidence of rhabdomyosarcoma in children is 4.3 out of 1 million annually. Two-thirds of the patients with rhabdomyosarcoma are under seven years of age. Rhabdomyosarcoma is more common in white ethnicities than in black ethnicities; in particular, it was shown that rhabdomyosarcoma occurs less frequently in black versus white girls. Additionally, the onset of rhabdomyosarcoma is slightly more common in boys than in girls. Multiple organ metastases occur in approximately 15–25% of children with rhabdomyosarcoma. The lung is the organ in which metastases most frequently occur, although metastases may also develop in the bone, bone marrow, and various lymph nodes. Uterine rhabdomyosarcoma consists of cells at various stages of differentiation. In uterine rhabdomyosarcoma, the expression of desmin, muscle-specific actin, myogenin, and MyoD1 is evident, and the expression status of these markers may be used as a reference for the diagnosis of uterine rhabdomyosarcoma [10].

Using immunohistochemical staining, strong expression of desmin, a molecular marker of muscle cells, was observed in the patient's uterine tumor and uterine leiomyosarcoma. Desmin expression was not observed in normal uterine smooth muscle tissue (Figure 4). Strong expression of myogenin, a molecular marker of muscle cells, was observed in the uterine tumor; however, no expression of myogenin was observed in uterine leiomyosarcoma (Figure 4). The expression status of other epithelial cell and neuroendocrine markers was evaluated in the patient's tumor. Based on these molecular pathological results, the uterine tumor was diagnosed as a pleomorphic rhabdomyosarcoma.

Rhabdomyosarcoma may be classified histopathologically into a fetal type, alveolar type, and pleomorphic type. Most rhabdomyosarcomas are fetal or alveolar, and occur most often in the head and neck, limbs, and genitourinary system of children. The pleomorphic type is believed to be more likely to occur in the limbs of the elderly [26]. For children, the International Rhabdomyosarcoma Study, which was established in the United States in 1972, has recommended combination therapy with surgery, chemotherapy, and radiation therapy [27].

According to recent data from the rhabdomyosarcoma study group in Europe, the United States, and Japan, the three-year progression-free survival rate is 80–100% in the low-risk group, 50–80% in the intermediate-risk group, and 30–50% in the high-risk group. Chemotherapy for fetal and alveolar rhabdomyosarcoma includes VAC therapy with vincristine (VCR), actinomycin D (ACD), and cyclophosphamide (CPA) as standard treatment. However, in adults, pleomorphic rhabdomyosarcoma often develops, and standard treatment has not been established. In particular, elderly people that do not respond to VAC therapy have a poor prognosis in many cases. Unfortunately, this case (Case 1: Supplementary Material S1) was a pleomorphic rhabdomyosarcoma and no response to VAC therapy was observed (Supplementary Material S1, Supplementary Material S3). In contrast, the case of embryonal rhabdomyosarcoma (Case 2: Supplementary Material S1) responded to VAC therapy (Supplementary Material S3).

Vimentin, cytokeratin, and ethylmalonic-adipicaciduria (EMA) are often used to distinguish epithelial tumors from non-epithelial soft tissue tumors. Vimentin is positive in many soft tissue tumors and negative in epithelial tumors. Cytokeratin and EMA are positive in epithelial tumors, but these markers tend to be positive in synovial sarcoma and epithelioid sarcoma, which have epithelial-like characteristics in soft tissue tumors. For pathological diagnosis, desmin, myoglobin, myogenin, MyoD1, α-smooth muscle actin, and HHF-35 are used as markers for myogenic tissues. The expression of desmin and HHF-35 is clearly observed in both striated and smooth muscle tumor tissue. Thus, the expression of desmin and HHF-35 is also observed in leiomyoma tissue, rhabdomyosarcoma tissue, benign leiomyoma, and nodular fasciitis tissue. Myogenin, MyoD1, and myoglobin are markers specific to striated muscle tissue. In particular, myogenin is useful for surgical pathological diagnosis because of its high sensitivity and specificity in rhabdomyosarcoma tissue, whereas α-smooth muscle actin is a marker specific for smooth muscle tissue.

Sarcomas are rare and usually display no specific line of differentiation, although rhabdomyosarcoma and leiomyosarcoma have been described [28,29]. Recent study shows that NT5DC2 is aberrantly upregulated in uterine leiomyosarcoma, and the expression of cyclin B1, cyclin A2, cyclin E1 is dependent on the expression of NT5DC2 [30]. However, the expression status of NT5DC2 in various mesenchymal tumors, including benign uterine leiomyoma, has not been clarified. Therefore, it is not clear whether NT5DC2 is a candidate biomarker for differentiating uterine leiomyosarcoma or rhabdomyosarcoma from other mesenchymal tumors. As pathogenesis for uterine leiomyosarcoma, the most frequently mutated genes include *TP53*, *ATRX*, and *MED12*; however no specific pathogenic variant has been identified [31,32]. On the other hand, molecular studies of a single case of pleomorphic rhabdomyosarcoma revealed *PIK3CA* and *TP53* mutations [33]. Therefore, it is inappropriate to distinguish between uterine leiomyosarcoma and uterine rhabdomyosarcoma based on the analysis results of pathological variants.

Previous research studies have indicated that the spontaneous onset of uterine leiomyosarcoma is observed in mice lacking LMP2/β1i, which is a subunit of the immunoproteasome [17–19]. In human uterine leiomyosarcoma, the expression of LMP2/β1i is significantly reduced [17–19]. However, as with normal uterine smooth muscle tissue and uterine leiomyoma, strong expression of LMP2/β1i was observed in the patient's uterine rhabdomyosarcoma (Figures 1 and 2, Table 1). Therefore, LMP2/β1i may be useful as a marker for differentiating uterine rhabdomyosarcoma from uterine leiomyosarcoma and other malignant mesenchymal tumors. The cytogenetic similarities detected thus far between leiomyoma and malignant muscle tumors (i.e., leiomyosarcoma and rhabdomyosarcoma) are few, which complicates the diagnosis of uterine leiomyoma and uterine rhabdomyosarcoma [34].

There are various theories regarding the origin of the development of uterine rhabdomyosarcoma [35], including Dr. Pfennenstiel's theory (stromal cell metaplasia), Dr. Giorke and Nehrkorn's theory (development of adult striated muscle in the bottom of the uterine), Dr. Wilms' theory (development of lumbar mesenchymal cells along the Wolff canal), and the theory of Dr. Lahn and colleagues (origin of the Muller duct). Dr. Silverberg reported that rhabdomyosarcoma mixed with mesodermal components may develop from the mesenchymal tissue around the Muller duct [36]; however, the origin has not yet been determined [37].

From clinical studies to date, it is not uncommon to observe the development of malignant uterine leiomyosarcoma over the course of follow-up for benign tumor uterine leiomyoma. We experienced a case involving the development of uterine rhabdomyosarcoma from a benign tumor uterine leiomyoma. In this case, when making a surgical pathological diagnosis, the use of candidate biomarkers for uterine leiomyosarcoma assisted us in the differential diagnosis of a large uterine tumor. Currently, no clinical treatment for adult rhabdomyosarcoma has been established [38,39]. Further clinical studies should be conducted to improve the diagnosis and treatment of uterine rhabdomyosarcoma.

5. Conclusions

In uterine mesenchymal tumors, cells with various histological types and cell morphologies are mixed. Furthermore, the components contained within the cells also vary. Therefore, surgical pathological diagnosis for uterine mesenchymal tumor is not straight forward. Therefore, the information obtained by the molecular pathological diagnosis using putative biomarkers for uterine smooth muscle tumor is useful for the differential diagnosis of other uterine mesenchymal tumors. The case in the present study was diagnosed as uterine pleomorphic rhabdomyosarcoma by molecular pathological diagnosis using candidate biomarkers for uterine smooth muscle tumors.

Supplementary Materials: The following are available online at https://www.mdpi.com/article/10.3390/curroncol29040190/s1. Material S1: Case 1 and Case 2; Material S2: Results of surgical pathological diagnosis; Material S3: Primary Uterine rhabdomyosarcoma.

Author Contributions: S.T., T.H. and T.I. performed most of the clinical work and coordinated the project. T.H. and I.K. conducted the diagnostic pathological studies. S.T. and T.H. conceptualized the study and wrote the manuscript. K.A., N.Y. and I.K. and carefully reviewed this manuscript and commented on the aspects of medical science. I.K. shared information on clinical medicine and oversaw the entirety of the study. All authors have read and agreed to the published version of the manuscript.

Funding: This clinical research was performed with research funding from the following: the Japan Society for Promoting Science for T.H. (Grant No. 19K09840) and for K.A. (No. 20K16431); the START-program Japan Science and Technology Agency for T.H. (Grant No. STSC20001); and the National Hospital Organization Multicenter clinical study for T.H. (Grant No. 2019-Cancer in general-02).

Institutional Review Board Statement: The study was conducted according to the guidelines of the Declaration of Helsinki, and approved by the Central Ethics Review Board of the National Hospital Organization Headquarters in Japan (Tokyo, Japan) and Shinshu University (Nagano, Japan). Ethical approval was obtained on 17 August 2019, and the code was NHO H31-02.

Informed Consent Statement: Informed consent was obtained from all subjects involved in the study. Written informed consent has been obtained from the patient(s) to publish this paper.

Data Availability Statement: The data presented in this study are available on request from the corresponding author.

Acknowledgments: We thank Yasuaki Amano for providing medical care to this patient at the National Hospital Organization Kyoto Medical Center.

Conflicts of Interest: The authors declare no potential conflict of interest.

Abbreviations

αSMA, alpha smooth muscle actin; CA125, ovarian carcinoma antigen-125; CD, clusters of differentiation; CT, computed tomography; DAPI, 4′,6-diamidino-2-phenylindole; EMA, ethylmalonic-adipicaciduria; ER, estrogen receptor; IHC, immunohistochemistry; HHF-35, familial hyperinsulinemic hypoglycemia-35; LDH, lactic acid dehydrogenase; LMP2/β1i, large multifunctional peptidase 2/β1i; LMS, leiomyosarcoma; LYVE-1, lymphatic vessel endothelial hyaluronan receptor 1; MyoD1, myogenic differentiation antigen 1; PgR, progesterone receptor; WHO, World Health Organization.

References

1. WHO Classification of Tumours Editorial Board. Mesenchymal tumours of the lower genital tract. In *Female Genital Tumours WHO Classification of Tumours*, 5th ed.; World Health Organization: Geneva, Switzerland, 2020; pp. 478–526.
2. WHO Classification of Tumours Editorial Board. Uterine leiomyosarcoma. In *Female Genital Tumours*; World Health Organization: Geneva, Switzerland, 2020; pp. 272–276.
3. Kaku, T.; Silverberg, S.G.; Major, F.J.; Miller, A.; Fetter, B.; Brady, M.F. Adenosarcoma of the uterus: A Gynecologic Oncology Group clinicopathologic study of 31 cases. *Int. J. Gynecol. Pathol.* **1992**, *11*, 75–88. [CrossRef]
4. Arend, R.; Bagaria, M.; Lewin, S.N.; Sun, X.; Deutsch, I.; Burke, W.M.; Herzog, T.J.; Wright, J.D. Long-term outcome and natural history of uterine adenosarcomas. *Gynecol. Oncol.* **2010**, *119*, 305–308. [CrossRef]
5. Clement, P.B.; Scully, R.E. Mullerian adenosarcoma of the uterus: A clinicopathologic analysis of 100 cases with a review of the literature. *Hum. Pathol.* **1990**, *21*, 363–381. [CrossRef]
6. Nathenson, M.J.; Ravi, V.; Fleming, N.; Wang, W.L.; Conley, A. Uterine Adenosarcoma: A Review. *Curr. Oncol. Rep.* **2016**, *18*, 68. [CrossRef] [PubMed]
7. Oliva, E. Practical issues in uterine pathology from banal to bewildering: The remarkable spectrum of smooth muscle neoplasia. *Mod. Pathol.* **2016**, *29* (Suppl. S1), S104–S120. [CrossRef] [PubMed]
8. Soslow, R.A.; Ali, A.; Oliva, E. Mullerian adenosarcomas: An immunophenotypic analysis of 35 cases. *Am. J. Surg. Pathol.* **2008**, *32*, 1013–1021. [CrossRef]

9. Marcus, J.Z.; Klobocista, M.; Karabakhtsian, R.G.; Prossnitz, E.; Goldberg, G.L.; Huang, G.S. Female Sex Hormone Receptor Profiling in Uterine Adenosarcomas. *Int. J. Gynecol. Cancer* **2018**, *28*, 500–504. [CrossRef] [PubMed]
10. Cytopathology Glossary—Edited Cytopathology Glossary Committee of the Japanese Society of Clinical Cytology, 27 May 2016. p. 15. Available online: http://jscc.or.jp/wp-content/uploads/2015/05/kaisetsu.pdf (accessed on 27 May 2016).
11. WHO Classification of Tumours Editorial Board. Rhabdomyosarcoma. In *Female Genital Tumours*; World Health Organization: Geneva, Switzerland, 2020; pp. 512–514.
12. Hayashi, T.; Kobayashi, Y.; Kohsaka, S.; Sano, K. The mutation in the ATP binding region of JAK1, identified in human uterine leiomyosarcomas, results in defective interferon-gamma inducibility of TAP1 and LMP. *Oncogene* **2006**, *25*, 4016. [CrossRef]
13. Hayashi, T.; Ichimura, T.; Yaegashi, N.; Shiozawa, T.; Konishi, I. Expression of CAVEOLIN 1 in uterine mesenchymal tumors: No relationship between malignancy and CAVEOLIN 1 expression. *Biochem. Biophys. Res. Commun.* **2015**, *463*, 982. [CrossRef] [PubMed]
14. Watanabe, K.; Hayashi, T.; Katsumata, M.; Sano, K.; Abiko, K.; Konishi, I. Development of Uterine Leiomyosarcoma During Follow-up After Caesarean Section in a Woman with Uterine Leiomyoma. *Anticancer Res.* **2021**, *41*, 3001–3010. [CrossRef]
15. Tamura, S.; Hayashi, T.; Tokunaga, H.; Yaegashi, N.; Abiko, K.; Konishi, I. Oncological Features of Intravenous Leiomyomatosis: Involvement of Mesenchymal Tumor Stem-Like Cells. *Curr. Issues Mol. Biol.* **2021**, *43*, 1188–1202. [CrossRef]
16. Aggarwal, N.; Bhargava, R.; Elishaev, E. Uterine adenosarcomas: Diagnostic use of the proliferation marker Ki-67 as an adjunct to morphologic diagnosis. *Int. J. Gynecol. Pathol.* **2012**, *31*, 447–452. [CrossRef] [PubMed]
17. Hayashi, T.; Faustman, D.L. Development of spontaneous uterine tumors in low molecular mass polypeptide-2 knockout mice. *Cancer Res.* **2002**, *62*, 24–27.
18. Hayashi, T.; Horiuchi, A.; Sano, K.; Hiraoka, N.; Kanai, Y.; Shiozawa, T.; Tonegawa, S.; Konishi, I. Mice-lacking LMP2, immunoproteasome subunit, as an animal model of spontaneous uterine leiomyosarcoma. *Protein Cell* **2010**, *1*, 711–717. [CrossRef]
19. Hayashi, T.; Horiuchi, A.; Sano, K.; Hiraoka, N.; Kasai, M.; Ichimura, T.; Sudo, T.; Tagawa, Y.; Nishimura, R.; Ishiko, O.; et al. Potential role of LMP2 as tumor-suppressor defines new targets for uterine leiomyosarcoma therapy. *Sci. Rep.* **2011**, *1*, 180. [CrossRef] [PubMed]
20. Patent: Detection of Uterine Leiomyosarcoma Using LMPApplication JP2007548042A Events. Available online: https://upload.umin.ac.jp/cgi-open-bin/ctr/ctr_view.cgi?recptno=R000044182 (accessed on 4 December 2019).
21. Hayashi, T.; Sano, K.; Ichimura, T.; Tonegawa, S.; Yaegashi, N.; Konishi, I. Diagnostic biomarker candidates including NT5DC2 for human uterine mesenchymal tumors. *Int. J. Trend Sci. Res. Dev.* **2021**, *5*, 604–606. Available online: https://www.ijtsrd.com/papers/ijtsrd38686.pdf (accessed on 1 April 2021).
22. WHO Classification of Tumours Editorial Board. Smooth muscle tumor of uncertain malignant potential of the uterine corpus. In *Female Genital Tumours*; World Health Organization: Geneva, Switzerland, 2020; pp. 279–280.
23. Hayashi, T.; Ichimura, T.; Kasai, M.; Sano, K.; Zharhary, D.; Shiozawa, T.; Yaegashi, N.; Konishi, I. Characterization of Leiomyomatoid Angiomatous Neuroendocrine Tumour (LANT)-like Tumour in the Myometrium with Histopathological Examination. *Anticancer Res.* **2017**, *37*, 1765–1772. [CrossRef]
24. Cessna, M.H.; Zhou, H.; Perkins, S.L.; Tripp, S.R.; Layfield, L.; Daines, C.; Coffin, C.M. Are myogenin and myoD1 expressionspecific for rhabdomyosarcoma? A study of 150 cases, with emphasis on spindle cell mimics. *Am. J. Surg. Pathol.* **2001**, *25*, 1150–1157. [CrossRef] [PubMed]
25. Watanabe, M.; Ansai, S.I.; Iwakiri, I.; Fukumoto, T.; Murakami, M. Case of pleomorphic rhabdomyosarcoma arising on subcutaneous tissue in an adult patient: Review of the published works of 13 cases arising on cutaneous or subcutaneous tissue. *J. Dermatol.* **2017**, *44*, 59–63. [CrossRef] [PubMed]
26. Yoshida, S.; Wakisaka, M. Rhabdomyosarcoma. *Pediatrics* **2011**, *52*, 985–992.
27. Crist, W.M.; Gehan, E.A.; Ragab, A.H.; Dickman, P.S.; Donaldson, S.S.; Fryer, C.; Hammond, D.; Hays, D.M.; Herrmann, J.; Heyn, R. The third intergroup rhabdomyosarcoma study. *J. Clin. Oncol.* **1995**, *13*, 610–630. [CrossRef]
28. Baergen, R.N.; Rutgers, J.L. Mural nodules in common epithelial tumors of the ovary. *Int. J. Gynecol. Pathol.* **1994**, *13*, 62–72. [CrossRef] [PubMed]
29. WHO Classification of Tumours Editorial Board. Mucinous borderline tumour. In *Female Genital Tumours*; World Health Organization: Geneva, Switzerland, 2020; pp. 50–52.
30. Hu, B.; Zhou, S.; Hu, X.; Zhang, H.; Lan, X.; Li, M.; Wang, Y.; Hu, Q. NT5DC2 promotes leiomyosarcoma tumour cell growth via stabilizing unpalmitoylated TEAD4 and generating a positive feedback loop. *J. Cell. Mol. Med.* **2021**, *25*, 5976–5987. [CrossRef] [PubMed]
31. An, Y.; Wang, S.; Li, S.; Zhang, L.; Wang, D.; Wang, H.; Zhu, S.; Zhu, W.; Li, Y.; Chen, W.; et al. Distinct molecular subtypes of uterine leiomyosarcoma respond differently to chemotherapy treatment. *BMC Cancer* **2017**, *17*, 639. [CrossRef]
32. Ravegnini, G.; Mariño-Enriquez, A.; Slater, J.; Eilers, G.; Wang, Y.; Zhu, M.; Nucci, M.R.; George, S.; Angelini, S.; Raut, C.P.; et al. MED12 mutations in leiomyosarcoma and extrauterine leiomyoma. *Mod. Pathol.* **2013**, *26*, 743–749. [CrossRef] [PubMed]
33. Pinto, A.; Kahn, R.M.; Rosenberg, A.E.; Slomovitz, B.; Quick, C.M.; Whisman, M.K.; Huang, M. Uterine rhabdomyosarcoma in adults. *Hum. Pathol.* **2018**, *74*, 122–128. [CrossRef] [PubMed]
34. Nibert, M.; Heim, S. Uterine leiomyoma cytogenetics. *Genes Chromosomes Cancer* **1990**, *2*, 3–13. [CrossRef] [PubMed]
35. Kulka, E.W.; Doglas, G.W. Rhabdomyosarcoma of the corpus uteri: Report of a case, associated with adenocarcinoma of the cervix, with review of the literature. *Cancer* **1952**, *5*, 727–736. [CrossRef]

36. Silverberg, S.G. Malignant mixed mesodermal tumor of the uterus: An ultrastructural study. *Am. J. Obstet. Gynecol.* **1971**, *10*, 702–712. [CrossRef]
37. Kikuchi, K.; Rubin, B.P.; Keller, C. Developmental origins of fusion-negative rhabdomyosarcomas. *Curr. Top. Dev. Biol.* **2011**, *96*, 33–56. [CrossRef]
38. Li, Z.J.; Li, C.L.; Wang, W.; Fu, X.Y.; Zhen, Y.Q. Diagnosis and treatment of pleomorphic rhabdomyosarcoma of the uterus: A rare case report and review of the literature. *J. Int. Med. Res.* **2021**, *49*, 3000605211014360. [CrossRef] [PubMed]
39. Chrisinger, J.S.A.; Wehrli, B.; Dickson, B.C.; Fasih, S.; Hirbe, A.C.; Shultz, D.B.; Zadeh, G.; Gupta, A.A.; Demicco, E.G. Epithelioid and spindle cell rhabdomyosarcoma with FUS-TFCP2 or EWSR1-TFCP2 fusion: Report of two cases. *Virchows Arch.* **2020**, *477*, 725–732. [CrossRef] [PubMed]

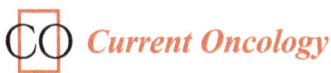

Article

P144 a Transforming Growth Factor Beta Inhibitor Peptide, Generates Antifibrogenic Effects in a Radiotherapy Induced Fibrosis Model

Sebastián Cruz-Morande [1,*], Javier Dotor [2] and Mikel San-Julian [3]

[1] Orthopaedic Surgery and Traumatology Department, Clínica San Miguel, Beloso Alto 36, 31006 Pamplona, Spain
[2] DISIT Biotech, Fuenlabrada Hospital, 28942 Madrid, Spain; jdotor@disitbiotech.com
[3] Orthopaedic Surgery and Traumatology Department, Clínica Universidad de Navarra, Av. Pio XII 36, 31008 Pamplona, Spain; msjulian@unav.es
* Correspondence: scruz@alumni.unav.es; Tel.: +34-948-296000 (ext. 1014)

Abstract: Radiation-induced fibrosis (RIF) is a severe side effect related with soft tissues sarcomas (STS) radiotherapy. RIF is a multicellular process initiated primarily by TGF-β1 that is increased in irradiated tissue, whose signaling leads to intracellular Smad2/3 phosphorylation and further induction of profibrotic target genes. P144 (Disetertide©) is a peptide inhibitor of TGF-β1 and is proposed as a candidate compound for reducing RIF associated wound healing problems and muscle fibrosis in STS. Methods: A treatment and control group of WNZ rabbits were employed to implement a brachytherapy animal model, through catheter implantation at the lower limb. Two days after implantation, animals received 20 Gy isodosis, intended to induce a high RIF grade. The treatment group received intravenous P144 administration following a brachytherapy session, repeated at 24–72 h post-radiation, while the control group received placebo. Four weeks later, affected muscular tissues underwent histological processing for collagen quantification and P-Smad2/3 immunohistochemistry through image analysis. Results: High isodosis Brachytherapy produced remarkable fibrosis in this experimental model. Results showed retained macro and microscopical morphology of muscle in the P144 treated group, with reduced extracellular matrix fibrosis, with a lower area of collagen deposition measured through Masson's trichrome staining. Intravenous P144 also induced a significant reduction in Smad2/3 phosphorylation levels compared with the placebo group. Conclusions: P144 administration clearly reduces RIF and opens a new potential co-treatment approach to reduce complications in soft tissue sarcoma (STS) radiotherapy. Further studies are required to establish whether the dosage and timing optimization of P144 administration, in different RIF phases, might entirely avoid fibrosis associated with STS brachytherapy.

Keywords: soft tissue sarcomas; radio-induced fibrosis; brachytherapy; transforming growth factor-beta1 (TGF-β1); Disitertide; Smad 2/3

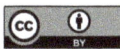

1. Introduction

Soft tissue sarcomas (STSs) are uncommon tumors of mesenchymal origin, with different subtypes having a different prognostic profile. STSs most commonly arise in the extremities, but can also occur in the trunk and retroperitoneum [1].

STSs account for 1% of all adult malignancies, with a global incidence of 180,000 cases per year and a mortality of 80,000 patients/year [2]. Extremity soft tissue sarcomas (ESTSs) are diagnosed frequently with a delay, due to the painless presentation and the rarity of the disease. For this reason, they often produce large tumor masses, with a mean tumor diameter of 10 cm at time of diagnosis [3].

Treatment includes surgical resection in combination with radiotherapy. Limb-preserving surgery combined with radiotherapy has dramatically improved the local control of soft tissue sarcoma patients [2,4,5]. However, it still carries a substantial risk of acute side effects, such as fatigue, nausea, vomitous, diarrhea, hair loss, or skin or mouth damage, and long-term side-effects that depend on the irradiated tissue and might include heart complications, breast size changes, damage in the lungs, brachial plexopathy, fertility problems together with changes in sexual life, and cystitis [6]. Post-radiotherapy fibrosis in the treatment of childhood soft tissue sarcomas occurs in 80% of patients, in different degrees of involvement [7], and 95% of patients have radiodermatitis, which has a similar pathophysiology [8].

Brachytherapy is a modality of radiotherapy used in the treatment of the soft tissue sarcomas [9,10]. This treatment frequently induces fibrotic processes in the tumor surrounding tissues like skin, the skeletal muscle and fascias [11,12], similar to other radiotherapy modalities. The administration of an early radiation within the first postoperative month is associated with the highest morbidity, whereas complication rates decrease with time. On the other hand, postponed radiation may lead to oncological compromises [13].

Although radio-induced fibrosis (RIF) closely resembles the chronic healing of a traumatic wound, it is subject to irradiation related disturbances, because all the cells and extracellular components of the irradiated volume tissues have been affected.

Fibrosis is essentially involved in the genesis of late reactions in slowly renewed healthy connective tissue with a non-compartmentalized structure, such as the dermis and subcutaneous tissues [14], or vasculo-connective parenchymal tissue [15].

Fibrosis is characterized by the activation and increase of an excessive number of activated fibroblasts, resulting in the deposition of extracellular matrix proteins such as collagen and impairment of normal tissue architecture. Although fibrosis is a physiological part of wound-healing processes, the excessive accumulation of collagen and other extracellular matrix components can lead to the destruction of normal tissue architecture and loss of function [11]. Recent studies have reported that cells other than fibroblasts also contribute very significantly to the appearance of fibrosis. Among these cells we find the macrophages resident in the connective tissue, which, as is well known, play a very important role in maintaining and amplifying the inflammatory response. This important role is due at least in part to the fact that macrophages are an important source of TGF-β and, in turn, this TGF-β contributes to the increased production of reactive oxygen species, which is closely linked to increased inflammation and the appearance of fibrosis [16,17].

Abnormal fibroblast proliferation and differentiation is considered central to fibrosis. RIF is a multicellular process that begins with the induction of and interaction between multiple growth factors and cytokines [18]. Among these factors, TGF-β1 levels are increased in irradiated mouse skin [19,20] and decrease slowly after irradiation in both pig and human skin [21,22].

Following microvascular hard or soft tissue transfer, TGF-β1 is again upregulated in a biphasic manner. The first expression peak on day 3 post operation is due to the enhanced activation of latent TGF-β1 by extracellular enzymes while the second peak of TGF–β1 expression between 14 and 28 days after surgery is the result of de novo synthesis cascade [23]. Its most important signaling receptor TGFBR2 is upregulated in irradiated graft beds as well [24]. TGFβ1 signaling leads to increased nucleoplasmatic shuttling of active Smad2/3 and induction of TGF-β1 target genes in fibrotic healing, which is mainly due to the decrease in cytoplasmatic levels of the inhibitory Smad7. As a consequence, the extracellular matrix is qualitatively and quantitatively altered [24,25]. Some of these alterations are related to Prolyl-hydroxyprolinase-β overexpression that promotes synthesis of collagen I, III, and IV, while the repression of degrading enzymes such as MMP-1 and induction of tissue inhibitors [24,26,27] suppress the degrading pathways. All these molecular events induced by active TGF-β1 generates the deposition of an excessive and dysfunctional extracellular matrix.

TGF-β is a cytokine with a very low half-life, around 2–3 min. It has been demonstrated that upon activation of its receptor, downstream phosphorylation of Smad 2/3 is a good marker of TGF-β pathway activity and it is better than direct measurement of latent/active TGF-β presence [28]. Some drug candidates, such as peptide P144 (Disitertide®—TSLDASIIWAMMQN), can inhibit TGβ-1 activity and have been successfully tested in clinical trials for pathological skin fibrosis conditions such as scleroderma [29]

P144 is a poorly soluble hydrophobic peptide derived from the sequence of the extracellular region of TGF-β type III receptor (Betaglycan) and specifically identified to block the interaction of TGF-β with its membrane receptors, blocking TGF-β1 biological activity in different in vitro and in vivo models [3,29–31]. P144 inhibits TGFβ1-dependent fibrosis [3] and also has the potential to present enhancing effects over antitumor immunotherapy [31].

In this study, it is proposed that targeting TGF-β1 with the synthetic peptide P144 (DISIT Biotech, Spain) could be an appropriate strategy for reducing the RIF of the muscle and thus reducing wound healing problems, which represent the major cause of complications related with limbs soft tissues sarcomas treatment [32].

2. Material and Methods

2.1. Animals

This study was approved by the Ethical Committee for Animal Experimentation of our institution (authorization number 032-07) and animal experimentation was conducted in accordance with Spanish and European legislation and approved by the Spanish National Research Council (CSIC).

For the study, adult female and male rabbits (aged 3–4 months, weighing 2.5–3 kg) were used. Rabbits were fed ad libitum with a standard diet and drinking water and controlled following FELASA (Federation of European Laboratory Animal Science Associations) recommendations.

The animals were randomly divided in three groups, namely the experimental model implementation group ($n = 5$), study group treated with P144 ($n = 6$), and placebo group treated with intra venomous (IV) saline vehicle ($n = 6$). Three rabbits were reserved as backup specimens if any complication occurs during the study.

2.2. Surgical Technique

The rabbits were intramuscularly anesthetized with a mixture of ketamine (Imalgene® 1000) (35 mg/kg) and Xylacine (Rompun® 2%) (5 mg/kg) before all surgical and irradiation procedures. Injections were administered with a 1 mL syringe and a 25-gauge needle and was repeat if required every 30 min, associated with 0.007 mg Fentanil (Fentanest®). After 2–4 min, adopting the aseptic technique, a longitudinal skin incision on the lateral aspect of the left leg was performed. The hamstrings muscle was recognized and a portion of muscle of 2 cm^3 was resected, then two 6F semiflexible high dose rate brachytherapy catheters were placed as parallel as possible at 1.0 cm in an intramuscular form in the hamstring. Passing in a subcutaneous way to the dorsal aspect of the rabbit thorax, the catheters were secured to the skin by suture stiches and protected with sterilized dressing. As postoperative analgesia, the animals received Ketoprofen (Ketofen® 10 mg/mL), 0.3 mL/kg intramuscularly every 24 h for three days.

2.3. Brachytherapy

After 48 h, a CT-guided brachytherapy planning was performed for each rabbit with the BrachyVision™ Brachytherapy Treatment Planning System (v.8.0, Varian, Palo Alto, CA, USA). Two rabbits of the model development group were irradiated with an Isodosis of 15 Gy, and two with 20 Gy with an Iridium 192 high dose rate (HDR) source in a constant volume of affected tissue (Figure 1). All the rabbits in the study and control group were irradiated with an Isodosis of 20 Gy. Immediately after brachytherapy procedures, the catheters were removed in all the rabbits

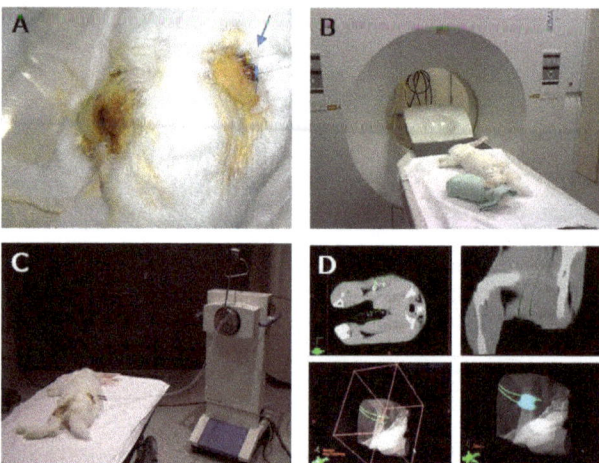

Figure 1. Images of rabbits undergoing brachytherapy procedure. (**A**) Catheters implantation in left posterior rabbit's limb as brachytherapy source applicator (blue arrow). (**B**) Imaging assurance of correct positioning of catheters through SOMATOM CT Sliding Ganty (**C**) Air pressure control of radioactive seeds delivery and positioning with a GammaMedplus IX (Varian Medical Systems). (**D**) 2D and 3D imaging guided axial visualization for virtual delivery of radioactive sources (BrachyVision™).

2.4. Drug Administration

Disitertide® (P144) was manufactured by Polypeptide Group (Strasbourg, France) as the lyophilized peptide was stored at −80 °C before the manipulation peptide vial was tempered to room temperature and then weighed, resuspended in buffer diazonium salt of carbonic acid 0.1 M pH 9.5, and sonicated until a homogeneous solution was obtained. Peptide was IV in the marginal ear veins of the rabbits at doses 10 mg per administration diluted in 10 mL of buffer (approximately 3.5 mg/Kg). As previously mentioned, this dose range was shown to be effective in prior published animal models of inflammation and fibrosis [3,29,33]. Placebo rabbits were injected IV with 10 mL of diazonium salt of carbonic acid 0.1 M pH 9.5.

The first dose was administrated immediately after the radiotherapy and repeated at 24 and 72 h after the first administration.

2.5. Sacrifice and Histological Examinations

After 4 weeks, the animals were sacrificed with a lethal dose of barbiturates, followed immediately by a resection of hamstring muscle of the irradiated leg, the muscle samples were embedded in paraffin after an overnight fixation in 4% polyformaldehyde solutions. A series of sections were routinely stained with hematoxylin and eosin, Massons trichrome. The immunohistochemical detection was performed with anti-phosphorylated Smad2/3 polyclonal antibody (Santa Cruz Biotechnology, Santa Cruz, California) adopting a biotin peroxidase-based method (ABC, Vector Laboratories, Burlingame, CA, USA).

2.6. Histomorphometric and Immunohistochemical Analysis

Semi-quantitative measurement of the total tissue area, collagen fibers, and positive P-Smad 2/3 cells area was performed using digital images obtained with a Zeiss Axio-CamICc3 camera (Plan-Neofluar objective with 0.50 NA) at 20× magnification with an AxioImager.M1 microscope (Zeiss, Oberkochen, Germany).

The quantification was based on collagen fibers stained in blue with Masson's Trichrome and immunohistochemical staining of P-Smad2/3. AxioVision software was used to conform a mosaic image of the whole muscle tissue sample with of different tissue pictures. We used four sections of each muscle tissue sample. Mosaic images were analyzed using an in-house developed plug-in for Fiji (a distribution of ImageJ) V1.46b. Individual Images were analyzed using an in-house developed plug-in for Fiji (a distribution of ImageJ) V1.48v. Then, images were subjected to threshold to measure the positive staining area of each marker. Mean intensity of staining value was also measured for all threshold areas. P144 effect over P-Smad 2/3 levels in RIF was presented as the positive stained area versus total area ratio in comparison with placebo treated group.

2.7. Statistics

The non-parametric Kruskal–Wallis test was used for comparisons between multiple groups and U Mann–Whitney tests were used for comparisons between two groups. A *p*-value of less than 0.05 was considered statistically significant. Statistical analyses of data were performed using GraphPad Prism 9 for Windows (GraphPad Software, San Diego, CA, USA).

3. Results

3.1. Animal Model

The proposed animal model presents a plausible manipulation and reproducibility. All the procedures were properly tolerated by experimental animals and no surgical related complications were detected. After four weeks placebo and P144 treated groups showed a weight mean increase of 10.4% and 14.1%, respectively, but without being statistically different.

3.2. Skin and Articular Range

Interestingly, all rabbits receiving P144 present less area and alopecia intensity in the skin region affected with brachytherapy application while the placebo group developed a marked and more extensive alopecia in the same region (Figure 2)

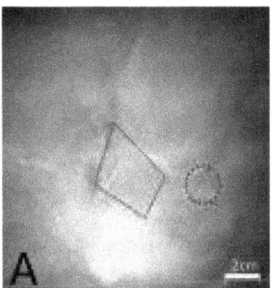
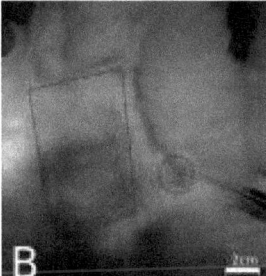

Figure 2. Rabbits skin regions expose to internal brachytherapy. (**A**) Representative picture of a rabbits treated with P144. (**B**) Representative picture of a rabbits treated with placebo. Skin area affected with post brachytherapy alopecia is indicated with discontinued red line square and catheters insertion point is indicated with a discontinued blue circle.

Post operated animals´ legs of all groups underwent a range of motion analysis, and no differences between contralateral legs, hip, and knee were found, discarding surgical affectation of surrounding joints, muscles, and tendons.

3.3. Muscle Fibrosis

In both animal groups, different amount of muscle disorganization and loss of the fibrillar patron of the muscle were detected, being qualitatively more evident in the placebo group. The P144 treated group presents more extensive areas with preserved muscle structure in the irradiated tissues associated with less necrosis and a lower presence of collagen deposition with respect to the placebo group (Figure 3).

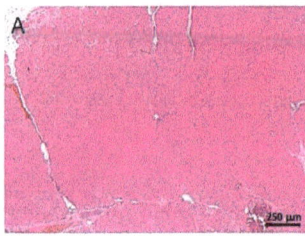 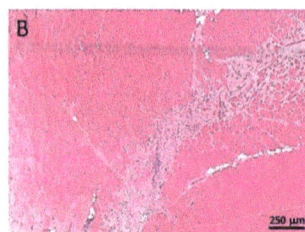 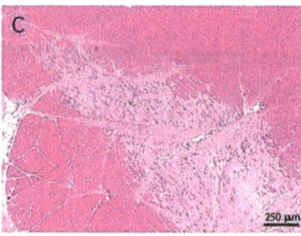

Figure 3. Hematoxylin and eosin staining example 5× showing the difference in muscular organization: (**A**) Normal Tissue, (**B**) P144 group (**C**) Placebo Group.

To evaluate the tissue collagen content in the muscles, a Masson's trichrome staining was performed, generating a mean collagen area of 11% in the P144 treated group with respect to a 24.9% of collagen-stained areas in muscle of the placebo group ($p < 0.007$) (Figures 4 and 5). The evaluation of collagen area in Masson's trichrome stained tissue where the brachytherapy catheters were placed showed only 2% of positive area with no differences between groups.

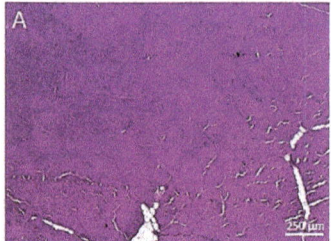 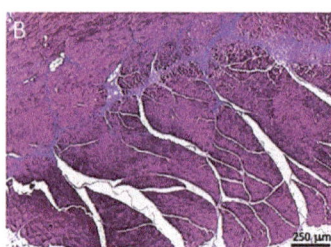 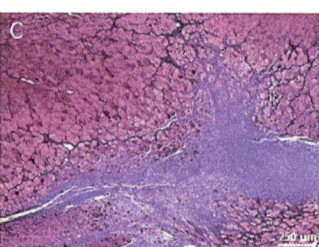

Figure 4. Masson´s Trichrome staining example 10×: (**A**) Normal Tissue, (**B**) P144 group, (**C**) Placebo group.

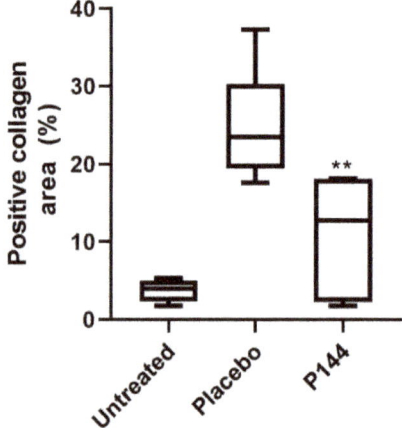

Figure 5. Histological collagen quantification in Masson's Trichrome stained slides in rabbits muscle tissue that underwent brachytherapy. Untreated, Placebo and P144 treated animals´ collagen tissue content. Statistical significance ** $p < 0.01$ vs. Placebo group.

3.4. P-Smad2/3 Immunohistochemical Staining

Intravenous administration of P144 induced a significant reduction in Smad2/3 phosphorylation levels compared to the placebo group ($p < 0.05$) four weeks after brachytherapy as demonstrated in the reduced levels of p-Smad2/3 in the P144 group vs. placebo group ($p < 0.01$) (Figures 6 and 7).

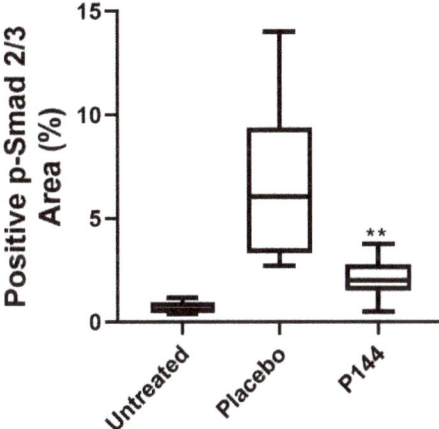

Figure 6. Immunohistochemical positive quantification of P-Smad2/3 in stained slides of rabbits' muscle tissue that underwent brachytherapy. Placebo vs. P144 treated animals' TGF-β signaling activation measured as positive detection of p-smad 2/3. Statistical significance ** $p < 0.01$.

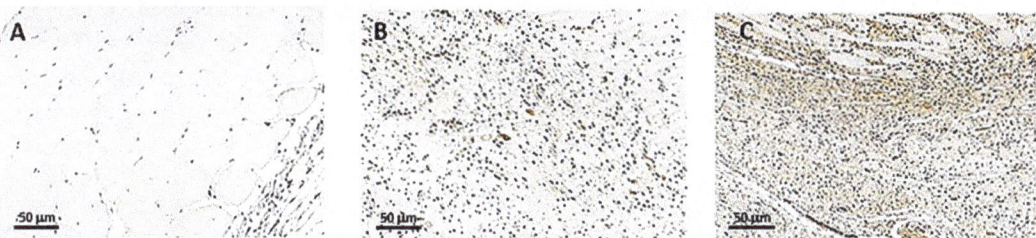

Figure 7. Representative Immunohistochemical positive p-Smad2/3 cells in stained slides of rabbits' muscle tissue Image 20×. (**A**) Normal Tissue example, (**B**) P144 group example, (**C**). Placebo group.

4. Discussion

Rodent models are often used to demonstrate the proof-of-principle tracer and therapeutic agent development, but their small size can make radiation dosing and tissue sampling collection challenging. The in vivo model obtained by the resection of muscle fragment and the radiation of the surgical area mimic a tumoral bed in rabbits, resulting in a plausible animal model for the study of the RIF in humans. Different animal models are described in the literature for radiation-induced fibrosis in rodents [34,35] or even in large animals [36], but there is no record in the literature describing an animal model similar to that pointed out in the present work and developed exclusively to evaluate muscular RIF.

In this work, the fibrotic response of limb muscles and surrender tissues to radiotherapy injury were monitored by histological methods, and according to other parameters that represent local and systemic damage cause by radiotherapy.

We found less alopecia in rabbits treated with P144 in the irradiated area, which may be due to the action of the peptide. P144 showed clear antifibrotic activity after topical application in a skin fibrosis mice model [29] and immunohistochemical studies in these P144-treated mice revealed a remarkable suppression of connective tissue growth factor expression, fibroblast SMAD2/3 phosphorylation, and alpha-smooth muscle actin positive myofibroblast development, whereas mast cell and mononuclear cell infiltration was not modified. These data suggested that the topical application of P144, a peptide inhibitor of TGF-β, is a feasible strategy to treat pathological skin scarring and skin fibrotic diseases for which there is no specific therapy. The systemic administration of the same active compound (P144) could exert a relevant antifibrotic effect in skin damage by radiotherapy. Moreover, P144 present anti-inflammatory properties that could protect hair follicles from the initial damage after a brachytherapy session [28].

Radiotherapy causes cellular injury by damaging the DNA and by generating free radicals [11]. Free-radical inactivation of anticoagulatory factors leads to rapid activation of the coagulation cascade following radiation injury. Endothelial cell apoptosis and slow regenerative proliferation result in increased vascular permeability and vessels denuded of endothelium which are prone to thrombosis, intimal proliferation, and eventually obliteration. Physical trauma results in the activation of an acute inflammatory response by stress-sensitive kinases and transcription factors. Pro-inflammatory cytokines, such as tumor necrosis factor-α (TNFα), interleukin (IL)-1, IL-8, and interferon-γ (IFNγ) are synthesized [15]. The termination of the inflammatory response results from the short half-life of these cytokines and anti-inflammatory cytokines, such as transforming growth factor-β (TGFβ), IL-4, IL-10, and IL-13. Inflammation does not resolve adequately following radiation injury because of the overproduction of pro-inflammatory cytokines leading to perturbed intercellular and cell–matrix interactions, uncontrolled matrix accumulation, and fibrosis [37]. This excessive fibrosis is characterized by collagen deposition and microvascular injury of the surrounding tumor healthy tissues, including skin, muscles, soft tissues, and internal organs (lungs, liver, etc.). In this context, collagen fibers represent the major component of the fibrotic extracellular matrix. Excessive collagen synthesis and accumulation was the rationale for pointing to collagen turnover as an activity and severity measure in radiotherapy induced fibrosis.

Collagen deposition is the final marker of the RIF pathophysiological process severely affecting irradiated organs and tissue in a mechanical and functional way. TGF-β/Smad signaling plays an essential role in the pathogenesis of muscular RIF. As P144 is a specific inhibitor of Smad intracellular activation by blocking extracellular TGF-β and inhibiting its interaction with membrane TGF-β receptors, the evaluation of P144 over Smad2/3 phosphorylation in RIF was performed. In this study, the efficacy of an inhibitor peptide of TGF β (P-144), intravenously administered, over irradiated tissue collagen content and TGF-β signaling activation, measured as P-Smad2/3 levels, show a significant lower phosphorylation of SMAD2 in the P144 group. Similar to our results, Disitertide induced significant inhibition of basal pSMAD2 in SNU449 cells [38]. Anscher et al. [35] demonstrated previously that direct interference with the actions of TGF-β can ameliorate the manifestations of the RIF on the lungs by using an anti-TGF-β antibody. Other authors show that black soybean anthocyanins inhibited radiation-induced fibrosis by downregulating TGF-β and Smad3 expression that resulted in a significant reduction in the level of skin injury, epidermal thickness, and collagen deposition after irradiation [39]. These findings are in the same line of our study, in that by the inhibition of the TGF-β, the final results constitute a reduction of collagen deposition in the extracellular matrix. Simultaneously, the direct correlation between P144, TGF-β biological activity inhibition, and fibrosis reduction confirms that intravenous administration of this compound is effective in the prevention for tissue affectation in an animal model representative of human radiotherapy induced fibrosis.

The peptide p144 has been used in different dermal fibrosis models, e.g., for the treatment of hypertrophic scars using a topical form [40] as an alternative route of administration in addition to the intravenous route [29], and also used intravitreally [41]. These results point out that there would be no limits in testing P-144 antifibrotic actions in other organs, such as the lung, where p17, a peptide similar to P144, has been tested showing good results [42]. On the other hand, it is well known that inflammation and fibrosis lead to transdifferentiation of fibroblast in myofibroblast and even favor the transition of epithelial to mesenchyme cells [43,44]. Thus, changes in the cellular profile of the connective tissue after treatment with P144 in RIF models needs to be evaluated in further studies.

These results confirm those obtained in previous research [3,30] regarding the efficacy of a systemic administration of P144 in fibrosis reduction in other kinds of fibrosis models and provide the basis for the clinical interest in a P144 intravenous formulation for further preclinical and clinical development of RIF protective therapy.

In vivo P144 activity against fibrosis is comparable or even superior to other TGF-β inhibitor compounds. In the work of Park et al., the effects of a small molecule inhibitor of TGF-β RI (SKI2162) activity in a model of skin RIF in mice were reported [45]. The effects were partial, and the dosage ranged from 10 to 30 mg/kg, while in the present study P144 is administered in a range of 2–3 mg/kg. Moreover, the intramuscular brachytherapy model is a more severe challenge in damage and tissue response respect skin irradiation. In a similar work, Flechsig et al. showed the effect of other small molecule (LY2109761) inhibitor in a lung RIF murine model, where effects were relevant but also partial and the dosage regimen was 50 mg/kg twice daily for four weeks [46].

There is not direct proof of how p144 may act against sarcomas yet. However, several studies in other type of cancers point out that it would be effective. Thus, in the case of glioblastoma, P144 has shown potential use by reducing proliferation, migration, invasiveness, and tumorigenicity [47]. On the other hand, it has also been seen that TGF-β is a mediator in the formation of metastases from the colon to the liver [48]. Furthermore, it has also been reported that the TGF-β is abundant in the environment of osteosarcomas and that inhibiting its production osteosarcoma progression is reduced [49]. Therefore, these collective findings support the idea that P144 could be effective in the treatment of sarcomas.

The proof of concept of a systemic formulation of Disitertide©, for the prevention of brachytherapy induced fibrosis, is validated in this work as a relevant strategy for future clinical applications that include other tissue locations tumors in relation with radiotherapy induced fibrosis. Furthermore, Disitertide© may have potential in radiotherapy-associated fibrosis in other organs and tissues, but this hypothesis should be confirmed in further studies with suitable animal models and different preclinical proof-of-concept studies. Further studies are necessary to elucidate whether the application of Disitertide© in the late phase of the radiotherapy induced fibrosis formation might avoid the excessive deposition of extracellular matrix components, hence acting as a preventive treatment.

5. Conclusions

In this work, we demonstrate that P144 treatment reduces RIF intensity and fibrotic tissue response in a rabbit model of brachytherapy, and this reduction is related to a decrease in the levels of Smad2/3 phosphorylation, as a representation of the canonical intracellular pathway activation of cells in response to TGF-β biological activity. These results invite the clinical consideration of a new potential co-treatment approach to reducing complications in soft tissue sarcomas treated with radiotherapy.

Author Contributions: Conceptualization, S.C.-M. and M.S.-J.; methodology, S.C.-M. and J.D.; software, J.D.; validation, S.C.-M. and M.S.-J.; formal analysis, J.D.; investigation, J.D.; resources, S.C.-M. and M.S.-J.; data curation, J.D. and S.C.-M.; writing—original draft preparation, S.C.-M. and J.D.; writing—review and editing, S.C.-M., J.D. and M.S.-J.; supervision, M.S.-J.; funding acquisition, M.S.-J. All authors have read and agreed to the published version of the manuscript.

Funding: This work was also partially supported by BITA (CIMA biomedicine project, S.L.) and by Clínica Universidad de Navarra.

Institutional Review Board Statement: This study was approved by the Ethical Committee for Animal Experimentation of University of Navarra (authorization number 032-07) and animal experimentation was conducted in accordance with Spanish and European legislation.

Data Availability Statement: The data presented in this study are available on request from the corresponding author.

Conflicts of Interest: Javier Dotor is CSO, co-founder and shareholder of DISITBiotech S.L. Private company focus on the development of clinical applications of Disitertide. The rest of the authors declare no conflict of interest.

References

1. Siegel, R.L.; Miller, K.D.; Fuchs, H.E.; Jemal, A. Cancer statistics, 2022. *CA Cancer J. Clin.* **2022**, *72*, 7–33. [CrossRef] [PubMed]
2. Gamboa, A.C.; Gronchi, A.; Cardona, K. Soft-tissue sarcoma in adults: An update on the current state of histiotype-specific management in an era of personalized medicine. *CA Cancer J. Clin.* **2020**, *70*, 200–229. [CrossRef] [PubMed]
3. Ezquerro, I.J.; Lasarte, J.J.; Dotor, J.; Castilla-Cortázar, I.; Bustos, M.; Peñuelas, I.; Blanco, G.; Rodríguez, C.; Lechuga, M.D.C.G.; Greenwel, P.; et al. A synthetic peptide from transforming growth factor β type III receptor inhibits liver fibrogenesis in rats with carbon tetrachloride liver injury. *Cytokine* **2003**, *22*, 12–20. [CrossRef]
4. Beane, J.D.; Yang, J.C.; White, D.; Steinberg, S.M.; Rosenberg, S.A.; Rudloff, U. Efficacy of adjuvant radiation therapy in the treatment of soft tissue sarcoma of the extremity: 20-Year follow-up of a randomized prospective trial. *Ann. Surg. Oncol.* **2014**, *21*, 2484–2489. [CrossRef] [PubMed]
5. Shah, C.; Verma, V.; Takiar, R.; Vajapey, R.; Amarnath, S.; Murphy, E.; Mesko, N.W.; Lietman, S.; Joyce, M.; Anderson, P.; et al. Radiation Therapy in the Management of Soft Tissue Sarcoma. *Am. J. Clin. Oncol. Cancer Clin. Trials* **2016**, *39*, 630–635. [CrossRef]
6. Habrand, J.L.; Le Pechoux, C. Radiation therapy in the management of adult soft tissue sarcomas. *Ann. Oncol.* **2004**, *15*, iv187–iv191. [CrossRef]
7. Paulino, A.C. Late effects of radiotherapy for pediatric extremity sarcomas. *Int. J. Radiat. Oncol. Biol. Phys.* **2004**, *60*, 265–274. [CrossRef]
8. Borrelli, M.R.; Shen, A.H.; Lee, G.K.; Momeni, A.; Longaker, M.T.; Wan, D.C. Radiation-Induced Skin Fibrosis: Pathogenesis, Current Treatment Options, and Emerging Therapeutics. *Ann. Plast. Surg.* **2019**, *83*, S59–S64. [CrossRef]
9. Martinez-Monge, R.; Cambeiro, M.; San-Julián, M.; Sierrasesúmaga, L. Use of brachytherapy in children with cancer: The search for an uncomplicated cure. *Lancet Oncol.* **2006**, *7*, 157–166. [CrossRef]
10. Martínez-Monge, R.; San Julián, M.; Amillo, S.; Cambeiro, M.; Arbea, L.; Valero, J.; González-Cao, M.; Martín-Algarra, S. Perioperative high-dose-rate brachytherapy in soft tissue sarcomas of the extremity and superficial trunk in adults: Initial results of a pilot study. *Brachytherapy* **2005**, *4*, 264–270. [CrossRef]
11. Dormand, E.L.; Banwell, P.E.; Goodacre, T.E.E. Radiotherapy and wound healing. *Int. Wound J.* **2005**, *2*, 112–127. [CrossRef] [PubMed]
12. Hopewell, J.W. The skin: Its structure and response to ionizing radiation. *Int. J. Radiat. Biol.* **1990**, *57*, 751–773. [CrossRef] [PubMed]
13. Abouarab, M.H.; Salem, I.L.; Degheidy, M.M.; Henn, D.; Hirche, C.; Eweida, A.; Uhl, M.; Kneser, U.; Kremer, T. Therapeutic options and postoperative wound complications after extremity soft tissue sarcoma resection and postoperative external beam radiotherapy. *Int. Wound J.* **2018**, *15*, 148–158. [CrossRef]
14. Archambeau, J.O.; Pezner, R.; Wasserman, T. Pathophysiology of irradiated skin and breast. *Int. J. Radiat. Oncol.* **1995**, *31*, 1171–1185. [CrossRef]
15. Denham, J.W.; Hauer-Jensen, M. The radiotherapeutic injury—A complex "wound". *Radiother. Oncol.* **2002**, *63*, 129–145. [CrossRef]
16. Binatti, E.; Zoccatelli, G.; Zanoni, F.; Donà, G.; Mainente, F.; Chignola, R. Phagocytosis of Astaxanthin-Loaded Microparticles Modulates TGFβ Production and Intracellular ROS Levels in J774A.1 Macrophages. *Mar. Drugs* **2021**, *19*, 163. [CrossRef]
17. Liu, R.M.; Desai, L.P. Reciprocal regulation of TGF-β and reactive oxygen species: A perverse cycle for fibrosis. *Redox Biol.* **2015**, *6*, 565–577. [CrossRef]
18. Burger, A.; Löffler, H.; Bamberg, M.; Rodemann, H.P. Molecular and cellular basis of radiation fibrosis. *Int. J. Radiat. Biol. Phys.* **1998**, *73*, 401–408. [CrossRef]
19. Randall, K. Long-term expression of transforming growth factor TGF beta1 in mouse skin after localized beta-irradiation. *Int. J. Radiat. Biol.* **1996**, *70*, 351–360. [CrossRef]
20. Randall, K.; Coggle, J.E. Expression of Transforming Growth Factor-β1 in Mouse Skin During the Acute Phase of Radiation Damage. *Int. J. Radiat. Biol.* **1995**, *68*, 301–309. [CrossRef]
21. Martin, M.; Lefaix, J.L.; Delanian, S. TGF-β1 and radiation fibrosis: A master switch and a specific therapeutic target? *Int. J. Radiat. Oncol. Biol. Phys.* **2000**, *47*, 277–290. [CrossRef]
22. Martin, M.; Lefaix, J.; Pinton, P.; Crechet, F.; Daburon, F. Temporal modulation of TGF-beta 1 and beta-actin gene expression in pig skin and muscular fibrosis after ionizing radiation—PubMed. *Radiat. Res.* **1993**, *134*, 63–70. [CrossRef] [PubMed]

23. Schultze-Mosgau, S.; Wehrhan, F.; Grabenbauer, G.; Amann, K.; Radespiel-Tröger, M.; Neukam, F.W.; Rodel, F. Transforming growth factor beta1 and beta2 (TGFbeta2 / TGFbeta2) profile changes in previously irradiated free flap beds. *Head Neck* **2002**, *24*, 33–41. [CrossRef] [PubMed]
24. Schultze-Mosgau, S.; Blaese, M.A.; Grabenbauer, G.; Wehrhan, F.; Kopp, J.; Amann, K.; Rodemann, H.P.; Rödel, F. Smad-3 and Smad-7 expression following anti-transforming growth factor beta 1 (TGFβ1)-treatment in irradiated rat tissue. *Radiother. Oncol.* **2004**, *70*, 249–259. [CrossRef] [PubMed]
25. Epstein, F.H.; Border, W.A.; Noble, N.A. Transforming Growth Factor β in Tissue Fibrosis. *N. Engl. J. Med.* **1994**, *331*, 1286–1292. [CrossRef]
26. Ulrich, D.; Lichtenegger, F.; Eblenkamp, M.; Repper, D.; Pallua, N. Matrix metalloproteinases, tissue inhibitors of metalloproteinases, aminoterminal propeptide of procollagen type III, and hyaluronan in sera and tissue of patients with capsular contracture after augmentation with Trilucent breast implants. *Plast. Reconstr. Surg.* **2004**, *114*, 229–236. [CrossRef]
27. Schultze-Mosgau, S.; Kopp, J.; Thorwarth, M.; Rödel, F.; Melnychenko, I.; Grabenbauer, G.G.; Amann, K.; Wehrhan, F. Plasminogen activator inhibitor-I-related regulation of procollagen I (α1 and α2) by antitransforming growth factor-β1 treatment during radiation-impaired wound healing. *Int. J. Radiat. Oncol. Biol. Phys.* **2006**, *64*, 280–288. [CrossRef]
28. Gallo-Oller, G.; Di Scala, M.; Aranda, F.; Dotor, J. Transforming growth factor beta (TGF-β) activity in immuno-oncology studies. In *Methods in Enzymology*; Academic Press: Cambridge, MA, USA, 2020; Volume 636, pp. 129–172, ISBN 9780128206676.
29. Santiago, B.; Gutierrez-Cañas, I.; Dotor, J.; Palao, G.; Lasarte, J.J.; Ruiz, J.; Prieto, J.; Borrás-Cuesta, F.; Pablos, J.L. Topical application of a peptide inhibitor of transforming growth factor-β1 ameliorates bleomycin-induced skin fibrosis. *J. Investig. Dermatol.* **2005**, *125*, 450–455. [CrossRef]
30. Dotor, J.; López-Vázquez, A.B.; Lasarte, J.J.; Sarobe, P.; García-Granero, M.; Riezu-Boj, J.I.; Martínez, A.; Feijoó, E.; López-Sagaseta, J.; Hermida, J.; et al. Identification of peptide inhibitors of transforming growth factor beta 1 using a phage-displayed peptide library. *Cytokine* **2007**, *39*, 106–115. [CrossRef]
31. Llopiz, D.; Dotor, J.; Casares, N.; Bezunartea, J.; Díaz-Valdés, N.; Ruiz, M.; Aranda, F.; Berraondo, P.; Prieto, J.; Lasarte, J.J.; et al. Peptide inhibitors of transforming growth factor-β enhance the efficacy of antitumor immunotherapy. *Int. J. Cancer* **2009**, *125*, 2614–2623. [CrossRef]
32. Beltrami, G.; Rüdiger, H.A.; Mela, M.M.; Scoccianti, G.; Livi, L.; Franchi, A.; Campanacci, D.A.; Capanna, R. Limb salvage surgery in combination with brachytherapy and external beam radiation for high-grade soft tissue sarcomas. *Eur. J. Surg. Oncol.* **2008**, *34*, 811–816. [CrossRef] [PubMed]
33. Hermida, N.; López, B.; González, A.; Dotor, J.; Lasarte, J.J.; Sarobe, P.; Borrás-Cuesta, F.; Díez, J. A synthetic peptide from transforming growth factor-β1 type III receptor prevents myocardial fibrosis in spontaneously hypertensive rats. *Cardiovasc. Res.* **2009**, *81*, 601–609. [CrossRef] [PubMed]
34. Schäffer, M.; Weimer, W.; Wider, S.; Stülten, C.; Bongartz, M.; Budach, W.; Becker, H.D. Differential expression of inflammatory mediators in radiation-impaired wound healing. *J. Surg. Res.* **2002**, *107*, 93–100. [CrossRef]
35. Anscher, M.S.; Thrasher, B.; Rabbani, Z.; Teicher, B.; Vujaskovic, Z. Antitransforming growth factor-β antibody 1D11 ameliorates normal tissue damage caused by high-dose radiation. *Int. J. Radiat. Oncol. Biol. Phys.* **2006**, *65*, 876–881. [CrossRef]
36. Collie, D.; Murchison, J.T.; Wright, S.H.; McLean, A.; Howard, L.; Del-Pozo, J.; Smith, S.; McLachlan, G.; Lawrence, J.; Kay, E.; et al. Nebulisation of synthetic lamellar lipids mitigates radiation-induced lung injury in a large animal model. *Sci. Rep.* **2018**, *8*, 13316. [CrossRef]
37. Herskind, C.; Bamberg, M.; Rodemann, H.P. The role of cytokines in the development of normal-tissue reactions after radiotherapy. *Strahlenther. Onkol.* **1998**, *174*, 12–15.
38. Hanafy, N.A.N.; Fabregat, I.; Leporatti, S.; Kemary, M. El Encapsulating TGF-β1 inhibitory peptides P17 and P144 as a promising strategy to facilitate their dissolution and to improve their functionalization. *Pharmaceutics* **2020**, *12*, 421. [CrossRef]
39. Park, S.W.; Choi, J.; Kim, J.; Jeong, W.; Kim, J.S.; Jeong, B.K.; Shin, S.C.; Kim, J.H. Anthocyanins from black soybean seed coat prevent radiation-induced skin fibrosis by downregulating TGF-β and Smad3 expression. *Arch. Dermatol. Res.* **2018**, *310*, 401–412. [CrossRef]
40. Qiu, S.S.; Dotor, J.; Hontanilla, B. Effect of P144®(Anti-TGF-β) in an "in Vivo" Human Hypertrophic Scar Model in Nude Mice. *PLoS ONE* **2015**, *10*, e0144489. [CrossRef]
41. Zarranz-Ventura, J.; Fernández-Robredo, P.; Recalde, S.; Salinas-Alamán, A.; Borrás-Cuesta, F.; Dotor, J.; García-Layana, A. Transforming Growth Factor-Beta Inhibition Reduces Progression of Early Choroidal Neovascularization Lesions in Rats: P17 and P144 Peptides. *PLoS ONE* **2013**, *8*, e0065434. [CrossRef]
42. Arribillaga, L.; Dotor, J.; Basagoiti, M.; Riezu-Boj, J.I.; Borrás-Cuesta, F.; Lasarte, J.J.; Sarobe, P.; Cornet, M.E.; Feijoó, E. Therapeutic effect of a peptide inhibitor of TGF-β on pulmonary fibrosis. *Cytokine* **2011**, *53*, 327–333. [CrossRef] [PubMed]
43. Kalluri, R.; Weinberg, R.A. The basics of epithelial-mesenchymal transition. *J. Clin. Investig.* **2009**, *119*, 1420–1428. [CrossRef] [PubMed]
44. Kramann, R.; Dirocco, D.P.; Humphreys, B.D. Understanding the origin, activation and regulation of matrix-producing myofibroblasts for treatment of fibrotic disease. *J. Pathol.* **2013**, *231*, 273–289. [CrossRef]
45. Park, J.H.; Ryu, S.H.; Choi, E.K.; Ahn, S.D.; Park, E.; Choi, K.C.; Lee, S.W. SKI2162, an inhibitor of the TGF-ß type I receptor (ALK5), inhibits radiation-induced fibrosis in mice. *Oncotarget* **2015**, *6*, 4171–4179. [CrossRef] [PubMed]

46. Flechsig, P.; Dadrich, M.; Bickelhaupt, S.; Jenne, J.; Hauser, K.; Timke, C.; Peschke, P.; Hahn, E.W.; Grone, H.J.; Yingling, J.; et al. LY2109761 attenuates radiation-induced pulmonary murine fibrosis via reversal of TGF-β and BMP-associated proinflammatory and proangiogenic signals. *Clin. Cancer Res.* **2012**, *18*, 3616–3627. [CrossRef]
47. Gallo-Oller, G.; Vollmann-Zwerenz, A.; Meléndez, B.; Rey, J.A.; Hau, P.; Dotor, J.; Castresana, J.S. P144, a Transforming Growth Factor beta inhibitor peptide, generates antitumoral effects and modifies SMAD7 and SKI levels in human glioblastoma cell lines. *Cancer Lett.* **2016**, *381*, 67–75. [CrossRef] [PubMed]
48. Gonzalez-Zubeldia, I.; Dotor, J.; Redrado, M.; Bleau, A.M.; Manrique, I.; de Aberasturi, A.L.; Villalba, M.; Calvo, A. Co-migration of colon cancer cells and CAFs induced by TGFβ1 enhances liver metastasis. *Cell Tissue Res.* **2015**, *359*, 829–839. [CrossRef]
49. Zhang, L.; Lu, X.Q.; Zhou, X.Q.; Liu, Q.B.; Chen, L.; Cai, F. NEAT1 induces osteosarcoma development by modulating the miR-339-5p/TGF-β1 pathway. *J. Cell. Physiol.* **2019**, *234*, 5097–5105. [CrossRef]

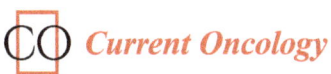

Article

Primary Angiosarcoma of the Breast: A Single-Center Retrospective Study in Korea

Yeon-Jin Kim, Jai-Min Ryu, Se-Kyung Lee, Byung-Joo Chae, Seok-Won Kim, Seok-Jin Nam, Jong-Han Yu * and Jeong-Eon Lee *

Division of Breast Surgery, Department of Surgery, Samsung Medical Center, Sungkyunkwan University School of Medicine, Seoul 06351, Korea; yeonjin.kim@samsung.com (Y.-J.K.); jaimin.ryu@samsung.com (J.-M.R.); sekyung.lee@samsung.com (S.-K.L.); bj.chae@samsung.com (B.-J.C.); seokwon1.kim@samsung.com (S.-W.K.); seokjin.nam@samsung.com (S.-J.N.)
* Correspondence: jonghan.yu@samsung.com (J.-H.Y.); jeongeon.lee@samsung.com (J.-E.L.); Tel.: +82-2-3410-0260 (J.-H.Y.); +82-2-3410-3479 (J.-E.L.); Fax: +82-2-3410-6982 (J.-H.Y.); +82-2-3410-6982 (J.-E.L.)

Abstract: Due to the rarity of primary angiosarcoma of the breast, optimal management is based on expert opinion. The aim of this study was to review all primary angiosarcomas of the breast obtained from a single center in terms of clinicopathologic characteristics, treatment, and survival outcomes. From 1997 to 2020, 15 patients with primary angiosarcoma of the breast underwent either mastectomy or wide excision. We analyzed the clinicopathologic data to assess disease-free survival and overall survival. Fifteen women with primary angiosarcoma of the breast were identified. The mean age at diagnosis was 33 years (range: 14–63 years). The overall mean tumor size was 7.7 cm (range 3.5–20 cm). Upon histological grading, there were three cases of low grade, five intermediate grade, six high grade, and one unidentified grade. The five-year disease-free survival rate was 24.4%, and the five-year survival rate was 37.2%. The survival rate of the low-grade patient group was statistically higher than that of the intermediate- or high-grade patient groups ($p = 0.024$). Primary angiosarcoma of the breast is a rare aggressive tumor characterized by high grade and poor outcome. Histologic grade appears to be a reliable predictor of survival. There are no standard treatment guidelines; thus, optimal R0 surgical resection remains the best approach. The roles of neoadjuvant, adjuvant chemotherapy, and radiotherapy remain unclear.

Keywords: primary angiosarcoma of the breast; breast angiosarcoma; primary sarcoma; angiosarcoma

1. Introduction

Angiosarcoma of the breast is a rare entity with poor prognosis, comprising less than 1% of all soft-tissue tumors [1–3]. Breast angiosarcoma commonly is divided into two types, primary and secondary angiosarcoma. Primary angiosarcoma of the breast develops de novo with no prior breast radiation. It occurs within the breast parenchyma, usually affecting women in their 30s to 50s [2,4]. Secondary angiosarcoma of the breast occurs in the setting of radiation therapy as part of breast-conservative treatment of breast cancer and is typically seen in older patients. [1,4]

Primary angiosarcoma of the breast is rarer than secondary angiosarcoma and has no known risk factors [5]. It usually is derived from the endothelial cell lining of the vascular channels and does not involve the regional lymph nodes [6]. However, angiosarcoma is aggressive and tends to have a high risk of local and distant metastases [1,7].

Due to the rarity of these tumors, optimal management is based on expert opinion. Complete surgical resection with optical margins (R0 resection) is the most common treatment [2]. The best surgical methods for resection are uncertain due to lack of long-term outcome data comparing wide excision and mastectomy.

The role of radiotherapy and chemotherapy remains unclear. Some studies have insisted that radiotherapy before surgery is not recommended, and that adjuvant radiotherapy conveys better local control [8,9]. However, one study showed no effect of radiotherapy on overall survival [10]. According to the meta-analysis study, it was revealed that adjuvant radiation therapy after surgery for primary angiosarcoma of the breast had a statistically significant effect on recurrence-free survival [2]. A prior study showed that adding chemotherapy to the treatment of angiosarcoma has a significant benefit on reduced risk of local recurrence [11]. However, other studies showed that adjuvant chemotherapy has no statistically significant benefit for breast angiosarcoma [2,12]. The effectiveness of the adjuvant treatment is uncertain.

The aim of this study was to review all cases of primary angiosarcoma of the breast diagnosed from 1997 to 2020, in a single center, and to describe a single-institution experience with primary angiosarcoma of the breast, including clinicopathologic characteristics, treatment, and survival outcomes.

2. Materials and Methods

This retrospective study included 15 patients with primary angiosarcoma of the breast who were treated at Samsung Medical Center from 1997 to 2020, accessed through the electronic medical recoding system of the institute. This study was approved by the institutional review board (Approval number: 2021-09-037) of the Samsung Medical Center.

We reviewed the demographic data, tumor size, histologic grades, treatment modality, and survival data. Tumor size was defined as the largest dimension recorded on the pathology report. If excisional biopsy was performed and followed by operation at Samsung Medical Center, the largest length was recorded by adding to the previous excision size. Tumor grade was categorized as low, intermediate, or high.

Overall survival (OS) was measured from the date of surgery to the date of last follow-up or the date of death, as recorded in Statistics Korea records. Disease-free survival was measured from the date of surgery to the date of any recurrence or death. Overall survival and disease-free survival (DFS) were evaluated using the Kaplan–Meier method with the log-rank test. All statistical analyses were carried out using IBM SPSS v 27.0 (SPSS, Inc., Chicago, IL, USA).

3. Results

From 1997 to 2020, 15 patients who were diagnosed with primary angiosarcoma of the breast were treated at Samsung Medical Center. All patients presented with a palpable mass and were diagnosed with a core needle biopsy. Radiologic imaging such as via mammograms, ultrasound and MRI, was performed for patients

All cases were defined as primary angiosarcoma without prior diagnosis of breast cancer or radiation treatment. All patients were female, and the mean age at diagnosis was 33 years (range: 14–63 years).

The overall mean tumor size was 7.7 cm (range 3.0–25 cm). For histological grade, there were three patients of low grade, five of intermediate grade, six of high grade, and one unidentified grade (Table 1).

Table 1. Patient Demographics and Characteristics (*n* = 15).

Clinicopathological Features		No. of Patients (%)
Age		
Median (range)	33 years (range 14–63 years)	
Grade	Low	3 (20.0)
	Intermediate	5 (33.3)
	High	6 (40.0)
	Unknown	1 (6.7)
Tumor size (cm)	>5 cm	11 (73.3)
	≤5 cm	4 (26.7)
Operation	Mastectomy	13 (86.7)
	Wide excision	2 (13.3)
Adjuvant chemotherapy	Yes	4 (26.7)
	No	11 (73.3)
Adjuvant Radiotherapy	Yes	8 (53.3)
	No	7 (46.7)

Thirteen patients underwent mastectomy, eight of whom also received axillary surgery (Table 2). However, no node metastasis was present in the axillary surgery group. Wide excision was performed in only two patients (13.3%). Surgical margin was negative in all patients.

Table 2. Summary of Cases (*n* = 15).

Patient	Age	Grade	Tumor Size (cm)	Surgery (Date, Type)	Adjuvant Chemotherapy	Adjuvant Radiotherapy	Recurrence	Treatment of 1st Recurrence
1	35	3	6.0	27 November 1997 Lt. Total mastectomy	No	Yes	Local (Lt. chest skin)	Wide excision
2	31	2	10.0	27 October 1999 Rt. Total mastectomy	No	Yes	Distant (Bone)	Palliative chemoTx.
3	29	3	4.2	02 December 1999 Lt. Total mastectomy	No	Yes	Local (Lt. chest skin)	Palliative chemoTx.
4	19	2	11.2	27 February 2001 Rt. Total mastectomy	No	Yes	Local (Rt. chest skin)	Wide excision
5	21	2	10.0	02 April 2004 Lt. Total mastectomy +ALND	No	No	Distant (Bone)	Palliative chemoTx.
6	44	1	3.5	24 December 2009 Lt. wide excision	No	No	No	
7	28	2	8.0	30 March 2010 Rt. Total mastectomy +ALND	Yes AI # 4 + paclitaxel # 4	Yes	Local contralateral breast (Lt. chest skin)	Wide excision
8	14	unidentified	25.0	17 February 2011 Rt. Total mastectomy	Yes EI (# 45)	No	Distant (Bone)	Palliative chemoTx.
9	47	3	5.5	22 April 2011 Rt. Total mastectomy +ALND	No	No	Local contralateral breast (Lt. chest skin)	Wide excision

Table 2. Cont.

Patient	Age	Grade	Tumor Size (cm)	Surgery (Date, Type)	Adjuvant Chemotherapy	Adjuvant Radiotherapy	Recurrence	Treatment of 1st Recurrence
10	63	1	1.0	20 August 2013 Rt. wide excision	No	No	No	
11	14	3	9.0	28 February 2014 Lt. Total mastectomy + SLNBx, Rt. Wide excision	No	No	Local +Distant (Lt.chest skin, Lung)	Palliative chemoTx.
12	47	1	5.5	25 August 2015 Lt. Total mastectomy +ALND	Neoadjuvant Tx. AC # 4+ D # 4	No	Local (Lt. chest skin)	Wide excision
13	43	2	5.5	21 December 2017 Rt. Total mastectomy + SLNBx	No	Yes	No	
14	25	3	7.5	24 August 2018 Rt. Skin sparing mastectomy +SLNBx	Yes AC # 4	Yes	No	
15	41	3	3.0	22 May 2020 Lt. Total mastectomy + SLNBx	Yes AC # 4	Yes	No	

Abbreviations: ALND, axillary lymph node dissection; SLNBx, sentinel lymph node biopsy; Tx, treatment; A, Adriamycin; C, Cyclophosphamide; D, Docetaxel; I, ifosfamide; E, Etoposide.

Recurrence was detected in 10 patients (66.7%). We described the site of the first recurrence. Some patients were found to have distant metastasis after first local recurrence. The median follow-up period was 29 months (5.6–89 months). The last follow-up was observed in July 2021. Local recurrence occurred in four patients and local contralateral breast recurrence was observed in two patients. Distant recurrence was noted in three patients and one who had both local and distant recurrence. In distant metastasis, one was pulmonary, three were bone metastases (Tables 2 and 3). Wide excision was performed in patients with local recurrence and palliative chemotherapy was performed in patients with distant metastases. Two patients with contralateral breast recurrence underwent wide excision and one patient with synchronous local and distant metastases received palliative chemotherapy (Table 2).

Table 3. Outcomes of Primary Breast Angiosarcoma (n = 15).

Outcomes		No. of Patients (%)
Recurrence	Local	4 (26.7)
	Local contralateral breast	2 (13.3)
	Distant	3 (20.0)
	Local + Distant	1 (6.7)
	No recurrence	5 (33.3)
Survival	Alive	6 (40.0)
	Death	9 (60.0)

As shown in Table 2, one patient was diagnosed with angiosarcoma on both sides and underwent bilateral breast surgery.

In terms of adjuvant therapy after surgery, three patients received both chemotherapy and radiation therapy, five patients received radiation therapy only, and one patient received chemotherapy alone. Only one patient underwent mastectomy after neoadjuvant chemotherapy (Table 2). The adjuvant chemotherapy regimen in Samsung Medical Center was Adriamycin combined with alkylating agents (ifosfamide), followed by taxane agent (paclitaxel) or Adriamycin combined with alkylating agents (cyclophosphamide). The pediatric chemotherapy regimen in the center was etoposide combined with ifosfamide.

Overall survival and disease-free survival are shown in Figure 1. The five-year survival rate was 37.2%, and the five-year disease-free survival rate 24.4%. Overall survival according to tumor size is shown in Figure 2. The five-year survival rate was 28.3% in the group with tumor 5 cm or more in size and 66.7% in the group with tumors smaller than 5 cm. There was no significant difference ($p = 0.096$).

Overall survival by tumor grade is shown in Figure 3. The five-year survival rate was 100% in the low-grade group, 30% in the intermediate-grade group, and 0% in the high-grade group. The survival rate of the low-grade patient group was statistically higher than that of the intermediate- or high-grade patient groups ($p = 0.024$)

At the time of last follow-up, six patients were alive without distant metastatic disease. Only one of the 6 patients experienced local recurrence and was alive until the last follow-up (Table 3).

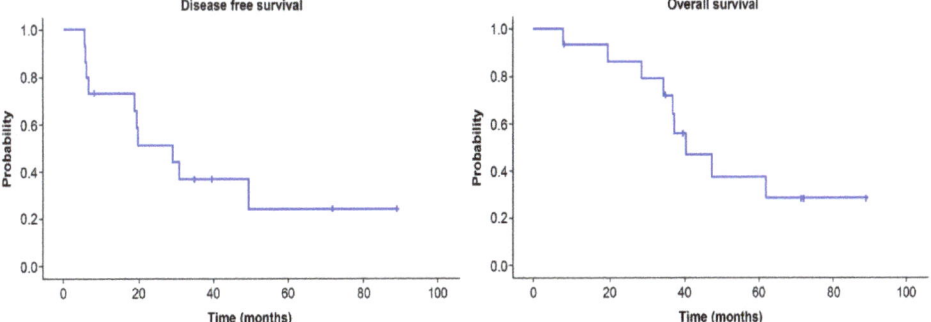

Figure 1. Disease-free survival and overall survival of primary angiosarcoma of the breast. The 5-year disease-free survival rate was 24.4% and the 5-year survival rate was 37.2%.

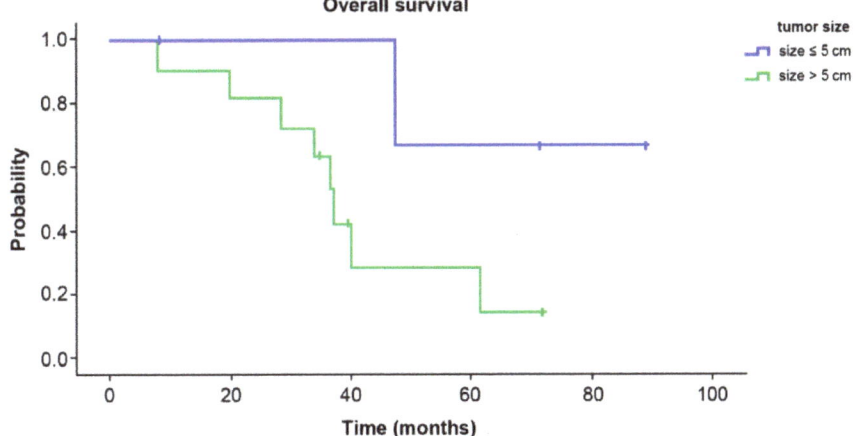

Figure 2. Overall survival according to tumor size. The 5-year survival rate was 28.3% in the group with tumor size ≥5 cm and 66.7% in the group with tumor size <5 cm. There was no significant difference between groups ($p = 0.096$).

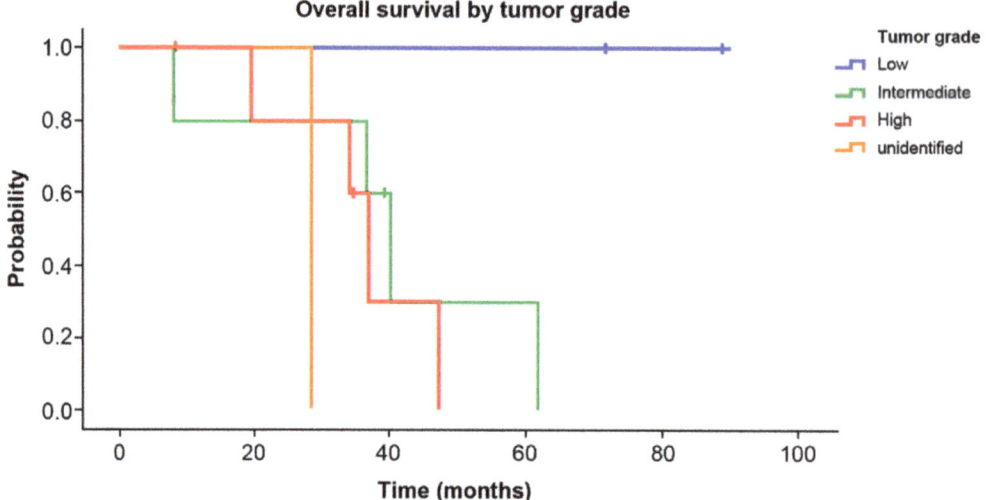

Figure 3. Overall survival by tumor grade. The 5-year survival rate was 100% in the low-grade group, 30% in the intermediate-grade group, and 0% in the high-grade group. The survival rate of the low-grade group was significantly higher than that of the intermediate- and high-grade groups ($p = 0.024$).

Figure 4A,B shows the overall survival and disease-free survival according to type of adjuvant 15 patients, including one patient with neoadjuvant chemotherapy.

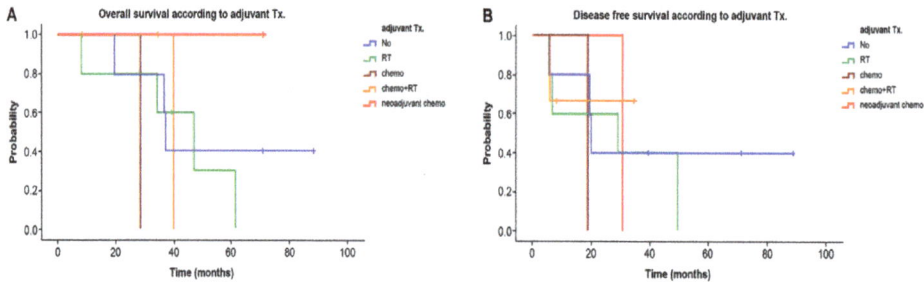

Figure 4. Overall survival (**A**) and disease-free survival (**B**) according to adjuvant treatment. There were no significant differences in 5-year overall survival ($p > 0.05$, Figure 4A) and 5-year disease-free survival ($p > 0.05$, Figure 4B) between groups according to adjuvant treatment. Abbreviations: adjuvant Tx, adjuvant chemotherapy; RT, radiotherapy; chemo, chemotherapy; neoadjuvant chemo, neoadjuvant chemotherapy.

4. Discussion

As in previous studies [2,4,5,13], primary angiosarcoma of the breast occurs in younger females between 30 and 50 years and can arise de novo with no risk factors. Primary angiosarcoma of the breast usually develops in the lining of the endothelial cell of the vascular channels and often involves the breast parenchyma without triggering factors [6]. Therefore, angiosarcoma appears mostly as a palpable mass, and the age at diagnosis is lower than the average age for invasive breast cancer [5]. This is consistent with our study. We found the average age at diagnosis of primary angiosarcoma of the breast was 33 years, which is younger (range: 14–63 years) than that of invasive breast cancer occurring in the 40–49-year age group, according to the Korea Breast Cancer Society registry data (KBCS) [14]. The minimum age of onset of primary angiosarcoma of the breast was 14 years in our study.

Several studies reported breast angiosarcoma as a more aggressive malignancy of the vascular endothelium, and the overall prognosis is poor compared to that of other invasive breast cancers [15,16]. In our study, the five-year overall survival rate of primary angiosarcoma of the breast was 37.2%, while the five-year overall survival rate of invasive breast cancer was 93.2% according to the KBCS [14].

Several studies suggested that the grade seemed to be the most consistent prognostic factors for primary angiosarcoma of the breast in regard to both OS and DFS [2,17,18]. In total, 6 of the 15 patients had high-grade disease on histopathology, and the median overall survival was 40 months (range: 8.2–71.6 months). We revealed a significantly higher survival rate of low-grade tumor than that of intermediate or high grade ($p = 0.024$). Other studies reported that histological grade was associated strongly with clinical presentation and overall prognosis. They noted an improved DFS for low- and intermediate-grade tumors compared to high-grade ones [18–20].

Several studies have suggested that tumor size is a prognostic factor [2,15,18,21,22]. Other studies have also revealed increased risk of local recurrence and decreased overall survival with larger tumor size [2,18,22]. In contrast to those studies, our study showed lower survival rates in groups with larger tumor sizes, though the difference was not significant (28.3% for size $\geq$ 5 cm vs. 66.7% for < 5 cm, $p = 0.096$). Although we did not find statistical difference of survival rate related to tumor size due to our small sample size, we did find the trend of the difference in survival rate according to size.

In terms of adjuvant treatment, survival was associated not favorably with administration of adjuvant chemotherapy or radiation therapy in our study. Other studies reported unclear roles of neoadjuvant and combined adjuvant chemotherapy and radiotherapy [13,19]. However, one author suggested that adjuvant radiotherapy can reduce local recurrence [1]. Another author reported that tumor size > 5 cm can predict patients at higher risk of local recurrence, who are more likely to obtain benefit from adjuvant radiation therapy [23]. In the analysis from one study, adjuvant radiation therapy seemed to have a significantly positive impact on recurrence-free survival when both primary angiosarcoma of the breast and secondary angiosarcoma of the breast were analyzed together. Despite concerns about radiation-induced etiology and complications in the re-irradiation environment, this study found that the local recurrence rate in primary and secondary angiosarcoma was lower when patients received surgery and adjuvant radiotherapy; this was in contrast to the lack of significant difference reported in our study [2]. So, the role of adjuvant radiotherapy remains controversial. Additionally, it was reported that chemotherapy is beneficial in high-grade lesions and in the metastatic setting [15]. Based on the results of previous studies, the lack of an association of survival with adjuvant therapy in the present study might be due to the retrospective study design and the relatively small number of patients.

The best treatment for primary angiosarcoma of the breast is surgery with R0 resection [2,18,22]. In our study, 13 patients underwent mastectomy, and only two underwent wide excision, both of whom had negative resection margins. One study revealed that patients who underwent breast-conserving surgery did not have worse prognosis than those who underwent mastectomy [24].

The role of axillary lymph node dissection in primary angiosarcoma of the breast is unknown, as breast angiosarcoma is due primarily to hematogenous spread [25]. According to one study, all 13 patients who underwent axillary staging showed absence of involved nodes. There also was no node metastases in the patients with axillary staging in our study. Based on these results, axillary surgery is not suitable in patients with breast angiosarcoma.

This study is limited by the very small sample of breast angiosarcoma and retrospective nature of this analysis, which prevents any definite conclusions. Some findings that failed to reach statistical significance might be due to lack of statistical power.

5. Conclusions

In conclusion, breast angiosarcoma is a rare aggressive tumor characterized by high grade and poor outcome. Histologic grade appears to be a reliable predictor of survival. There are no standard treatment guidelines, and optimal R0 surgical resection remains the best approach. The roles of neoadjuvant, adjuvant chemotherapy, and radiotherapy remain unclear.

Author Contributions: Conceptualization, J.-E.L. and J.-H.Y.; methodology, Y.-J.K.; software, Y.-J.K.; validation, J.-E.L. and J.-H.Y.; formal analysis, S.-K.L. and B.-J.C.; investigation, S.-K.L., B.-J.C. and J.-M.R.; data curation, S.-W.K. and S.-J.N.; writing—original draft preparation, Y.-J.K.: J.-E.L. and J.-H.Y.; writing—review and editing, Y.-J.K., J.-E.L. and J.-H.Y.; visualization, J.-E.L.; supervision, J.-H.Y.; project administration, S.-W.K. and S.-J.N. All authors have read and agreed to the published version of the manuscript.

Funding: This research received no external funding.

Institutional Review Board Statement: The study was conducted according to the guidelines of the Declaration of Helsinki and approved by the Institutional Review Board of Samsung Medical Center (Approval number: 2021-09-037).

Informed Consent Statement: Based on the retrospective character of the study, informed consent was not obtained.

Data Availability Statement: The data presented in this study are available on request from the corresponding author.

Acknowledgments: Authors' efforts towards the work described herein have been supported by the kind donation of Yong-Seop Lee and Sun-Hee Kang.

Conflicts of Interest: The authors declare no conflict of interest.

References

1. Hodgson, N.C.; Bowen-Wells, C.; Moffat, F.; Franceschi, D.; Avisar, E. Angiosarcomas of the breast: A review of 70 cases. *Am. J. Clin. Oncol.* **2007**, *30*, 570–573. [CrossRef] [PubMed]
2. Abdou, Y.; Elkhanany, A.; Attwood, K.; Ji, W.; Takabe, K.; Opyrchal, M. Primary and secondary breast angiosarcoma: Single center report and a meta-analysis. *Breast Cancer Res. Treat.* **2019**, *178*, 523–533. [CrossRef] [PubMed]
3. Im, S.; Chae, B.J.; Kim, S.H.; Kang, B.J.; Song, B.J.; Lee, A. Primary angiosarcoma of the breast: A case report. *Int. J. Clin. Exp. Pathol.* **2019**, *12*, 664–668. [PubMed]
4. Hui, A.; Henderson, M.; Speakman, D.; Skandarajah, A. Angiosarcoma of the breast: A difficult surgical challenge. *Breast* **2012**, *21*, 584–589. [CrossRef]
5. Bae, S.Y.; Choi, M.Y.; Cho, D.H.; Lee, J.E.; Nam, S.J.; Yang, J.H. Large clinical experience of primary angiosarcoma of the breast in a single Korean medical institute. *World J. Surg.* **2011**, *35*, 2417–2421. [CrossRef]
6. Biswas, T.; Tang, P.; Muhs, A.; Ling, M. Angiosarcoma of the breast: A rare clinicopathological entity. *Am. J. Clin. Oncol.* **2009**, *32*, 582–586. [CrossRef]
7. Russo, D.; Campanino, M.R.; Cepurnaite, R.; Gencarelli, A.; De Rosa, F.; Corvino, A.; Menkulazi, M.; Tammaro, V.; Fuggi, M.; Insabato, L. Primary High-Grade Angiosarcoma of the Breast in a Young Woman with Breast Implants: A Rare Case and a Review of Literature. *Int. J. Surg. Pathol.* **2020**, *28*, 906–912. [CrossRef]
8. Johnson, C.M.; Garguilo, G.A. Angiosarcoma of the breast: A case report and literature review. *Curr. Surg.* **2002**, *59*, 490–494. [CrossRef]
9. Johnstone, P.A.; Pierce, L.J.; Merino, M.J.; Yang, J.C.; Epstein, A.H.; DeLaney, T.F. Primary soft tissue sarcomas of the breast: Local-regional control with post-operative radiotherapy. *Int. J. Radiat. Oncol. Biol. Phys.* **1993**, *27*, 671–675. [CrossRef]
10. Pandey, M.; Mathew, A.; Abraham, E.K.; Rajan, B. Primary sarcoma of the breast. *J. Surg. Oncol.* **2004**, *87*, 121–125. [CrossRef]
11. Torres, K.E.; Ravi, V.; Kin, K.; Yi, M.; Guadagnolo, B.A.; May, C.D.; Arun, B.K.; Hunt, K.K.; Lam, R.; Lahat, G.; et al. Long-term outcomes in patients with radiation-associated angiosarcomas of the breast following surgery and radiotherapy for breast cancer. *Ann. Surg. Oncol.* **2013**, *20*, 1267–1274. [CrossRef] [PubMed]
12. Depla, A.L.; Scharloo-Karels, C.H.; de Jong, M.A.A.; Oldenborg, S.; Kolff, M.W.; Oei, S.B.; van Coevorden, F.; van Rhoon, G.C.; Baartman, E.A.; Scholten, R.J.; et al. Treatment and prognostic factors of radiation-associated angiosarcoma (RAAS) after primary breast cancer: A systematic review. *Eur. J. Cancer* **2014**, *50*, 1779–1788. [CrossRef] [PubMed]
13. Sher, T.; Hennessy, B.T.; Valero, V.; Broglio, K.; Woodward, W.A.; Trent, J.; Hunt, K.K.; Hortobagyi, G.N.; Gonzalez-Angulo, A.M. Primary angiosarcomas of the breast. *Cancer* **2007**, *110*, 173–178. [CrossRef] [PubMed]

14. Kang, S.Y.; Kim, Y.S.; Kim, Z.; Kim, H.Y.; Kim, H.J.; Park, S.; Bae, S.Y.; Yoon, K.H.; Lee, S.B.; Lee, S.K.; et al. Breast Cancer Statistics in Korea in 2017: Data from a Breast Cancer Registry. *J. Breast Cancer* **2020**, *23*, 115–128. [CrossRef] [PubMed]
15. Wang, X.Y.; Jakowski, J.; Tawfik, O.W.; Thomas, P.A.; Fan, F. Angiosarcoma of the breast: A clinicopathologic analysis of cases from the last 10 years. *Ann. Diagn. Pathol.* **2009**, *13*, 147–150. [CrossRef]
16. Yin, M.; Wang, W.; Drabick, J.J.; Harold, H.A. Prognosis and treatment of non-metastatic primary and secondary breast angiosarcoma: A comparative study. *BMC Cancer* **2017**, *17*, 295. [CrossRef]
17. Donnell, R.M.; Rosen, P.P.; Lieberman, P.H.; Kaufman, R.J.; Kay, S.; Braun, D.W., Jr.; Kinne, D.W. Angiosarcoma and other vascular tumors of the breast. *Am. J. Surg. Pathol.* **1981**, *5*, 629–642. [CrossRef]
18. Kunkiel, M.; Maczkiewicz, M.; Jagiello-Gruszfeld, A.; Nowecki, Z. Primary angiosarcoma of the breast-series of 11 consecutive cases-a single-centre experience. *Curr. Oncol.* **2018**, *25*, e50–e53. [CrossRef]
19. Arora, T.K.; Terracina, K.P.; Soong, J.; Idowu, M.O.; Takabe, K. Primary and secondary angiosarcoma of the breast. *Gland Surg.* **2014**, *3*, 28–34. [CrossRef]
20. Bousquet, G.; Confavreux, C.; Magné, N.; de Lara, C.T.; Poortmans, P.; Senkus, E.; de Lafontan, B.; Bolla, M.; Largillier, R.; Lagneau, E.; et al. Outcome and prognostic factors in breast sarcoma: A multicenter study from the rare cancer network. *Radiother. Oncol.* **2007**, *85*, 355–361. [CrossRef]
21. Vorburger, S.A.; Xing, Y.; Hunt, K.K.; Lakin, G.E.; Benjamin, R.S.; Feig, B.W.; Pisters, P.W.T.; Ballo, M.T.; Chen, L.; Trent, J., III; et al. Angiosarcoma of the breast. *Cancer* **2005**, *104*, 2682–2688. [CrossRef] [PubMed]
22. Fields, R.C.; Aft, R.L.; Gillanders, W.E.; Eberlein, T.J.; Margenthaler, J.A. Treatment and outcomes of patients with primary breast sarcoma. *Am. J. Surg.* **2008**, *196*, 559–561. [CrossRef] [PubMed]
23. Ghareeb, E.R.; Bhargava, R.; Vargo, J.A.; Florea, A.V.; Beriwal, S. Primary and Radiation-induced Breast Angiosarcoma: Clinicopathologic Predictors of Outcomes and the Impact of Adjuvant Radiation Therapy. *Am. J. Clin. Oncol.* **2016**, *39*, 463–467. [CrossRef] [PubMed]
24. Toesca, A.; Spitaleri, G.; De Pas, T.; Botteri, E.; Gentilini, O.; Bottiglieri, L.; Rotmentsz, N.; Sangalli, C.; Marrazzo, E.; Cassano, E.; et al. Sarcoma of the breast: Outcome and reconstructive options. *Clin. Breast Cancer* **2012**, *12*, 438–444. [CrossRef]
25. Ragavan, S.; Lim, H.J.; Tan, J.W.; Hendrikson, J.; Chan, J.Y.; Farid, M.; Chia, C.S.; Tan, G.H.C.; Soo, K.C.; Teo, M.C.C.; et al. Axillary Lymph Node Dissection in Angiosarcomas of the Breast: An Asian Institutional Perspective. *Sarcoma* **2020**, *2020*, 4890803. [CrossRef]

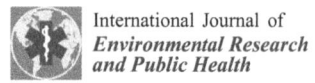

Article

A New Nonlinear Photothermal Iterative Theory for Port-Wine Stain Detection

Na Cao, Hongtao Liang, Ruoyu Zhang, Yanhua Li and Hui Cao *

Shaanxi Key Laboratory of Ultrasound, School of Physics and Information Technology, Shaanxi Normal University, Xi'an 710062, China; caona@snnu.edu.cn (N.C.); li-yanhua@snnu.edu.cn (H.L.); zhangruoyu@snnu.edu.cn (R.Z.); wangyajun@cau.edu.cn (Y.L.)
* Correspondence: caohui@snnu.edu.cn

Abstract: The development of appropriate photothermal detection of skin diseases to meet complex clinical demands is an urgent challenge for the prevention and therapy of skin cancer. An extensive body of literature has ignored all high-order harmonics above the second order and their influences on low-order harmonics. In this paper, a new iterative numerical method is developed for solving the nonlinear thermal diffusion equation to improve nonlinear photothermal detection for the noninvasive assessment of the thickness of port-wine stain (PWS). First, based on the anatomical and structural properties of skin tissue of PWS, a nonlinear theoretical model for photothermal detection is established. Second, a corresponding nonlinear thermal diffusion equation is solved by using the new iterative numerical method and taking into account harmonics above the second-order and their effects on lower-order harmonics. Finally, the thickness and excitation light intensity of PWS samples are numerically simulated. The simulation results show that the numerical solution converges faster and the physical meaning of the solution is clearer with the new method than with the traditional perturbation method. The rate of change in each harmonic with the sample thickness for the new method is higher than that for the conventional perturbation method, suggesting that the proposed numerical method may provide greater detection sensitivity. The results of the study provide a theoretical basis for the clinical treatment of PWS.

Keywords: nonlinear thermal diffusion equation; new numerical iterative method; port-wine stain; sensitivity

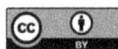

1. Introduction

Port-wine stain (PWS), also known as nevus flammeus, is a congenital telangiectasia deformity. It is the most common type of benign vascular malformation and is difficult to cure [1,2]. Wine discoloration often occurs on the head, face, and neck, and severe cases are accompanied by overgrowth of soft tissues and bones in the lesion area, resulting in local enlargement and deformation [3]. These lesions greatly affect the patient's appearance, decrease their quality of life, and cause considerable mental stress [4,5]. Therefore, early and effective intervention is particularly important.

Currently, the evaluation and prediction of PWS treatment consist of invasive and noninvasive approaches. Although biopsy has long been considered the gold standard for treatment, it is invasive and not widely performed. Noninvasive treatments include chromatography [6], dermoscopy [7], high−frequency ultrasound [8,9], and laser scatter imaging [10]. However, none of these commonly used imaging techniques provide adequate imaging depth and contrast to accurately assess PWS. A recent trial has shown that the use of photoacoustic techniques for the clinical evaluation of PWS disorders provides a new method for the quantitative evaluation of PWS [11].

Due to combining the advantages of both deep penetration provided by ultrasound imaging [12,13] and high contrast provided by optical imaging [14], photoacoustic technology [15,16] has become a research frontier and hot spot in the field of biomedical imaging. Most studies of photoacoustic techniques ignore the effect of the local temperature increase of the medium caused by light absorption on the thermodynamic parameters of the medium (e.g., thermal conductivity, density, and isobaric specific heat capacity) and assume that the thermodynamic parameters are constant. However, a statistically significant increase in the local temperature can change the values of thermodynamic parameters of the medium, and contribute to nonlinear photoacoustic conversion. The nonlinearity describing the thermal conductivity problem of laser irradiated tissue can be caused by various physical reasons, e.g., laser−induced formation of bubbles due to temperature dependence of gas solubility [17,18]; temperature dependence of thermodynamic parameters [19], etc. The nonlinear photoacoustic effect has attracted increasing attention as a possible means of selective detection of contrast agents by heat accumulation and local temperature increase thus enhancing the photoacoustic signal, and it is necessary to consider the nonlinearity of the thermal parameters in the thermal diffusion equation [20,21].

Therefore, this paper investigates the theory of thermal field imaging of PWS using nonlinear photoacoustic effect in the frequency domain by introducing nonlinear thermal conductivity coefficients. Based on previous work [22,23], a new semianalytic numerical iterative method is proposed in this paper. First, the temperature field is expanded in a Fourier series in the frequency domain to separate time variables and spatial coordinates. Then, the nonlinear diffusion equation is solved by selecting the appropriate high−frequency harmonics according to the specific requirements for calculation accuracy. Finally, the thickness and excitation light intensity are numerically simulated in light absorbers of different thicknesses using the new iterative numerical method and the conventional perturbation method. The results show that the solution by the numerical method has greater sensitivity and bandwidth than that of the perturbation method and can better distinguish between PWS samples of different thicknesses. This work extends the application of nonlinear thermal field theory in clinical medicine and contributes to a better understanding of PWS in lesions during different stages of development.

2. Theoretical Analysis

2.1. Theoretical Model

The skin is the largest and most important tissue in the human body. Anatomically, the skin can be divided into the epidermis, dermis, hypodermis, and muscle layers, as shown in Figure 1a. The epidermis consists of the high-fat, low-water stratum corneum and the melanin-containing living epidermis. Similarly, the dermis has two sublayers: the papillary dermis and the reticular dermis, which contain two vascular plexuses; the upper and deep blood plexuses are located in the upper and lower reticular layers of the dermis. The subcutaneous tissue consists mainly of fat cells.

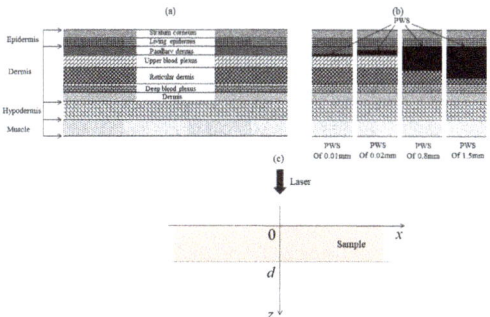

Figure 1. (**a**) Schematic of multilayered skin; (**b**) schematic of skin with different growth phases of a cancerous lesion; (**c**) theoretical model for photoacoustic detection of skin tissue.

In human dermatology, PWS is one of the most common benign tumors involving vascular malformations, with an incidence of between approximately 0.3 and 0.5% in the general population. PWS are mainly located in the papillary layer of the dermis and the upper layer of the reticular layer, with a diameter of approximately 0.01~0.15 mm and a thickness of approximately 0.001~1.5 mm [24]. Lesions can expand in size to cover a larger dermal area over time, as shown in Figure 1b.

Based on the anatomical and structural properties of skin tissue lesions, this paper constructs a nonlinear photothermal detection model for PWS, as shown in Figure 1c. Based on the optical attenuation, imaging depth, and other information reported by Chen et al., a laser pulse with a wavelength of 840 nm was chosen for PWS detection in this study. The parameters of each skin layer at a wavelength of 840 nm are shown in Table 1 [11,25–27].

Table 1. Thickness, optical and thermal parameters of the skin model at 840 nm [11,25–27].

Layers	d (mm)	β (mm^{-1})	σ (mm^{-1})	g	ρ (g/cm^{-3})	C (J/(g. K))	K$_0$ (mW/(cm. K))
Stratum corneum	0.01	0.00091	18.95	0.8	1.2	3.59	2.4
Living epidermis	0.08	0.13	18.95	0.8	1.2	3.59	2.4
Papillary dermis	0.10	0.105	11.65	0.8	1.09	3.35	4.2
Upper blood plexus	0.08	0.15875	15.485	0.818	1.09	3.35	4.2
Reticular dermis	1.50	0.105	11.65	0.8	1.09	3.35	4.2
Deep blood plexus	0.07	0.4443	46.165	0.962	1.09	3.35	4.2
Dermis	0.16	0.105	11.65	0.8	1.09	3.35	4.2
Hypodermis	3.00	0.009	11.44	0.9	1.21	2.24	1.97
Muscle tissues	3.00	0.029	7.13	0.9	1.075	3.5	4.5
PWS	0.001~1.5	0.15875	46.7	0.99	1.0	3.6	5.3

2.2. Nonlinear Thermal Diffusion Equation

A wave pulsed laser $I(t) = 2\sqrt{\frac{\ln(2)}{\pi}}\frac{w_P}{\tau}\exp\left\{-4\ln(2)(\frac{t-t_0}{\tau})^2\right\}$ irradiates the sample, and light is absorbed by the sample and converted into heat, generating a photoacoustic signal through thermal expansion, where τ is the pulse width, t_0 is the pulse center, and w_P is the luminous flux (mJ/cm^2). The fundamental equation of the photoacoustic imaging theory is based on the thermal diffusion equation; therefore, the thermal diffusion equation and boundary conditions in the sample are [28,29]:

$$T_{s,zz}(z,t) = \frac{1}{\alpha}T_{,t}(z,t) - \frac{Q(z,t)}{K_s}, \tag{1}$$

$$\begin{cases} K_s T_{s,z}(0,t) = K_g T_{g,z}(0,t) - \beta' w_P[1+\exp(j\omega t)] + H[T_s(0,t) - T_g(0,t)], z = 0, \\ K_s T_{s,z}(d,t) = K_g T_{g,z}(d,t) - \beta'(1-\beta')w_P\exp(-\beta d)[1+\exp(j\omega t)] + H[T_s(d,t) - T_g(d,t)], z = d. \end{cases} \tag{2}$$

where $T_s(z,t)$, $T_g(z,t)$ are the temperature rise and fall of the sample and air, respectively, $\alpha = K_s/(\rho C_P)$ is the thermal diffusion coefficient, ρ and C_p are the density and isobaric specific heat capacity of the sample, respectively, $H = h + 4\varepsilon\sigma T^3$, h is the convection coefficient and $4\varepsilon\sigma T^3$ is the heat radiation exchange term. According to $4\varepsilon\sigma T^3 \ll h$ [30], the heat radiation exchange term can be neglected. Subscripts behind the comma mean the calculation of partial derivatives for the corresponding subscripts. The endothermic source in the sample is $Q(z,t)$, which can be expressed as [28]:

$$Q(z,t) = \beta(1-\beta')w_P\exp(-\beta z)[1+\exp(j\omega t)], \tag{3}$$

where β is the bulk absorption coefficient of the sample, β' is the surface absorption rate of the sample, ω is the modulation angular frequency, and K_s, K_g is the thermal conductivity of the sample and air.

In linear theory, K_s is generally assumed to be constant; however, when the local temperature rise is significantly higher than the average temperature, K_s this assumption is not valid. Therefore, this paper introduces nonlinear thermal conductivity coefficients into the nonlinear thermal diffusion equation to investigate the theory of nonlinear photothermal imaging.

In nonlinear thermal diffusion theory, the dependence of thermal conductivity on the temperature is usually considered to be linear to simplify the problem [31]:

$$K_s = K_0[1 + bT_s(z,t)], \quad (4)$$

where K_0 is the thermal conductivity of the sample at steady−state temperature, b is the temperature coefficient of thermal conductivity, and in general, $b \ll 1$ [32]. Substituting Equation (4) into Equation (1), the one−dimensional nonlinear thermal diffusion equation is obtained as follows:

$$T_{s,zz}(z,t) = \frac{1}{\alpha_b} T_{s,t}(z,t) - bT_s(z,t)T_{s,zz}(z,t) - b[T_{s,z}(z,t)]^2 - \frac{Q(z,t)}{K_0}, \quad (5)$$

where $\alpha_b = K_0/(\rho C_P)$. Subscripts z and t behind the comma mean the calculation of partial derivatives for the corresponding subscripts.

2.3. Iterative Numerical Method for Solving the Nonlinear Heat Diffusion Equation

Because it is difficult to obtain a general solution of the one−dimensional nonlinear thermal diffusion equation, a new numerical method is proposed in this paper as follows. In many cases, it is advantageous to separate the variables t and z in $T(z,t)$. In general, the Fourier series expansion $T(z,t)$ in the frequency domain can be expressed as [33]:

$$T_s(z,t) = A_0/2 + \sum_{n=1}^{\infty}(1/2)A_n \exp(jn\omega t) + \sum_{n=1}^{\infty}(1/2)A_n^* \exp(-jn\omega t), \quad (6)$$

where j is an imaginary unit, A_0 is a real field variable, and $A_0/2$ represents the DC component of the sound wave. When $A_n(n \geq 1)$ is the complex field variable (i.e., complex amplitude) of the nth−order harmonic, the real part of $A_n \exp(jn\omega t)$ is the real displacement of the nth-order harmonic, and $A_n^*(n \geq 1)$ is the complex conjugate field variable of A_n. Note that A_n and A_n^* no longer contain the time variable t, which is a function of the spatial coordinate z.

Generally, higher−order harmonics are weaker, and some higher−order harmonics can be ignored according to the requirements for calculation accuracy. To simplify the theoretical description, only harmonics of the order less than or equal to $N(N \leq 5)$ are considered in this paper, and other higher−order harmonics are ignored; this is referred to as an $N - order$ approximation.

Substituting Equation (6) into Equation (5), the following equation can be obtained by orthogonality:

$$A_{i,zz} - i\omega\alpha_b^{-1} A_i j = -\frac{b}{2} F_i, (i = 0, \pm 1, \pm 2, \pm 3, \pm 4, \pm 5), \quad (7)$$

where,

$$\begin{aligned}F_0 &= A_0 A_{0,zz} + A_1^* A_{1,zz} + A_2^* A_{2,zz} + A_3^* A_{3,zz} + A_4^* A_{4,zz} + A_5^* A_{5,zz} + A_1 A_{1,zz}^* + A_2 A_{2,zz}^* + A_3 A_{3,zz}^* \\ &+ A_4 A_{4,zz}^* + A_5 A_{5,zz}^* + A_{0,z} A_{0,z} + 2A_{1,z} A_{1,z}^* + 2A_{2,z} A_{2,z}^* + 2A_{3,z} A_{3,z}^* + 2A_{4,z} A_{4,z}^* + 2A_{5,z} A_{5,z}^*,\end{aligned} \quad (8)$$

$$\begin{aligned}F_1 &= A_{0,zz} A_1 + A_{1,zz} A_0 + A_1^* A_{2,zz} + A_2^* A_{3,zz} + A_3^* A_{4,zz} + A_4^* A_{5,zz} + A_{1,zz}^* A_2 + A_{2,zz}^* A_3 + A_{3,zz}^* A_4 + \\ & A_{4,zz}^* A_5 + A_{0,z} A_{1,z} + 2A_{2,z} A_{1,z}^* + 2A_{3,z} A_{2,z}^* + 2A_{4,z} A_{3,z}^* + 2A_{5,z} A_{4,z}^* \\ &- \beta(1-\beta')w_P \exp(-\beta z)/K_0,\end{aligned} \quad (9)$$

$$F_2 = A_{0,zz}A_2 + A_{1,zz}A_1 + A_{2,zz}A_0 + A_{3,zz}A_1^* + A_{4,zz}A_2^* + A_{5,zz}A_3^* + A_{1,zz}^*A_3 + A_{2,zz}^*A_4 + A_{3,zz}^*A_5 + \\ A_{1,z}A_{1,z} + 2A_{2,z}A_{0,z} + 2A_{3,z}A_{1,z}^* + 2A_{4,z}A_{2,z}^* + 2A_{5,z}A_{3,z}^*, \tag{10}$$

$$F_3 = A_{0,zz}A_3 + A_{1,zz}A_2 + A_{2,zz}A_1 + A_{3,zz}A_0 + A_{4,zz}A_1^* + A_{5,zz}A_2^* + A_{1,z}^*A_4 + A_{2,zz}^*A_5 + 2A_{0,z}A_{3,z} + \\ 2A_{1,z}A_{2,z} + 2A_{2,z}A_{1,z} + 2A_{1,z}^*A_{4,z} + 2A_{2,z}^*A_{5,z}, \tag{11}$$

$$F_4 = A_{0,zz}A_4 + A_{1,zz}A_3 + A_{2,zz}A_2 + A_{3,zz}A_1 + A_{4,zz}A_0 + A_{5,zz}A_1^* + A_{1,zz}^*A_5 + 2A_{0,z}A_{4,z} + 2A_{1,z}A_{3,z} + \\ 2A_{2,z}A_{2,z} + 2A_{3,z}A_{1,z} + 2A_{4,z}A_{0,z} + 2A_{5,z}A_{1,z}^*, \tag{12}$$

$$F_5 = A_{0,zz}A_5 + A_{1,zz}A_4 + A_{2,zz}A_3 + A_{3,zz}A_2 + A_{4,zz}A_1 + A_{5,zz}A_0 + 2A_{0,z}A_{5,z} + 2A_{1,z}A_{4,z} + 2A_{2,z}A_{3,z}. \tag{13}$$

Notably, Equation (7) gives only an equation of field variables and not an equation of conjugate field variables. The equation of conjugate field variables can be obtained by taking the complex conjugate of Equation (7); therefore, Equation (7) is complete. Substituting $i = 0, \pm 1, \pm 2, \pm 3, \pm 4, \pm 5$ into Equation (7) yields a set of nonlinear equations. However, it is difficult to solve these equations directly. Therefore, a simple iterative method for solving these equation is proposed, where $A^{*(m)}$ and $A^{(m)}$ denotes the field quantities obtained from the $m - th$ iterative calculation. In the iterative calculation, the following method is used. First, the field quantities on the left side of Equation (7) are taken as $A_i^{(m)}$ and the constants on the right side are taken as $A_i^{(m-1)}$ and $A_i^{*(m-1)}$. Second, A_i and A_i^* in F_i are replaced with $A_i^{(m-1)}$ and $A_i^{*(m-1)}$, respectively. Third, the result obtained is $F_i^{(m-1)}$. Therefore, the following equation is used in the $m - th$ iterative calculation:

$$A_{i,zz}^{(m)} - i\omega \alpha_b^{-1} A_i^{(m)} j = -\frac{b}{2} F_i^{(m-1)}, \tag{14}$$

when $i = 0, \pm 1, \pm 2, \pm 3, \pm 4, \pm 5$, an uncoupled set of equations can be obtained from (14). Therefore, $A_i^{(m)}$ can be calculated separately and independently from the other iterations, which means that the computational effort does not increase dramatically when higher-order harmonics are involved.

Outputting results $A_i^{(m)}$ of the 1 iteration calculation are same with those predicted by the linear approximation theory. Outputting results $A_i^{(2)} (i \neq 1)$ of the 2 iteration calculation are same with those predicted by the perturbation theory. The depletion of pump waves has already been taken into account in the 2 interaction calculation. However, it is not taken into account in the perturbation theory [31].

In the iterative calculation, this study let $A_i^{(0)} = 0$ and $A_i^{*(0)} = 0$, and this paper uses the boundary excitation conditions to generate nonzero values of $A_i^{(m)}$ and $A_i^{*(m)}$. At both endpoints $z = 0$ and $z = d$, this work considers that the photothermal radiation signal is mainly due to the alternating temperature field. To simplify the calculation, this paper ignores the DC term and the effect of other layers and convective radiation on the temperature

3. Numerical Results and Discussion

In this section, we numerically calculate the solution to Equation (5) using the new numerical iterative method and the conventional perturbation method and discuss the effect of different sample parameters on the amplitude of the posterior surface of the sample. Table 1 lists the physical parameters used in the calculation of the PWS samples. The thermal conductivity is $K_0 = 121.5$ W/m and the thermal diffusion coefficient is $\alpha_b = 5.9419 \times 10^{-5}$ m^2/s for the 2219 aluminum alloy sample.

The amplitude of the signal from the posterior surface of PWS samples of different thicknesses obtained by the two numerical methods decreases with increasing frequency in the low−frequency and high−frequency ranges as shown in Figures 2 and 3, respectively. In the low−frequency range, Figure 2 shows that the amplitude of each order harmonic of the signal from the posterior surface of the PWS samples obtained by both numerical methods decreases with increasing frequency when other parameters are constant and the sample thicknesses are $d = 0.5$ mm and $d = 0.8$ mm. In the high−frequency range, Figure 3 reveals that the amplitude of each order harmonic of the signal from the posterior surface of the PWS samples obtained by both numerical methods decreases with increasing frequency when other parameters are constant and the thickness of the samples is $d = 0.01$ mm and $d = 0.02$ mm.

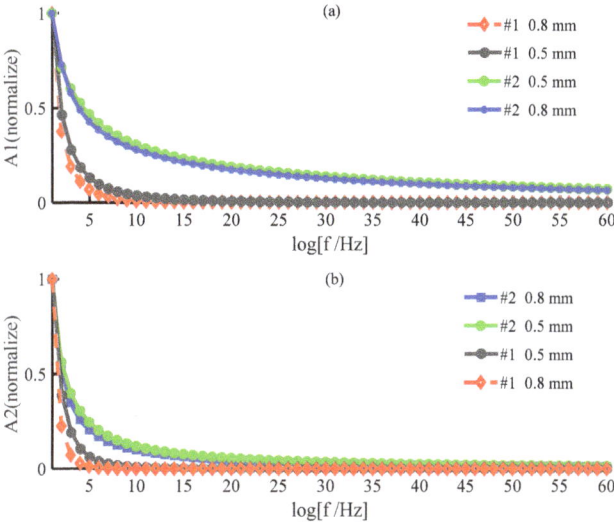

Figure 2. Variation in the amplitude with frequency on the posterior surface of a wine−discolored sample when the sample thickness varies: (**a**) fundamental frequency wave; (**b**) second harmonic (low frequency).

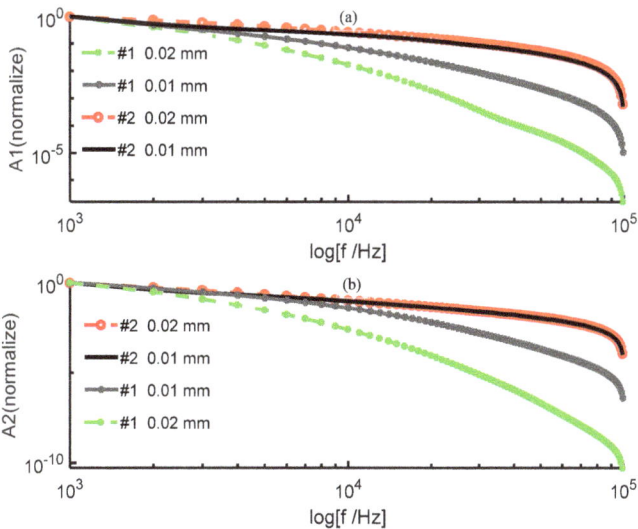

Figure 3. Variation in the amplitude of the posterior surface of the wine−discolored samples with frequency for different sample thicknesses: (**a**) fundamental frequency wave; (**b**) second harmonic (high frequency).

As seen in Figures 2 and 3, the results obtained by the new numerical iterative method are more sensitive to thickness than those obtained by the conventional perturbation method. Figure 2 shows the results in the low−frequency range PWS samples with thicknesses $d = 0.5$ mm and $d = 0.8$ mm. Both the fundamental and second harmonics on the posterior surface of the samples obtained by the two numerical methods decrease with increasing thickness, which is in good agreement with the results predicted in the literature [28,29]. For the fundamental and second harmonics obtained by the conventional perturbation method, there is no significant change in the effect of the sample thickness on the results, and there is no significant difference between the fundamental and second harmonics. However, the fundamental and second harmonics obtained by the new numerical method have a statistically significant effect on the results due to the change in the sample thickness, and the change is more pronounced in the second harmonic, so that it is necessary to consider the second harmonic. Figure 3 shows the results in the high-frequency range for the PWS samples with the thicknesses of $d = 0.01$ mm and $d = 0.02$ mm. Both fundamental frequency waves and second harmonics on the posterior surface of the samples obtained by the new method decrease with increasing thickness. However, both fundamental frequency waves and second harmonics on the posterior surface of the samples obtained by the conventional perturbation method increase with thickness, contradicting the literature predictions. Therefore, it is possible that the conventional perturbation method is not applicable at high frequencies. Additionally, the new numerical method shows a more pronounced change in the second harmonic than in the fundamental frequency wave when a weak change in the sample thickness occurs. Therefore, the second harmonic has stronger sensitivity to thickness, and the new method has the potential for important applications in the noninvasive assessment of PWS thickness.

Reference [31] applied the perturbation method to the solution of the nonlinear thermal diffusion equation to theoretically study the nonlinear photoacoustic effect; while the physical meaning of its simple method and solution is clear, Reference [31] considers only the effect of lower−order harmonics on higher−order harmonics and ignores the inverse effect. Figures 2 and 3 show that the sensitivity of the perturbation method to the sample thickness and the applicable frequency range is slightly lower effective than that of the new method.

In Figure 4, the solid line shows the thickness of the PWS sample inv $d = 0.01$ mm, and the marked dashed line shows the thickness of the PWS sample in $d = 0.02$ mm. The numbers 1−5 indicate the fundamental frequency wave and second through fifth harmonics, respectively.

Figure 4 shows the variation in the amplitude of each order of harmonics the frequency on the posterior surface of PWS samples at different thicknesses obtained by the new method. From Figure 4, the following conclusion can be drawnwhile other parameters held constant. First, each order of harmonic decreases with increasing frequency. Second, each order of harmonic decreases with increasing thickness. Third, the rate of change with thickness is larger for higher−order harmonics than lower−order harmonics, indicating that the effects of higher−order harmonics are more sensitive to the change in the sample thickness than those of the lower−order harmonics. Therefore, it is necessary to consider higher−order harmonics. In addition, the difference between the rates of change of the fourth and fifth harmonics with thickness is not very obvious. Therefore, the choice $N \leq 5$ is appropriate in the theoretical derivation.

Figure 5 shows the variation of each order of harmonics with light energy on the posterior surface of the PWS samples at different thicknesses obtained with the new method. Figure 5 shows that the amplitude of each order of harmonics increases with increasing light energy when other parameters are constant. Additionally, when other parameters are constant, the amplitude of each order of harmonic decreases with increasing thickness. As observed from Figure 5a, the fundamental frequency amplitude is proportional to the optical energy w_p, which is consistent with the results of linear theory. As observed from

Figure 5b,c, the amplitudes of the higher−order harmonics are proportional to the square of the light energy, which is consistent with the theoretical derivation.

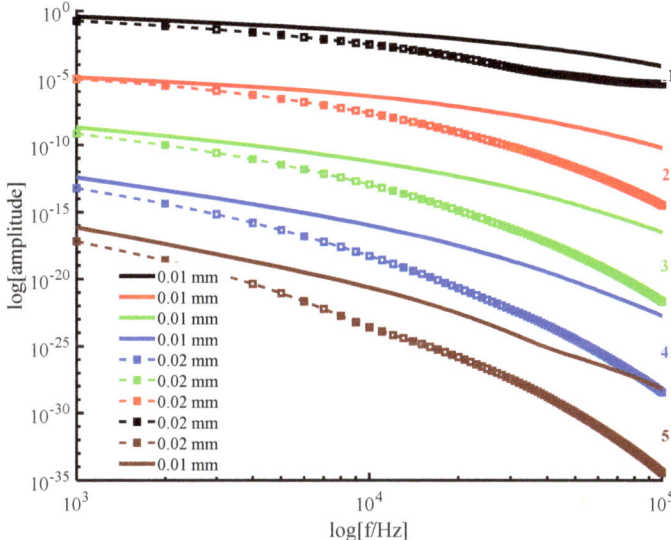

Figure 4. Variation in the harmonic amplitude with frequency for each order of harmonic for different sample thicknesses.

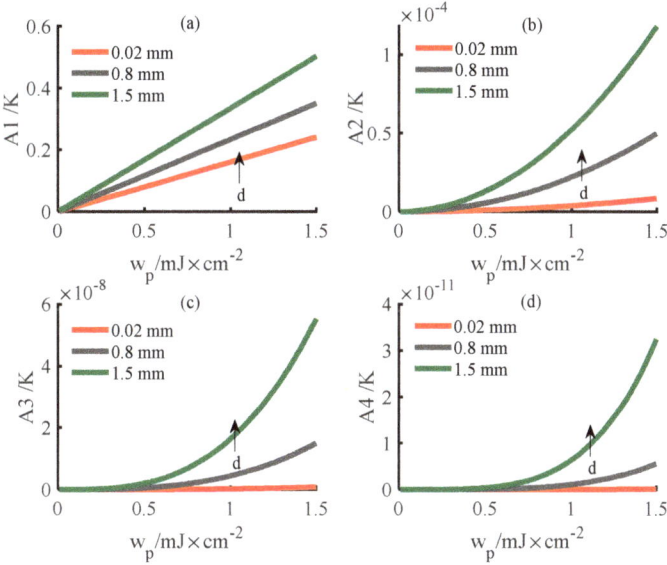

Figure 5. Variation in the harmonic amplitude with light energy for different sample thicknesses. (**a**) Fundamental frequency wave; (**b**) second harmonic; (**c**) third harmonic; (**d**) fourth harmonic.

To demonstrate the validity of the new theory, two numerical methods were used to analyze and compare the results for the variation in the amplitude with sample thickness on the posterior surface of 2219 aluminum alloy samples. The two methods are the new iterative numerical method and the conventional perturbation method [28,29].

The effectiveness of the new iterative numerical method for solving the nonlinear heat diffusion equation is demonstrated in Figures 6 and 7. Numerical simulations of the nonlinear heat diffusion equation for the 2219 aluminum alloy sample using the new numerical iterative method show two effects. First, the amplitude of each order of harmonics decreases with increasing frequency. Second, the second−order harmonic amplitude decreases with increasing thickness. The above conclusions are consistent with those obtained by the conventional perturbation method, and Figure 6 shows that the fundamental frequency wave results obtained by the two methods are very consistent. Therefore, the effectiveness of the method is demonstrated in Figures 6 and 7.

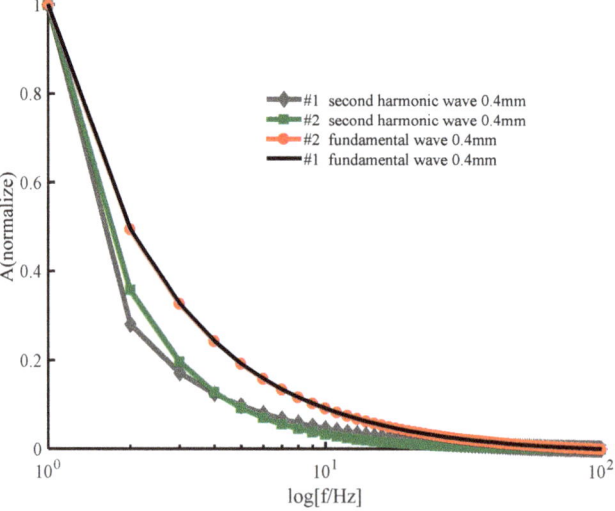

Figure 6. Variation in the fundamental frequency wave and second harmonic with frequency.

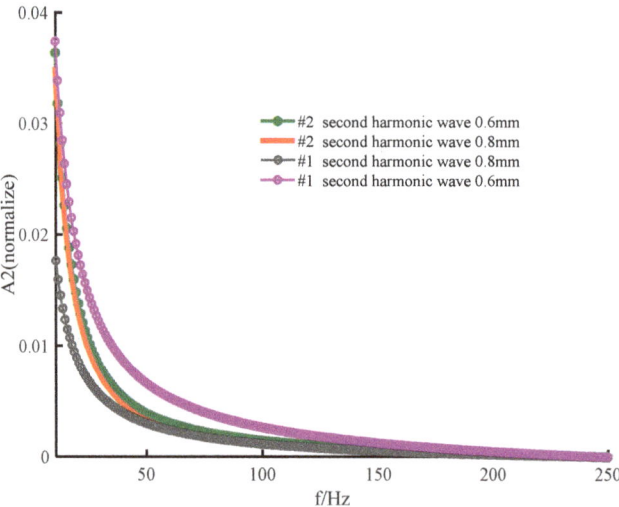

Figure 7. Variation in the second harmonic with frequency for different sample thicknesses.

An examination of Figures 6 and 7 shows the superiority of the new numerical method. For the 2219 aluminum alloy sample, the rate of change with the frequency of the second harmonic is larger than that of the fundamental frequency wave, and the rate of change of the results obtained by the new numerical method is larger than that of the second harmonic results obtained by the traditional perturbation method. Additionally, Figure 7 shows that the rate of change of the second harmonic amplitude with increasing thickness with other parameters unchanged is greater with the new method than with the traditional method. Therefore, the new numerical method is better than the traditional perturbation method. This comparison reflects the greater sensitivity of the results to the sample thickness obtained by the proposed method compared to the traditional method.

Figure 8 describes the relationship between the second harmonic amplitude on the posterior surface of the 2219 aluminum alloy sample and the iteration frequency m when the light energy w_p differs. Figure 8 shows that when the light energy is 5 mJ/cm^2 and the number of iterations is greater than or equal to 6, the fundamental frequency amplitude converges to 7.6485 K. In addition, when the light energy is 8 mJ/cm^2 and the number of iterations is greater than or equal to 10, the fundamental frequency amplitude converges to 19.8287 K. Moreover, when the light energy is 10 mJ/cm^2 and the number of iterations is greater than or equal to 12, the fundamental frequency amplitude converges to 31.3493 K. These results imply that the proposed method is converges well.

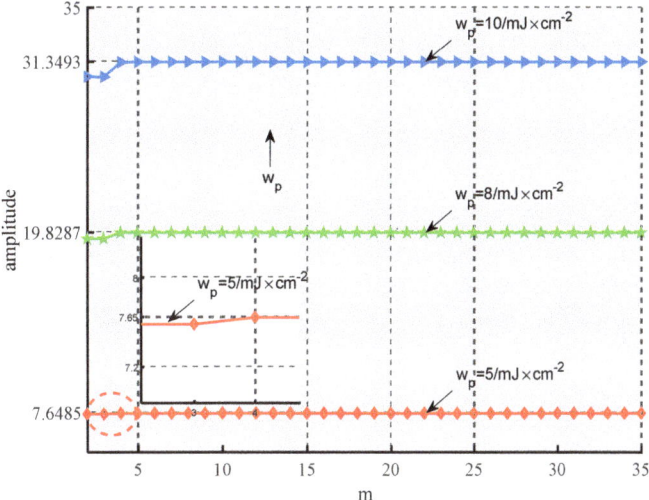

Figure 8. The variation in the second harmonic amplitude with number of iterations for different light energies.

4. Conclusions

In this paper, a theoretical model for thermal nonlinear photoacoustic detection related to port-wine stain samples is constructed. A new numerical iteration approach is developed and compared to the perturbation method for analyzing the thickness and absorption coefficient of PWS samples. The main conclusions are as follows:

(1) The rates of change with frequency, thickness, and optical energy intensity are larger for higher−order harmonics than lower-order harmonics; higher−order harmonics are more sensitive to sample detection than lower-order harmonics.

(2) For the same parameter values, the proposed new numerical iterative method has greater sensitivity and a wider frequency band than the perturbation method. Fur-

thermore, the calculation time of our proposed method will not drastically increase when additional high−order harmonics are included.

Author Contributions: N.C. initiated the idea; H.C. advised on the study design and the analysis plan; N.C. facilitated the study design, specifically the integration of disciplines, and wrote the first draft of the paper, which was reviewed and edited by H.L., R.Z. and Y.L. All authors have read and agreed to the published version of the manuscript.

Funding: The study was supported by the National Natural Science Foundation of China, grant number 11074159, and the Fundamental Research Funds for the Central Universities, grant number 2021TS088.

Institutional Review Board Statement: The study received ethical approval from the Shaanxi Normal University Institutional Review Board, and all procedures performed in studies involving human participants were following the 1964 Helsinki declaration and its later amendments.

Informed Consent Statement: Informed consent was obtained from all subjects involved in the study.

Data Availability Statement: The data that support the findings of this study are available from the corresponding author (H.C.), upon reasonable request.

Acknowledgments: The authors acknowledge the financial support from the National Natural Science Foundation of China under grant 11074159, and the Fundamental Research Funds for the Central Universities under grant 2021TS088. And authors would like to thank all reviewers and editors who provided extensive invaluable comments and suggestions.

Conflicts of Interest: This work is original research and approved by all authors. The authors declare that they have no conflict of interest.

References

1. Raath, M.; Chohan, S.; Wolkerstorfer, A.; van der Horst, C.M.A.M.; Heger, M. Port wine stain treatment outcomes have not improved over the past three decades. *J. Eur. Acad. Dermatol.* **2019**, *33*, 1369–1377. [CrossRef] [PubMed]
2. Raath, M.; Amesfoort, J.; Hermann, M.; Ince, Y.; Heger, M. Site-specific pharmaco-laser therapy: A novel treatment modality for refractory port wine stains. *J. Clin. Transl. Res.* **2019**, *5*, 1–24. [PubMed]
3. Lee, J.W.; Chung, H.Y.; Cerrati, E.W.; Teresa, M.O.; Waner, M. The natural history of soft tissue hypertrophy, bony hypertrophy, and nodule formation in patients with untreated head and neck capillary malformations. *Dermatol. Surg.* **2015**, *41*, 1241–1245. [CrossRef] [PubMed]
4. Jiang, F.; Shao, J.; Chen, L.; Yang, N.; Li, Z. Influence of port-wine stains on quality of life of children and their parents. *Acta. Derm.-Venereol.* **2021**, *101*, adv00516. [CrossRef]
5. Hagen, S.L.; Grey, K.R.; Korta, D.Z.; Kelly, K.M. Quality of life in adults with facial port-wine stains. *J. Am. Acad.* **2016**, *76*, 695–702. [CrossRef]
6. Han, Y.; Ying, H.; Zhang, X.J. Retrospective study of photodynamic therapy for pulsed dye laser-resistant port-wine stains: PDT for PDL-resistant port-wine stains. *J. Dermatol.* **2020**, *47*, 348–355. [CrossRef]
7. Li, D.C.; Nong, X.; Hu, Z.Y.; Fang, T.W.; Ye, L.I. Efficacy and related factors analysis in hmme-pdt in the treatment of port wine stains. *Photodiagn. Photodyn.* **2020**, *29*, 101649–101668. [CrossRef]
8. Alexander, H.; Miller, D.L. Determining skin thickness with pulsed ultra sound. *J. Investig. Dermatol.* **1979**, *72*, 17–19. [CrossRef]
9. John, P.R. Klippel-Trenaunay Syndrome. *J. Vasc. Interv. Radiol.* **2019**, *22*, 100634. [CrossRef]
10. Eriksson, S.; Nilsson, J.; Lindell, G.; Sturesson, C. Laser speckle contrast imaging for intraoperative assessment of liver microcirculation: A clinical pilot study. *Med. Devies.-Evid. Res.* **2014**, *7*, 257–261. [CrossRef]
11. Cheng, Q.; Qian, M.L.; Wang, X.L.; Zhang, H.N.; Wang, P.R. LED-Based Photoacoustic Imaging. Diagnosis and Treatment Monitoring of Port-Wine Stain Using LED-Based Photoacoustics: Theoretical Aspects and First In-Human Clinical Pilot Study; Mithun, K.A.S., Ed.; Springer: Singapore, 2020; Volume 7, pp. 351–377.
12. Goh, J.H.L.; Tan, T.L.; Aziz, S.; Rizuana, I.H. Comparative Study of Digital Breast Tomosynthesis (DBT) with and without Ultrasound versus Breast Magnetic Resonance Imaging (MRI) in Detecting Breast Lesion. *Int. J. Environ. Res. Public Health* **2022**, *19*, 759. [CrossRef] [PubMed]
13. Valera-Calero, J.A.; Fernández-de-Las-Peñas, C.; Varol, U.; Ortega-Santiago, R.; Gallego-Sendarrubias, G.M.; Arias-Buría, J.L. Ultrasound Imaging as a Visual Biofeedback Tool in Rehabilitation: An Updated Systematic Review. *Int. J. Environ. Res. Public Health* **2021**, *18*, 7554. [CrossRef] [PubMed]
14. Hazer, A.; Yildirim, R. A review of single and multiple optical image encryption techniques. *J. Opt.* **2021**, *23*, 113501. [CrossRef]
15. Khokhlova, T.D.; Pelivanov, I.M.; Karabutov, A.A. Methods of optoacoustic diagnostics of biological tissues. *Acoust. Phys.* **2009**, *55*, 672–683. [CrossRef]

16. Estrada, H.; Sobol, E.; Baum, O.; Razansky, D. Hybrid optoacoustic and ultrasound biomicroscopy monitors' laser-induced tissue modifications and magnetite nanoparticle impregnation. *Laser Phys. Lett.* **2014**, *11*, 125601. [CrossRef]
17. Craig, D.W.; Diebold, G.; Calasso, I.G. Photoacoustic point source. *Phys. Rev. Lett.* **2001**, *86*, 3550–3553.
18. Inkov, V.N.; Karabutov, A.A.; Pelivanov, I.M. A theoretical model of the linear thermo-optical response of an absorbing particle immersed in a liquid. *Laser Phys.* **2001**, *11*, 1283–1291.
19. Baum, O.; Wachsmann-Hogiu, S.; Milner, T.; Sobol, E. Laser-assisted formation of micropores and nanobubbles in sclera promote stable normalization of intraocular pressure. *Laser Phys. Lett.* **2017**, *14*, 065601. [CrossRef]
20. Danielli, A.; Maslov, K.; Favazza, C.P.; Xia, J.; Wang, L.V. Nonlinear photoacoustic spectroscopy of hemoglobin. *Appl. Phys. Lett.* **2015**, *106*, 203701. [CrossRef]
21. Gao, R.K.; Xu, Z.Q.; Ren, Y.G.; Song, L. Nonlinear mechanisms in photoacoustics—Powerful tools in photoacoustic imaging. *J. Am. Acad. Dermatol.* **2012**, *67*, 100343. [CrossRef]
22. Ms Ma, A.B.; Klb, C.; Mhab, C.; Eb, D.; Eai, E. Electromagnetic hall current effect and fractional heat order for microtemperature photo-excited semiconductor medium with laser pulses. *Results Phys.* **2020**, *17*, 103161.
23. Lotfy, K.H.; Hassan, W.; El-Bary, A.A.; Mona, A.K. Response of electromagnetic and thomson effect of semiconductor medium due to laser pulses and thermal memories during photothermal excitation. *Results Phys.* **2020**, *16*, 102877. [CrossRef]
24. Jennifer, K.C.; Pedram, G.; Guillermo, A.; Anne, M.V.D.; Albert, W.; Kristen, M.K.; Michal, H. An overview of clinical and experimental treatment modalities for port wine stains. *J. Am. Acad. Dermatol.* **2012**, *67*, 289–304.
25. Bashkatov, A.N.; Genina, E.A.; Tuchin, V.V. Optical properties of skin, subcutaneous, and muscle tissues: A review. *J. Innov. Opt. Health Sci.* **2011**, *4*, 9–38. [CrossRef]
26. Wang, S.; Zhao, J.; Lui, H.; He, Q.; Zeng, H. Monte carlo simulation of near infrared autofluorescence measurements of in vivo skin. *J. Photochem. Photobiol. B* **2011**, *105*, 183–189. [CrossRef]
27. Iorizzo, T.W.; Jermain, P.R.; Salomatina, E.; Muzikansky, A.; Yaroslavsky, A.N. Temperature induced changes in the optical properties of skin in vivo. *Sci. Rep.* **2021**, *11*, 754–762. [CrossRef]
28. Wang, Q.H.; Li, P.Z. Study on the characteristics of second harmonic in PTR. *Acta. Phys. Sin.-Ch. Ed.* **1993**, *13*, 878–882. (In Chinese)
29. Wang, Q.H.; Li, P.Z. Nonlinear theory and experiment of photothermal radiometry. *J. Infrared Millim. Waves* **1993**, *12*, 281–286. (In Chinese)
30. Yan, C.C.; Liu, C.; Yang, C.Y.; Xue, G.G. Research on the 3-D and 1-D theories of photothermal radiometry. *Appl. Laser* **2004**, *24*, 399–401. (In Chinese)
31. Du, G.H. Nonlinear theory of photoacoustic effect of restricted beam. *Acta. Phys. Sin.* **1988**, *37*, 769–775. (In Chinese)
32. Gusev, V.E.; Karabutov, A.A. *Laser Optoacoustics*; American Institute of Physics: New York, NY, USA, 1993; pp. 135–172.
33. Zhang, X.H. *Signals and Systems*, 2nd ed.; Xidian University Press: Xi'an, China, 2008; pp. 81–102. (In Chinese)

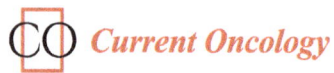

Article

Treatment Outcomes for Primary Hepatic Angiosarcoma: National Cancer Database Analysis 2004–2014

Ankit Mangla [1,*], Gino Cioffi [2], Jill S. Barnholtz-Sloan [2] and Richard T. Lee [1]

1. Seidman Cancer Center, University Hospitals, Cleveland, OH 44106, USA; rtl24@case.edu
2. Department of Population and Quantitative Health Sciences, Case Western Reserve University School of Medicine, Cleveland, OH 44106, USA; gino.cioffi@nih.gov (G.C.); jill.barnholtz-sloan@nih.gov (J.S.B.-S.)
* Correspondence: ankit.mangla@uhhospitals.org

Simple Summary: Primary hepatic angiosarcoma is a rare tumor of the liver. The prognosis and treatment of this rare tumor remains an enigma. Despite being the most common liver tumor of mesenchymal origin, the prognosis of patients diagnosed with primary hepatic angiosarcoma has never been compared with that of the most common liver tumor which is hepatocellular carcinoma. In this manuscript, we have analyzed all the recorded cases in the National Cancer Center Database and determine the best approach to treat this rare tumor. We have also conducted a brief review of the literature to guide the reader toward the finer nuances of managing patients diagnosed with primary hepatic angiosarcoma, especially in the context of a liver transplant.

Abstract: Background: To determine the risk of mortality and factors associated with survival amongst patients diagnosed with primary hepatic angiosarcoma (PHA). Methods: All patients diagnosed with hepatocellular carcinoma (HCC) or PHA from 2004 to 2014 were identified from the National Cancer Database (NCDB). Further analysis was performed within the cohort of patients with PHA to assess the impact of surgery, chemotherapy, radiation, and facility type on overall survival (OS). A multivariable analysis using the Cox proportional methods and a survival analysis using the Kaplan–Meier method were used. Results: A total of 117,633 patients with HCC were identified, out of whom 346 patients had PHA. Patients with PHA had a mean age of 62.9 years (SD 13.7), the majority were men (64.7%), white (85.8%), and had a Charlson comorbidity index (CCI) of zero (66.2%). A third of the patients with PHA (35.7%) received chemotherapy, and 14.6% underwent a surgical resection. The median survival was 1.9 months (1.8–2.4 months) compared to patients with HCC (10.4 months, 10.2–10.5) (aHR-2.41, 95% CI: 2.10–2.77, $p < 0.0001$). Surgical resection was associated with a higher median survival (7.7 versus 1.8 months, aHR-0.23, 95% CI: 0.15–0.37, $p < 0.0001$). A receipt of chemotherapy was associated with a higher median survival than no chemotherapy (5.1 versus 1.2 months, aHR-0.44, 95% CI: 0.32–0.60, $p < 0.0001$), although the survival benefit did not persist long term. Conclusion: PHA is associated with poor outcomes. A surgical resection and chemotherapy are associated with improved survival outcomes; however, the long-term benefits of chemotherapy are limited.

Keywords: angiosarcoma; database; surgery; chemotherapy; academic medical center

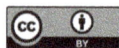

1. Introduction

Primary hepatic angiosarcoma (PHA) is an extremely rare malignancy with an estimated incidence of 0.5–2.5 cases per 10 million people [1,2]. Despite being rare, PHA is the most common mesenchymal tumor of the liver [3]. Several chemical compounds such as vinyl chloride, colloidal thorium dioxide, androgenic steroids, and phenylhydrazine are implicated in the development of PHA. Hereditary conditions such as hemochromatosis and neurofibromatosis are also associated with PHA [3,4]. A latency period of 10–40 years is noted between exposure to a carcinogen and the development of PHA [1,3,4]. A clinical diagnosis of PHA requires a high index of suspicion as most patients will present with non-specific symptoms, such as abdominal pain, weight loss, and fatigue. Imaging is needed to differentiate PHA from benign lesions and other malignant tumors. Contrast-enhanced computed tomography (CT) of the liver shows a multifocal, heterogenous, vascular tumor with internal hemorrhage in larger lesions and a disordered patchy arterial phase enhancement which is progressive in later phases [5,6]. Histopathology shows large pleomorphic sinusoidal cells. Immunohistochemistry is positive for endothelial markers (von Willebrand factor, *Ulex europaeus* agglutinin 1, and CD 31 are the most reliable markers amongst several others) [3,7,8].

PHA is an aggressive malignancy and tends to metastasize quickly within the liver or distant organs. Surgical resection is offered to patients with localized disease. In patients with localized PHA, resection of the tumor with an R0 margin (microscopic negative margin) is associated with the best survival outcomes [9–11]. Patients diagnosed with metastatic PHA are treated with systemic therapy only. However, neoadjuvant systemic therapy is sometimes offered to patients with localized disease to help increase the chances of achieving an R0 resection. Adjuvant therapy has also been used in patients undergoing surgical resection in an attempt to increase the progression-free survival [11,12]. Because PHA is a rare disease, most data in the literature come from case reports and short case series. We conducted this study utilizing the National Cancer Database (NCDB) to explore the real-world outcomes of patients diagnosed with this extremely rare tumor. Although hepatocellular carcinoma (HCC) and PHA are two different malignancies, they are aggressive and associated with poor outcomes. There has never been a formal comparison of the difference in outcomes of the two cancers. Hence, we also incorporated data from patients with hepatocellular carcinoma (HCC) as a reference to patients with PHA to compare the outcomes of the two malignancies.

2. Materials and Methods

Adults (ages 18+) diagnosed with HCC or PHA were identified in the National Cancer Database (NCDB) from 2004 to 2014. International Classification of Diseases for Oncology, Third Edition (ICD-O-3) codes were used for the identification of HCC (8170/3) and PHA (9120/3). Descriptive statistics for clinical and sociodemographic characteristics were obtained. Chi-square test was used to assess differences in categorical variables, and t-tests were performed to assess differences in continuous variables. These tests were also performed within PHA patients to compare characteristics between surgery status and chemotherapy status. The Kaplan–Meier method with log-rank test was used to calculate survival for HCC and PHA patients. Additional analyses were performed on the PHA cohort to assess the impact of surgery and facility type on overall survival. Univariate and multivariable Cox proportional hazards models were performed to assess differences in survival. Multivariable analyses were adjusted for age, sex, Charlson–Deyo comorbidity index (CCI) score, race, and ethnicity, urbanicity, insurance status, facility location and type, treatment received (surgery, chemotherapy, or RT) were performed, and adjusted hazard ratios (aHR) are reported. Statistical significance was set at <0.05. All analyses were performed using SAS version 9.4 (SAS institute, Cary, NC, USA). The study was approved by the institutional review board at Case Western Reserve University. The study was performed in accordance with relevant guidelines and regulations.

3. Results

A total of 117,633 patients with HCC and 346 patients with PHA were identified in the database. PHA was diagnosed in patients with a mean age of 62.9 years (SD: 13.7 years) and had male preponderance (male versus female: 64.7% versus 35.3%, respectively). Most patients belonged to the white race (85.8%), and most were treated either in an academic/research program or in a comprehensive community cancer program (49.8% and 31.6%, respectively). Only 14.6% of patients received surgery, 3.5% received RT, and 35.7% received chemotherapy (Table 1). Twelve patients (3.47%) with PHA received chemotherapy and surgery, six patients (1.74%) received chemotherapy and RT, and two patients (0.58%) received surgery and RT. No patient recorded in the database received all three treatment modalities. Among the patients with PHA, those who received surgery had a median survival of 7.7 months (5.5–16.9), compared to 1.8 months (1.5–1.9) for those who did not receive surgery. When adjusted for demographic factors, such as age, sex, race, ethnicity, and location, and clinical factors, such as comorbidities and treatment, patients who received surgery had a 77% decrease in the risk of death compared to those who did not receive surgery (aHR-0.23, 95% CI: 0.15–0.37, $p < 0.0001$). There was a similar trend among those who received chemotherapy, having a median survival of 5.1 months (3.8–5.8) as compared to 1.2 months (0.9–1.6, $p < 0.0001$) without chemotherapy. Adjusting for the same factors as above, those patients who received chemotherapy had a 56% decrease in the risk of death than those who did not (aHR-0.44, 95% CI-0.32–0.60, $p < 0.0001$) (Table 2). Among patients diagnosed with PHA, those who received surgery were significantly younger than those who did not (55.9 years vs. 64.2 years, $p < 0.001$), as well as those who received chemotherapy (59.7 years vs. 65.0 years, $p < 0.001$). (Table 3). Patients treated at an academic center had a higher median survival (2.9 months, 95% CI: 2.2–4.1) than those treated at a non-academic center (1.9 months, 95% CI: 1.2–2.4). However, there was no significant difference in the overall survival of patients treated at an academic center (aHR-0.99, 95% CI: 0.74–1.34), $p = 0.97$).

Table 1. Descriptive statistics for Primary Hepatic Angiosarcoma and Hepatocellular Carcinoma. National Cancer Database 2004–2014.

	Histologic Type		
	Angiosarcoma	HCC	p
Overall n	346	118,066	
Age, Mean (SD)	62.9 (13.7)	62.4 (11.1)	0.458
Sex, n (%)			
Male	224 (64.7%)	90,367 (76.8%)	<0.0001
Female	122 (35.3%)	27,266 (23.2%)	
Race, n (%)			
White	290 (85.8%)	85,200 (7.4%)	<0.0001
Black	25 (7.4%)	18,712 (15.9%)	
American Indian	1 (0.3%)	839 (0.7%)	
Asian and Pacific Islander	22 (6.5%)	9477 (8.1%)	
Ethnicity, n (%)			
Non Spanish	284 (88.8%)	97,216 (86.5%)	0.245
Hispanic	36 (11.3%)	15,142 (13.5%)	
Metro Status, n (%)			
Metro	270 (81.1%)	99,948 (87.3%)	0.002
Urban	54 (16.2%)	12,986 (11.5%)	
Rural	9 (2.7%)	1470 (1.3%)	
Insurance Status, n (%)			
Not Insured	15 (4.5%)	7772 (6.8%)	<0.0001
Private Insurance	146 (43.7%)	38,481 (33.5%)	
Medicaid	22 (6.6%)	17,587 (15.3%)	
Medicare	145 (43.4%)	48,763 (42.5%)	
Other Government	6 (1.8%)	2120 (1.9%)	
Region, n (%)			
Northeast	63 (19.1%)	24,451 (21.1%)	<0.0001
Midwest	104 (31.6%)	22,811 (19.7%)	
South	98 (29.8%)	45,337 (39.1%)	
West	64 (19.5%)	23,382 (20.2%)	
Facility Type, n (%)			
Community Cancer Program	21 (6.4%)	6335 (5.5%)	0.141
Comprehensive Community Cancer Program	104 (31.6%)	32,083 (27.7%)	
Academic/Research Program	164 (49.8%)	65,237 (56.3%)	
Integrated Network Cancer Program	40 (12.2%)	12,326 (10.6%)	

Table 1. Cont.

	Histologic Type		
	Angiosarcoma	HCC	p
Charlson/Deyo Score			
0	229 (66.2%)	55,031 (46.8%)	<0.0001
1	57 (16.5%)	31,722 (27.0%)	
2	20 (5.8%)	12,403 (10.5%)	
≥3	40 (11.6%)	18,477 (15.7)	
Metastasis	43 (26.2%)	5407 (8.6%)	<0.0001
Bone	24 (13.0%)	2509 (3.8%)	
Lung	19 (10.3%)	2997 (4.5%)	
Treatment Modalities used			
Surgery, n (%)	50 (14.6%)	31,248 (26.7%)	<0.0001
Radiation, n (%)	12 (3.5%)	9946 (8.5%)	0.001
Chemotherapy, n (%)			
No	218 (64.3%)	56,023 (55.0%)	0.086
Yes (single agent)	82 (24.2%)	34,755 (34.1%)	
Yes (multi-agent)	39 (11.5%)	11,161 (11.0)	
Alive, n (%)	34 (9.8%)	31,158 (26.5%)	<0.0001

Table 2. Descriptive Statistics: National Cancer Database 2004–2014, Primary Hepatic Angiosarcoma stratified by Surgery and Chemotherapy Status.

	Received Surgery			Received Chemotherapy		
	No	Yes	p	No	Yes	p
Overall n	293 (85.4%)	50 (14.6%)		218 (64.3%)	121 (42.0%)	
Age, Mean (SD)	64.2 (13.4)	55.9 (13.4)	<0.0001	65.0 (13.7)	59.7 (12.6)	<0.0001
Sex, n (%)						
Male	198 (67.6%)	25 (50%)	0.016	140 (64.2%)	79 (65.3%)	0.84
Female	95 (32.4%)	25 (40%)		78 (35.8%)	42 (34.7%)	
Race, n (%)						
White	245 (83.6%)	44 (88.0%)	0.93	184 (84.4%)	100 (82.6%)	0.85
Black	21 (7.2%)	3 (6.0%)		14 (6.4%)	11 (9.1%)	
American Indian	1 (0.3%)	0 (0%)		1 (0.5%)	0 (0%)	
Asian and Pacific Islander	20 (6.8%)	2 (4.0%)		14 (6.4%)	7 (5.8%)	
Ethnicity, n (%)						
Non-Spanish	243 (89.7%)	39 (83.0%)	0.18	175 (87.5%)	102 (90.3%)	0.46
Hispanic	28 (10.3%)	8 (17.0%)		25 (12.5%)	11 (9.7%)	
Metro Status, n (%)						
Metro	231 (81.9%)	36 (75.0%)	0.51	166 (79.1%)	98 (84.5%)	0.28
Urban	44 (15.6%)	9 (20.8%)		39 (18.6%)	14 (12.0%)	
Rural	7 (2.5%)	2 (4.2%)		5 (2.4%)	4 (3.5%)	
Insurance Status, n (%)						
Not Insured	11 (3.9%)	3 (6.1%)	0.099	10 (4.7%)	4 (3.5%)	0.004
Private Insurance	118 (41.8%)	27 (55.1%)		79 (36.7%)	64 (56.6%)	
Medicaid	18 (6.4%)	4 (8.3%)		20 (9.3%)	2 (1.8%)	
Medicare	131 (46.5%)	13 (26.5%)		102 (47.4%)	41 (36.8%)	
Other Government	4 (1.4%)	2 (4.1%)		4 (1.9%)	2 (1.8%)	
Region, n (%)						
Northeast	54 (19.3%)	7 (15.2%)	0.18	39 (18.5%)	24 (21.2%)	0.004
Midwest	89 (31.8%)	15 (32.6%)		55 (216.1%)	47 (41.6%)	
South	78 (27.9%)	19 (41.3%)		66 (31.3%)	30 (26.6%)	
West	59 (21.1%)	5 (10.9%)		51 (24.2%)	12 (106%)	
Facility Type, n (%)						
Community Cancer Program	19 (6.8%)	1 (2.2%)	<0.0001	17 (8.1%)	4 (3.5%)	0.097
Comprehensive Community Cancer Program	99 (35.4%)	4 (8.7%)		73 (34.6%)	29 (25.7%)	
Academic/Research Program	127 (45.4%)	36 (78.3%)		98 (46.5%)	65 (57.5%)	
Integrated Network Cancer Program	35 (12.5%)	5 (10.9%)		23 (10.9%)	15 (13.3%)	

Table 2. Cont.

	Received Surgery			Received Chemotherapy		
	No	Yes	p	No	Yes	p
	Charlson/Deyo Score					
0	192 (65.5%)	34 (68.0%)	0.83	131 (60.1%)	94 (77.7%)	0.002
1	50 (17.1%)	7 (14.0%)		36 (16.5%)	18 (14.9%)	
2	16 (5.5%)	4 (8.0%)		17 (7.8%)	6 (5.0%)	
≥3	35 (12.0%)	5 (10%)		34 (15.6%)	33 (12.5%)	
Metastasis	42 (29.0%)	1 (5.3%)	0.027	16 (22.3%)	21 (37.5%)	0.073
Radiation, n (%)	10 (3.4%)	2 (4.0%)	0.84	5 (2.3%)	6 (5.0%)	0.39
Chemotherapy, n (%)	109 (45.6%)	12 (26.1%)	0.014	–	–	
Surgery, n (%)	–	–	–	34 (20.7%)	12 (9.9%)	0.014
Alive, n (%)	20 (6.8%)	13 (26.0%)	<0.001	23 (10.6%)	11 (9.1%)	0.44

Table 3. Median Survival and Cox Proportional Hazards Models for surgery and chemotherapy status for Primary Angiosarcoma of Liver. National Cancer Database 2004–2014.

		Median Survival	Cox Proportional Hazards			
		Median Survival (95% CI)	Univariate HR (95% CI)	p	Multivariable HR *,† (95% CI)	p
		Surgery Status				
	Yes	7.69 (5.46–16.92)	0.34 (0.24–0.49)	<0.0001	0.23 (0.15–0.37)	<0.0001
	No	1.77 (1.48–1.94)	Ref		Ref	
		Chemotherapy Status				
	Yes	5.09 (3.77–5.81)	0.59 (0.47–0.76)	0.001	0.44 (0.32–0.60)	<0.0001
	No	1.15 (0.85–1.61)	Ref		Ref	

* Surgery Status—Adjusted for Age, Race, Ethnicity, Sex, Urbanicity, Facility Location and Type, Charlson/Deyo Score, Chemotherapy, and Radiation. † Chemotherapy Status—Adjusted for Age, Race, Ethnicity, Sex, Urbanicity, Facility Location and Type, Charlson/Deyo Score, Surgery, and Radiation.

Primary Hepatic Angiosarcoma versus Hepatocellular Carcinoma

A notably larger proportion of female patients with PHA than those with HCC were recorded in the NCDB database (35.3% vs. 23.3%, $p < 0.0001$). A higher proportion of white patients with PHA than with HCC were recorded (85.8% vs. 74.6%, $p < 0.0001$). Overall, patients with PHA had fewer comorbidities, with 66.2% of patients having a Charlson/Deyo score of 0, compared to 46.9% for patients diagnosed with HCC ($p < 0.0001$). The demographics of the patients diagnosed with HCC and PHA are detailed in Table 1. The median survival for patients with HCC was 10.3 months (95% CI: 10.2–10.5) and 1.9 months (1.8–2.4) for patients with PHA (Figure 1), and this correlated with a higher risk of death for patients with PHA compared to those with HCC (aHR 2.41 (95% CI) (2.1–2.77), $p < 0.0001$) (Table 4).

Table 4. Median Survival and Cox Proportional Hazards Models for Primary Angiosarcoma and HCC of Liver. National Cancer Database 2004–2014.

	Median Survival (Months)	Cox Proportional Hazards			
	Median Survival (95% CI)	Univariate HR (95% CI)	p	Multivariable HR * (95% CI)	p
Cancer Type					
Angiosarcoma	1.94 (1.77–2.36)	2.39 (2.13–2.67)	<0.0001	2.41 (2.10–2.77)	<0.0001
HCC	10.35 (10.22–10.51)	Ref		Ref	

* Surgery Status—Adjusted for Age, Race, Ethnicity, Sex, Urbanicity, Facility Location and Type, Charlson/Deyo Score, Chemotherapy, and Radiation.

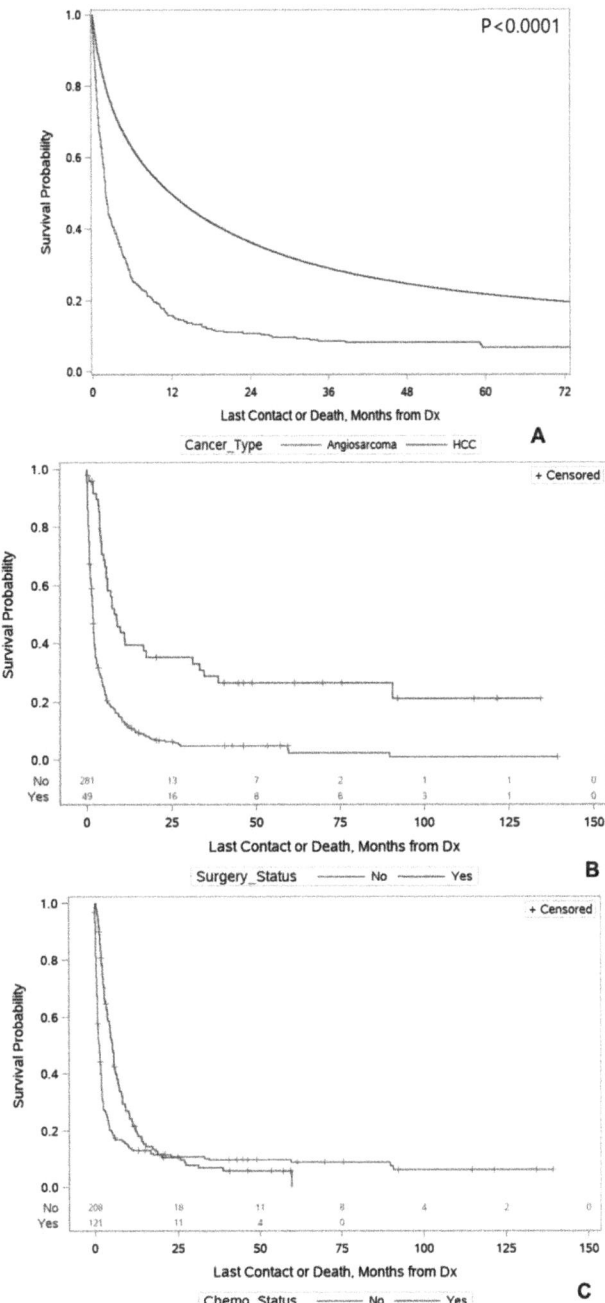

Figure 1. Panel (**A**): Kaplan–Meier Survival curves for patients diagnosed with primary hepatic angiosarcoma and hepatocellular carcinoma. Panel (**B**): Kaplan–Meier Survival curves for surgery status for patients diagnosed with primary hepatic angiosarcoma. Panel (**C**): Kaplan–Meier Survival curves for chemotherapy status for patients diagnosed with primary hepatic angiosarcoma, patients diagnosed with primary hepatic angiosarcoma. Data from National Cancer Database 2004–2014.

4. Discussion

4.1. Primary Hepatic Angiosarcoma

PHA is a rare disease whose pathogenesis, clinical characteristics, and treatment outcomes are described only in case reports and small case series [3,9,10,13]. Ours is the first database study exclusively addressing the demographics and treatment outcomes of patients diagnosed with PHA. The NCDB contains data from approximately 1500 participating centers, representing roughly 70% of all oncologic cases in the United States [14]. The incidence of PHAs amongst the primary hepatic tumors reported here is derived from the NCDB database (2004–2014). Individual cancer registries report a 0.04 to 2% incidence of PHAs amongst hepatic tumors [15,16]. We found the incidence of PHAs was 0.29% amongst all primary hepatic tumors. The majority of patients diagnosed with PHA identified themselves as white race (85.8%), and 11.3% of patients were of Hispanic race. Thus far, PHAs have been reported to exhibit a male preponderance (2–4:1 ratio favoring men) and occur between the fifth and seventh decades of life [10,11,15,17]. In our study, PHAs were diagnosed at a mean age of 62.9 years and showed a 2:1 male preponderance, which is congruent with the reported literature.

The median OS of patients with PHA in our study was 1.9 months. Retrospective studies and systematic reviews report a median OS of approximately six months in patients diagnosed with PHA [9,10,17]. Groeschl et al., in their analysis of the SEER database (1975–2007), reported an overall median OS of 1 month in the 207 patients with PHA [18]. Retrospective studies and case series report a median OS of 6 months for patients diagnosed with PHA. This discrepancy in results could be because individual case reports and case series are usually derived from academic centers where patients have access to tertiary care [9,11,12,19]. When treated at 'high-volume centers', patients diagnosed with sarcoma have a better outcome than those treated at non-academic centers [20,21]. Although our results show that the patients treated in academic centers had a numerically higher medical survival than those treated at non-academic centers, these results were not statistically significant. One probable reason for this result could be the difference in definitions of academic centers as defined in the NCDB vis-à-vis the definition used in other studies. Studies that had access to more granular data had strict criteria to define 'high-volume centers.' On the other hand, the NCDB dictionary defines an Academic Comprehensive Cancer Program (ACCP) as any facility that encounters more than 500 cancers per year and participates in post-graduate medical education in at least four subjects (hematology–oncology training is NOT a must). Sarcoma is a rare tumor, and it is hard to ascertain if all facilities falling under an ACCP, or even otherwise, have a multidisciplinary tumor board or not. Other authors have also reported such discrepancies in their cohorts, and it is a limitation of big-data analysis [22].

Our results show that patients who received surgery had improved survival compared to those who did not. These results are congruent with the general principles of managing patients with PHAs, where surgical resection affords the best survival outcomes [7,8,23–25]. The existing literature also reflects better survival outcomes for patients diagnosed with PHAs who undergo surgical resection with or without locoregional therapies, such as transarterial chemoembolization (TACE) [9–11,18,26]. In patients with lesser stage tumors (Stage 1b) who underwent surgery with or without TACE, the median survival can extend beyond five years [9,12,27–29]. Wilson et al. retrospectively reviewed 44 patients diagnosed with PHA. Six out of eight patients presenting with resectable disease underwent an R0 resection in this cohort. Only two patients who underwent an R0 resection were alive at the end of five years. Patients undergoing a surgical resection for PHA had a median OS of 33.4 months compared to a median OS of 9.3 months for those who underwent locoregional therapy and 7.7 months for those who received chemotherapy. The patients who did not receive any treatment had the worst median OS of 1.9 months [9]. In another cohort of 5 patients with solitary PHA who underwent surgical resection, the 1-, 3-, and 5-year survival was 100%, 80%, and 40%, respectively. Although four out of five patients had a tumor recurrence (death recorded between 23 to 69 months), the excellent 1-year survival validates the benefit of a surgical resection [12]. It is important to note that a surgical resection is usually offered to patients with localized disease in patients diagnosed with any soft-tissue sarcoma (STS) [7,30]. It is also known that patients with localized angiosarcoma have better survival than those with metastatic disease [7]. In the current study, it is challenging to ascertain if a possible early stage of presentation confounds the survival benefit seen with surgical resection or not.

Patients with PHA who received chemotherapy had better survival and a lower risk of death than those who did not receive any chemotherapy. Patients with metastatic disease and a locally advanced STS that are not amenable to curable surgery or RT are treated with cytotoxic chemotherapy [7,30]. However, the survival data in our study only indicate the initial benefit as the survival curves cross over by two years, indicating no long-term benefit. Many studies have shown an improvement in OS with chemotherapy in patients with angiosarcoma, especially in the metastatic stage [23–25]. Kim et al. retrospectively reviewed records of 11,415 patients with primary hepatic tumors, out of whom five were diagnosed with PHA. All five patients had metastatic disease at presentation in this cohort, and three died within three months of diagnosis. The other two patients, who were younger and had better performance status, received second and third lines of chemotherapy regimens and lived for 16 and 9 months, respectively [15]. Likewise, Wilson et al. also reported a better median OS in patients receiving chemotherapy than those who did not receive any treatment (7.7 months versus 1.9 months). A study by Huang et al. studied a cohort of 34 patients reported and noted a median OS of 41 months (IQR—20 months) among patients that received both surgery and chemotherapy ($n = 7$) compared to 3 months (IQR—9.35 months) for those who received chemotherapy only ($n = 5$) [11]. These results from individual cohorts of patients with PHA are consistent with our findings. More research is needed to understand the long-term outcomes of patients with systemic chemotherapy and if any additional benefit may arise from combining it with surgery.

4.2. Primary Hepatic Angiosarcoma versus Hepatocellular Carcinoma

HCC is the most common primary tumor of the liver and the fourth most common cause of tumor-related death worldwide [31]. The overall five-year survival for HCC is 18%, making it a lethal tumor [31]. On the other hand, PHA is reported to have only a 3% survival rate at the end of 2 years compared to cutaneous or extremity angiosarcoma [7]. Although both malignancies are associated with poor outcomes, no study has reported a head-to-head comparison of survival outcomes of patients with HCC and PHA. Ours is the first study to report a significantly worse survival for patients diagnosed with PHA than those diagnosed with HCC. Moreover, patients diagnosed with PHA are 2.23 times more likely to die from the diagnosis at any given point compared to those diagnosed with HCC. The data in this analysis extended to 2014, when significant advancements were being made in treating patients with HCC [32]. On the contrary, no significant advances came in the treatment of STS, except for the approval of pazopanib in 2014, which did not provide an OS benefit to patients diagnosed with any STS [33]. In the last five years, systemic options for angiosarcomas have increased with the inclusion of checkpoint inhibitors, and it would be interesting to see their impact on the survival of patients diagnosed with PHA.

A liver transplant is controversial in PHAs. Unlike HCC, where a liver transplant is an option for patients with limited tumor burden and satisfying the Milan Criteria [31], it is contraindicated in patients with PHA due to high rates of recurrence, infection, and high mortality. Orlando et al. reviewed 22 patients with PHA listed in the European Liver Transplant Registry who underwent a liver transplant [34]. The OS was reported at 7.2 ± 2.6 months, and all patients died by 23 months. The recurrence was recorded in 17 patients by 5.0 ± 2.6 months, all of whom were dead by 23 months. Five patients died from infection. In addition, multiple patients experienced transplant-related complications such as rejection (14 patients) and renal and respiratory failure (4 patients). A review of the published literature by the same authors also demonstrated the same dismal results. In a subset analysis of primary liver sarcomas recorded in the NCDB, the authors reported a trend toward better survival in patients with PHA who received a resection compared to those who received a liver transplant [35].

4.3. Limitations of the Study

This study has a few significant limitations. First, being a retrospective analysis, there is a potential to introduce selection bias. In addition to this, a large proportion of patients with missing records could potentially worsen this bias. Second, the NCDB dataset does not include many clinically relevant variables (such as performance status) and hence were not included in our model [14]. Third, we cannot account for miscoding or erroneous data that can be seen in large multi-institutional registries. In addition, it is challenging to ascertain the course of treatment beyond the first course of treatment from cancer registries, limiting our analysis to assess the impact of subsequent treatments on overall survival. Moreover, many treatment-related variables such as the extent of surgery or the use of RT did not meet our prespecified criteria and could not be included in the analysis.

5. Conclusions

PHA is an aggressive malignancy with a significantly worse prognosis compared to HCC. Surgery and chemotherapy are associated with better survival outcomes in patients with PHA; however, the long-term benefits of chemotherapy are not clear. More research is needed to help determine the optimal treatment approaches for this very rare disease.

Author Contributions: A.M. and R.T.L. formulated the concept, wrote the manuscript, and revised the manuscript. G.C. and J.S.B.-S. extracted data from the NCDB, analyzed the data and results, and helped to write the manuscript. All authors have read and agreed to the published version of the manuscript.

Funding: This research received no external funding.

Institutional Review Board Statement: The study used deidentified patient data from the National Cancer Database 2004–2014. The protocol was reviewed by the institutional review board (IRB) at University Hospitals, and it was exempt from IRB approval.

Informed Consent Statement: Patient consent was WAIVED as this study did not involve any protected health information.

Data Availability Statement: Not applicable.

Conflicts of Interest: The authors declare no conflict of interest.

References

1. Zocchetti, C. Liver angiosarcoma in humans: Epidemiologic considerations. *Med. Lav.* **2001**, *92*, 39–53.
2. Elliott, P.; Kleinschmidt, I. Angiosarcoma of the liver in Great Britain in proximity to vinyl chloride sites. *Occup. Environ. Med.* **1997**, *54*, 14–18. [CrossRef] [PubMed]
3. Chaudhary, P.; Bhadana, U.; Singh, R.A.; Ahuja, A. Primary hepatic angiosarcoma. *Eur. J. Surg. Oncol.* **2015**, *41*, 1137–1143. [CrossRef] [PubMed]
4. Block, J.B. Angiosarcoma of the Liver Following Vinyl Chloride Exposure. *JAMA* **1974**, *229*, 53–54. [CrossRef] [PubMed]
5. Gaballah, A.H.; Jensen, C.T.; Palmquist, S.; Pickhardt, P.J.; Duran, A.; Broering, G.; Elsayes, K.M. Angiosarcoma: Clinical and imaging features from head to toe. *Br. J. Radiol.* **2017**, *90*, 20170039. [CrossRef]
6. Pickhardt, P.J.; Kitchin, D.; Lubner, M.G.; Ganeshan, D.M.; Bhalla, S.; Covey, A.M. Primary hepatic angiosarcoma: Multi-institutional comprehensive cancer centre review of multiphasic CT and MR imaging in 35 patients. *Eur. Radiol.* **2015**, *25*, 315–322. [CrossRef]
7. Young, R.J.; Brown, N.J.; Reed, M.W.; Hughes, D.; Woll, P.J. Angiosarcoma. *Lancet Oncol.* **2010**, *11*, 983–991. [CrossRef]
8. Cao, J.; Wang, J.; He, C.; Fang, M. Angiosarcoma: A review of diagnosis and current treatment. *Am. J. Cancer Res.* **2019**, *9*, 2303–2313.
9. Wilson, G.C.; Lluis, N.; Nalesnik, M.A.; Nassar, A.; Serrano, T.; Ramos, E.; Torbenson, M.; Asbun, H.J.; Geller, D.A. Hepatic Angiosarcoma: A Multi-institutional, International Experience with 44 Cases. *Ann. Surg. Oncol.* **2019**, *26*, 576–582. [CrossRef]
10. Zheng, Y.W.; Zhang, X.W.; Zhang, J.L.; Hui, Z.Z.; Du, W.J.; Li, R.M.; Ren, X.B. Primary hepatic angiosarcoma and potential treatment options. *J. Gastroenterol. Hepatol.* **2014**, *29*, 906–911. [CrossRef]

11. Huang, I.H.; Wu, Y.-Y.; Huang, T.-C.; Chang, W.-K.; Chen, J.-H. Statistics and outlook of primary hepatic angiosarcoma based on clinical stage. *Oncol. Letters.* **2016**, *11*, 3218–3222. [CrossRef]
12. Duan, X.F.; Li, Q. Primary hepatic angiosarcoma: A retrospective analysis of 6 cases. *J. Dig. Dis.* **2012**, *13*, 381–385. [CrossRef]
13. Zhu, Y.P.; Chen, Y.M.; Matro, E.; Chen, R.B.; Jiang, Z.N.; Mou, Y.P.; Hu, H.J.; Huang, C.J.; Wang, G.Y. Primary hepatic angiosarcoma: A report of two cases and literature review. *World J. Gastroenterol.* **2015**, *21*, 6088–6096. [CrossRef]
14. Lerro, C.C.; Robbins, A.S.; Phillips, J.L.; Stewart, A.K. Comparison of cases captured in the national cancer data base with those in population-based central cancer registries. *Ann. Surg. Oncol.* **2013**, *20*, 1759–1765. [CrossRef]
15. Kim, H.R.; Rha, S.Y.; Cheon, S.H.; Roh, J.K.; Park, Y.N.; Yoo, N.C. Clinical features and treatment outcomes of advanced stage primary hepatic angiosarcoma. *Ann. Oncol.* **2009**, *20*, 780–787. [CrossRef]
16. Wang, Z.-B.; Yuan, J.; Chen, W.; Wei, L.-X. Transcription factor ERG is a specific and sensitive diagnostic marker for hepatic angiosarcoma. *World J. Gastroenterol.* **2014**, *20*, 3672. [CrossRef]
17. Molina, E.; Hernandez, A. Clinical manifestations of primary hepatic angiosarcoma. *Dig. Dis. Sci.* **2003**, *48*, 677–682. [CrossRef]
18. Groeschl, R.T.; Miura, J.T.; Oshima, K.; Gamblin, T.C.; Turaga, K.K. Does histology predict outcome for malignant vascular tumors of the liver? *J. Surg. Oncol.* **2014**, *109*, 483–486. [CrossRef]
19. Tripke, V.; Heinrich, S.; Huber, T.; Mittler, J.; Hoppe-Lotichius, M.; Straub, B.K.; Lang, H. Surgical therapy of primary hepatic angiosarcoma. *BMC Surg.* **2019**, *19*, 5. [CrossRef]
20. Gutierrez, J.C.; Perez, E.A.; Moffat, F.L.; Livingstone, A.S.; Franceschi, D.; Koniaris, L.G. Should soft tissue sarcomas be treated at high-volume centers? An analysis of 4205 patients. *Ann. Surg.* **2007**, *245*, 952–958. [CrossRef]
21. Martin-Broto, J.; Hindi, N.; Cruz, J.; Martinez-Trufero, J.; Valverde, C.; De Sande, L.M.; Sala, A.; Bellido, L.; De Juan, A.; Rubió-Casadevall, J.; et al. Relevance of Reference Centers in Sarcoma Care and Quality Item Evaluation: Results from the Prospective Registry of the Spanish Group for Research in Sarcoma (GEIS). *Oncologist* **2019**, *24*, e338–e346. [CrossRef] [PubMed]
22. Johnson, A.C.; Ethun, C.G.; Liu, Y.; Lopez-Aguiar, A.G.; Tran, T.B.; Poultsides, G.; Valerie Grignol, J.; Howard, H.; Bedi, M.T.; Gamblin, C.; et al. Studying a Rare Disease Using Multi-Institutional Research Collaborations vs Big Data: Where Lies the Truth? *J. Am. Coll. Surg.* **2018**, *227*, 357.e3–366.e3. [CrossRef] [PubMed]
23. Buehler, D.; Rice, S.R.; Moody, J.S.; Rush, P.; Hafez, G.R.; Attia, S.; Longley, B.J.; Kozak, K.R. Angiosarcoma outcomes and prognostic factors: A 25-year single institution experience. *Am. J. Clin. Oncol.* **2014**, *37*, 473–479. [CrossRef] [PubMed]
24. Ren, S.; Wang, Y.; Wang, Z.; Shao, J.; Ye, Z. Survival predictors of metastatic angiosarcomas: A surveillance, epidemiology, and end results program population-based retrospective study. *BMC Cancer* **2020**, *20*, 778. [CrossRef]
25. Fury, M.G.; Antonescu, C.R.; Van Zee, K.J.; Brennan, M.E.; Maki, R.G. A 14-year retrospective review of angiosarcoma: Clinical characteristics, prognostic factors, and treatment outcomes with surgery and chemotherapy. *Cancer J.* **2005**, *11*, 241–247. [CrossRef] [PubMed]
26. Matthaei, H.; Krieg, A.; Schmelzle, M.; Boelke, E.; Poremba, C.; Rogiers, X.; Knoefel, W.T.; Peiper, M. Long-term survival after surgery for primary hepatic sarcoma in adults. *Arch Surg.* **2009**, *144*, 339–344. [CrossRef] [PubMed]
27. Nakayama, H.; Masuda, H.; Fukuzawa, M.; Takayama, T.; Hemmi, A. Metastasis of hepatic angiosarcoma to the gastric vein. *J. Gastroenterol.* **2004**, *39*, 193–194. [CrossRef]
28. Timaran, C.H.; Grandas, O.H.; Bell, J.L. Hepatic angiosarcoma: Long-term survival after complete surgical removal. *Am. Surg.* **2000**, *66*, 1153–1157.
29. Özden, I.; Bilge, O.; Erkan, M.; Cevikbaş, U.; Acarlı, K. Five years and 4 months of recurrence-free survival in hepatic angiosarcoma. *J. Hepato Biliary Pancreat. Surg.* **2003**, *10*, 250–252. [CrossRef]
30. Mangla, A.; Yadav, U. *Cancer, Leiomyosarcoma*; StatPearls: Treasure Island, FL, USA, 2020.
31. Villanueva, A. Hepatocellular Carcinoma. *N. Engl. J. Med.* **2019**, *380*, 1450–1462. [CrossRef]
32. Chen, Z.; Xie, H.; Hu, M.; Huang, T.; Hu, Y.; Sang, N.; Zhao, Y. Recent progress in treatment of hepatocellular carcinoma. *Am. J. Cancer Res.* **2020**, *10*, 2993–3036. [PubMed]
33. Van der Graaf, W.T.; Blay, J.Y.; Chawla, S.P.; Kim, D.W.; Bui-Nguyen, B.; Casali, P.G.; Schöffski, P.; Aglietta, M.; Staddon, A.P.; Beppu, Y.; et al. Pazopanib for metastatic soft-tissue sarcoma (PALETTE): A randomised, double-blind, placebo-controlled phase 3 trial. *Lancet* **2012**, *379*, 1879–1886. [CrossRef]
34. Orlando, G.; Adam, R.; Mirza, D.; Soderdahl, G.; Porte, R.J.; Paul, A.; Burroughs, A.K.; Seiler, C.A.; Colledan, M.; Graziadei, I.; et al. Hepatic hemangiosarcoma: An absolute contraindication to liver transplantation—the European Liver Transplant Registry experience. *Transplantation* **2013**, *95*, 872–877. [CrossRef] [PubMed]
35. Konstantinidis, I.T.; Nota, C.; Jutric, Z.; Ituarte, P.; Chow, W.; Chu, P.; Singh, G.; Warner, S.G.; Melstrom, L.G.; Fong, Y. Primary liver sarcomas in the modern era: Resection or transplantation? *J. Surg. Oncol.* **2018**, *117*, 886–891. [CrossRef]

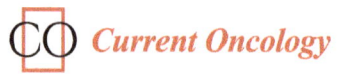

Article

Does Systemic Chemotherapy Influence Skeletal Growth of Young Osteosarcoma Patients as a Treatment-Related Late Adverse Effect?

Manabu Hoshi *, Naoto Oebisu, Tadashi Iwai, Yoshitaka Ban and Hiroaki Nakamura

Department of Orthopedic Surgery, Osaka Metropolitan University Graduate School of Medicine, 1-4-3 Asahi-Machi, Abeno-Ku, Osaka 545-8585, Japan; evis@med.osaka-cu.ac.jp (N.O.); qq329xpd@opal.ocn.ne.jp (T.I.); ychbanchan@gmail.com (Y.B.); hnakamura@med.osaka-cu.ac.jp (H.N.)
* Correspondence: manabu.hoshi.0205@omu.ac.jp; Tel.: +81-6-6645-3851

Abstract: The aim of this study was to investigate the influence of systemic chemotherapy on the skeletal growth of young osteosarcoma patients as a treatment-related late adverse effect. We reviewed the height data of 20 osteosarcoma patients (13 males and 7 females) aged ≤18 years. The average (±SD) age at diagnosis was 14.5 (±3.3) years. The average follow-up interval was 89.6 months. After wide resection of the affected bones, reconstruction with tumor prostheses and auto-bone grafting was carried out in 11 and 9 cases, respectively. Pearson's correlation coefficient was calculated to evaluate the association between actual and predicted (using Paley's multiplier method) heights. Z-scores were used to compare the initial and final heights with the Japanese national growth curve. Actual and predicted heights were correlated according to Pearson's correlation coefficient ($R = 0.503$). Z-analysis showed that statistical significance ($p = 0.04$) was noted for the height data Z-scores of patients between ≤10 years and >10 years at the final follow-up. Systemic chemotherapy did not reduce skeletal growth in young osteosarcoma patients as a late adverse effect based on two different evaluation methods. However, patients aged ≤10 years at diagnosis may develop a short stature after systemic chemotherapy.

Keywords: chemotherapy; osteosarcoma; height; skeletal growth; treatment-related late adverse effect

Citation: Hoshi, M.; Oebisu, N.; Iwai, T.; Ban, Y.; Nakamura, H. Does Systemic Chemotherapy Influence Skeletal Growth of Young Osteosarcoma Patients as a Treatment-Related Late Adverse Effect? *Curr. Oncol.* **2022**, *29*, 4081–4089. https://doi.org/10.3390/curroncol29060325

Received: 10 May 2022
Accepted: 4 June 2022
Published: 4 June 2022

Publisher's Note: MDPI stays neutral with regard to jurisdictional claims in published maps and institutional affiliations.

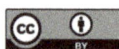

Copyright: © 2022 by the authors. Licensee MDPI, Basel, Switzerland. This article is an open access article distributed under the terms and conditions of the Creative Commons Attribution (CC BY) license (https://creativecommons.org/licenses/by/4.0/).

1. Introduction

Osteosarcoma is the most common primary malignant bone tumor in adolescents and young adults. The standard treatment for osteosarcoma is neoadjuvant systemic chemotherapy and limb-salvage surgery with wide resection [1,2]. Recent multidisciplinary therapies have remarkably improved the prognoses of osteosarcoma patients, reporting a 5-year survival rate of over 65% [3,4]. A study on survival rate improvement also reported that the treatments for young patients receiving systemic chemotherapy have generated various kinds of late adverse effects [5]. Therefore, the interest in treatment-related late adverse effects among young cancer patients has increased.

Osteosarcoma most commonly affects patients between 10 and 19 years of age [6], which is also the period of growth spurts in adolescents. Therefore, we speculate that systemic chemotherapy during this active development period may reduce skeletal growth as a treatment-related late adverse effect. Short stature after cancer treatment is relatively common as a treatment-related late adverse effect in pediatric cancer patients, especially in pediatric leukemia and brain cancer [7,8].

However, studies concerning skeletal growth after osteosarcoma treatment are few. Therefore, we investigated the influence of systemic chemotherapy on skeletal growth among osteosarcoma patients.

2. Materials and Methods

This was a retrospective study. Between September 1985 and December 2019, a total of 48 patients aged ≤18 years and diagnosed with high-grade osteosarcoma were treated at our hospital. The inclusion criteria for this study were diagnosis with high-grade osteosarcoma at the age of ≤18 years, systemic chemotherapy, and availability of clinical data on patient height during initial diagnosis and final follow-up. During the final follow-up, patient age was >18 years.

Clinical information, including sex, age at diagnosis, affected site, height data at diagnosis and final follow-up, chemotherapy protocol, and surgical procedure, were examined.

The height was routinely recorded without shoes within one week after definite diagnosis. At the final follow-up, the height was measured based on the standing position on the healthy side. If necessary, the soles of the feet were heightened and adjusted to compensate for the shortening of the affected lower limbs. Height was measured after confirming that the heights of the pelvis on both sides were parallel to the ground. The height data of 17 patients was collected during routine follow-up in the outpatient department of our hospital or in another hospital. We performed telephone surveys with three patients and asked them to correct their height as much as possible.

To determine whether the height of young osteosarcoma patients treated with systemic chemotherapy grew as expected, the final height was compared with values predicted using Paley's multiplier method [9]. These values were predicted according to a specific age and sex and were calculated using the formula $M = Hm/H$, where M is the sex and age-specific multiplier, Hm is the predicted height value at skeletal maturity, and H is the height at osteosarcoma diagnosis. At the time of final follow-up, the height of patients aged 18 years or older was substituted for the height value at the age of 18 years.

All patients included in this study are Japanese aged ≤18 years. Therefore, we used a registry based on Japanese data. The Z-scores of the height data at diagnosis and at final follow-up were determined based on Japanese national growth curve data [10]. Each Z-score was adjusted for age and sex.

The Z-scores at diagnosis and at final follow-up were compared among all patients, as well as between each sex and age group (≤10 years and >10 years).

This study protocol was approved by the Institutional Ethics Review Board of our hospital.

Statistical Analyses

Pearson's correlation coefficient (R) was calculated to compare the actual and predicted heights. Z-analyses were used for available data from the Japanese national growth curve, and the Z-scores were expressed as mean ($\pm$ SD). These Z-scores have a normal distribution (mean of 0 and standard deviation of 1). The Mann–Whitney U test was performed for statistical comparison of the two groups. Statistical analyses were performed using Excel statistics software (version 2020; Social Survey Research Information Co., Ltd., Tokyo, Japan) for Windows, and p values of <0.05 were considered statistically significant.

3. Results

Patients were excluded if they presented with metastasis at diagnosis ($n = 11$), were managed with additional chemotherapy for newly appearing metastatic lesion after conventional chemotherapy during the follow-up ($n = 7$), or had amputation surgery ($n = 2$). Seven patients were excluded because of incomplete clinical data. A total of 28 patients were excluded. One patient was followed up with for less than one year.

In total, 20 patients (13 males and 7 females) fulfilled the inclusion criteria and were enrolled in the study. The average age ($\pm$SD) at diagnosis was 14.5 ($\pm$3.3) years (range: 9–17 years). The average interval from the diagnosis to the last follow-up was 89.6 months (range 13–325 months).

The tumors were located in the femur in 13 patients (proximal, 1; mid-shaft, 2; and distal; 10), tibia in 5 (proximal, 4 and distal, 1), and humerus in two (proximal, 2).

The treatment protocol for patients included in this study consisted of preoperative chemotherapy, wide resection, and postoperative chemotherapy. After wide resection of the affected bones, reconstruction with tumor prostheses and auto-bone grafting had been carried out in 11 and 9 cases, respectively.

Chemotherapy was based on the Osaka University Osteosarcoma (OOS) D protocol [11] and Kanazawa (K)—2 protocols [12] in 18 and 2 cases, respectively. Both were modified with T12 protocols [1], and the treatments were composed mainly of doxorubicin, cisplatin, ifosfamide, methotrexate, and etoposide (Table 1).

Table 1. Chemotherapeutic protocol for osteosarcoma patients in this study.

Author	Year	Pre-Operative Chemotherapy	Post-Operative Chemotherapy
Kudawara, et al. [11]	2013	DOX 80–90 mg/m^2 + CDDP 120 mg/m^2: 2 courses IFM 15 g/m^2: 2 courses	MTX 10–12 g/m^2: 4 courses DOX 80–90 mg/m^2 + CDDP 120 mg/m^2: 2 courses IFM 15 g/m^2: 2 courses
Tsuchiya, et al. [12]	1999	DOX 60 mg/m^2 + CDDP 100–120mg/m^2: 3 courses IFM 9g/m^2 + ETP 180 mg/m^2: 2 courses	MTX 10–12 g/m^2: 3 courses DOX 60 mg/m^2 + CDDP 100–120 mg/m^2: 3 courses

DOX: Doxorubicin. CDDP: Cisplatin. MTX: Methtrexate. IFM: Ifosfamide. ETP: Etoposide.

Figure 1 shows the relationship between the actual and predicted heights among the 20 patients with osteosarcoma. R, which was calculated to determine the accuracy of heights predicted using Paley's multiplier method, is equal to 0.503. This means that the predicted height is correlated with the actual height.

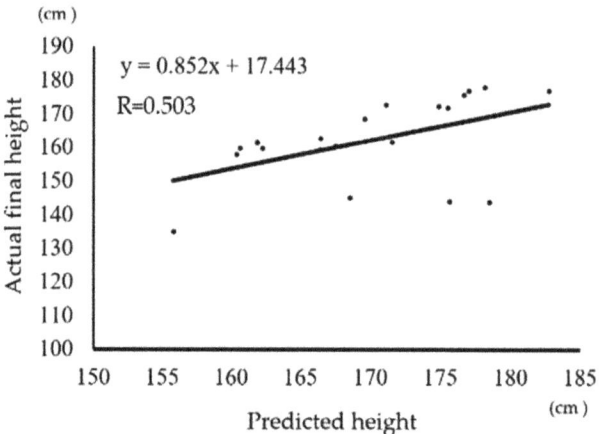

Figure 1. Relationship between actual and predicted height.

There was a statistical correlation between the actual and predicted (using Paley's multiplier method) heights, according to the calculated Pearson's correlation coefficient (R = 0.503).

The Z-scores were calculated from the Japanese national growth curve, and the scores were arranged from low to high (Figure 2). The scores at the time of diagnosis (Figure 2A) were compared with those at the time of final follow-up (Figure 2B). Decreasing Z-scores could be seen among the final follow-up height data, but no statistically significant difference was observed.

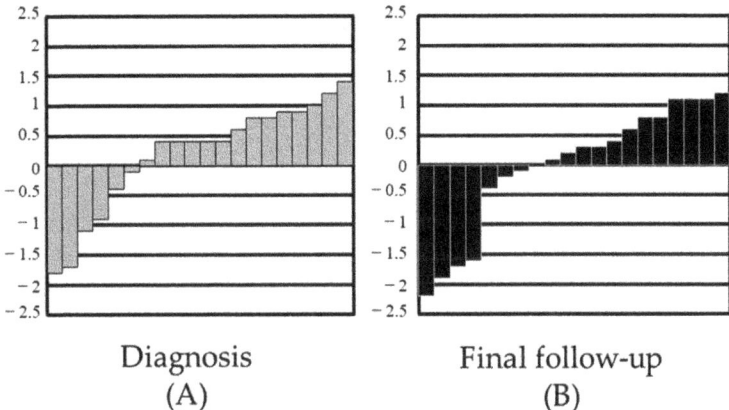

Figure 2. Distribution of standard deviations in height data: (**A**) standard deviation (SD) score at diagnosis; (**B**) SD score at final follow-up.

Among all patients, the Z-scores were 0.4 (±0.9) and 0.3 (±1.1) at diagnosis of osteosarcoma and at the final follow-up, respectively (Figure 3A). Among male patients, the values were 0.4 (±1.0) and 0.1 (±1.1) (Figure 3B), and, among female patients, the values were 0.6 (±0.8) and 0.4 (±0.9) (Figure 3C), respectively. There was no statistical significance observed among these three groups ($p = 0.48$, $p = 0.71$, and $p = 0.44$).

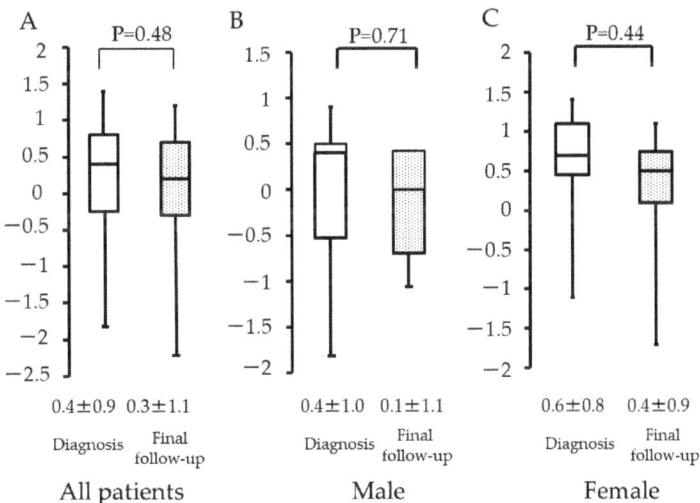

Figure 3. Height at diagnosis and final follow-up with respect to patient sex. (**A**) All patients. (**B**) Male patients. (**C**) Female patients.

Among patients aged ≤10 years, the Z-scores were 0.1 (±0.8) and −0.2 (±0.9) at diagnosis and at the final follow-up, respectively (Figure 4A). Among patients >10 years, the values were 0.4 (±1.0) and 0.4 (±1.1), respectively (Figure 4B). There was no statistical significance observed among these two groups ($p = 0.14$ and $p = 0.87$).

Among all patients with femur osteosarcoma, the Z-scores were 0.9 (±0.4) and 0.8 (±0.4) at diagnosis and at the final follow-up, respectively (Figure 5). There was no statistical significance observed between these two groups ($p = 0.48$).

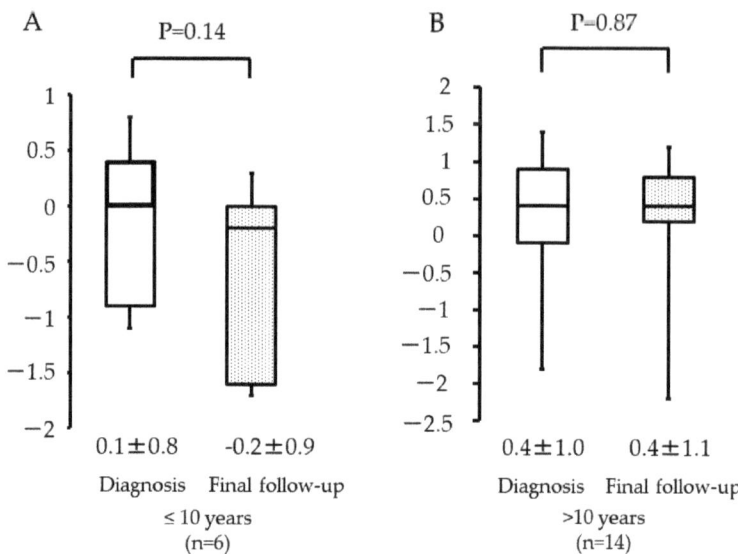

Figure 4. Height at diagnosis and final follow-up with respect to patient age: (**A**) ≤10 years; (**B**) >10 years.

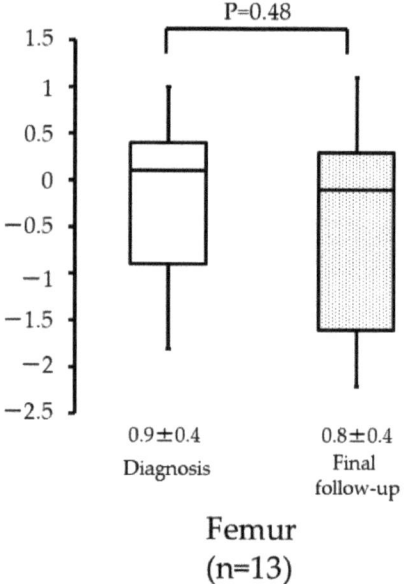

Figure 5. Height of patients with femur osteosarcoma at diagnosis and final follow-up.

The Z-scores at diagnosis were 0.3 (±0.6) and 0.5 (±1.0) for patients aged ≤10 years and >10 years, respectively (Figure 6A). The values at the final follow-up were −0.2 (±0.9) and 0.5 (±1.1), respectively (Figure 6B). There was no statistical significance observed at diagnosis ($p = 0.22$), but a statistical difference was observed at the final follow-up ($p = 0.04$).

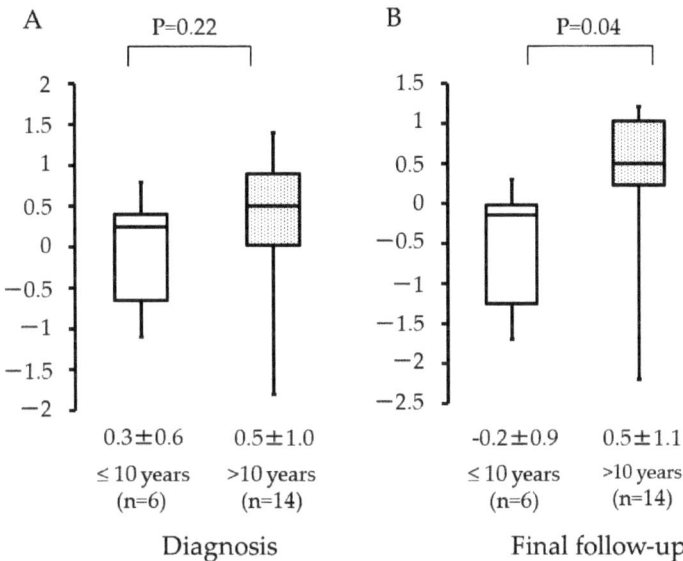

Figure 6. Height per patient age group, with respect to time: (**A**) Z-score of height at diagnosis for patients aged ≤10 years and >10 years; (**B**) Z-score of height at final follow-up for patients aged ≤10 years and >10 years.

4. Discussion

This study examined the influence of systemic chemotherapy on the skeletal growth of osteosarcoma patients aged ≤18 years at the time of diagnosis. We speculated that reduced height could be expected as a treatment-related adverse effect, since these young osteosarcoma patients underwent systemic chemotherapy during the active skeletal growth period. Based on our results, the height predicted by Paley's multiplier method was correlated with the actual height at the final follow-up, which means that the actual final height was relatively within the prediction. Additionally, the Z-analysis using data from the Japanese national growth curve showed no significant difference in the height data at diagnosis and at the final follow-up. This study failed to prove that systemic chemotherapy significantly reduced the skeletal growth of osteosarcoma patients as a treatment-related late adverse effect.

Short stature in pediatric leukemia and pediatric brain tumor patients after cancer treatment is among the common treatment-related adverse effects, especially when radiation therapy had been applied to the brain and spinal cord [13,14]. The treatment-related adverse effects of systemic chemotherapy on the skeletal maturation of patients with malignant primary bone tumors have been previously investigated (Table 2). Glasser et al. demonstrated that patients with osteosarcoma and Ewing's sarcoma who were treated with systemic chemotherapy did have height impairments when compared to the normal population [15]. Cool et al. also reported that 72 osteosarcoma patients had no significant difference in height at their last follow-up after systemic chemotherapy when compared to healthy individuals [16]. In contrast, Glig et al. showed that patients with osteosarcoma and Ewing's sarcoma had shorter statures compared to predicted height values after systemic chemotherapy [17].

Table 2. Previous studies concerning the skeletal maturity of patients with primary malignant bone tumours after cancer treatment.

Author	Year	Diagnosis	N	Reference	Outcome
Glasser, et al. [15]	1990	Osteosarcoma	68	United Kingdim cross sectional reference data	The final height was not affected.
		Ewing sarcoma	54		
Cool, et al. [16]	1998	Osteosarcoma	72	National Cancer for Health Statistic data	The final height was not affected.
This study	2020	Osteosacoma	24	Paley's multiplier method	The final height was not affected.
				Japanese national growth curve data	

The prediction of height at skeletal maturity has been advocated by Bayley and Pinneau [18], Tanner et al. [19], and Roche et al. [20]. These previously reported prediction methods require complex data comprising radiographs measuring skeletal age, nude height, occurrence of menarche, and mid-parent height. In contrast, Paley's multiplier method [9] is simple and purely based on sex and chronological age data. In our study, we compared predicted and actual height values. R was calculated to be 0.503, which means that the height predicted by Paley's multiplier method is correlated with the actual height at the final follow-up. This result supports the idea that the final height of young osteosarcoma patients is not affected by systemic chemotherapy.

Paley's multiplier method was based on height data from the National Center for Health Statistics. The population data were composed of healthy and multiethnic children [9]. However, our study involved Japanese patients; hence, we also needed to compare our data with the Japanese registry. The Japanese national growth curve was designed and is available for the evaluation of short stature among patients of various pediatric diseases. According to our results, there were no significant differences among the factors of sex and age for height data at the time of diagnosis and the final follow-up. These findings illustrate that skeletal growth in osteosarcoma patients was not affected by systemic chemotherapy.

A statistical significance was observed among the Z-scores of patients at the final follow-up (-0.2 (± 0.9) and 0.5 (± 1.1) for patients aged ≤ 10 years and >10 years, respectively). This result suggests that ages ≤ 10 years seem to be an important factor in predicting future short statue, when compared to patients aged >10 years who received the same systemic chemotherapy regimen. Previous studies have identified some factors as significant for predicting the risk of short stature after cancer chemotherapy, such as sex and age. Vinnna [7] and Sklar [21] reported that systemic chemotherapy for leukemia significantly reduced height especially in female patients. Moreover, height increase after treatment for leukemia has been suppressed in younger patients. Daiton et al. [13] reported that patients between 5 and 8 years had short statures after systemic chemotherapy. Similarly, Vilela et al. [14] reported that treatment for acute lymphocytic leukemia induced short stature in patients younger than 4 years.

The femur, which is the longest bone in humans, is also the most common location of osteosarcoma. Therefore, we speculate that the affected femur has a significant impact on the final height of osteosarcoma patients because skeletal growth may be interrupted by chemotherapy; however, no significant difference was observed in the height values at the time of diagnosis and the final follow-up.

Chemotherapy-induced short stature is thought to be the result of direct and indirect mechanisms. The direct effect may be growth plate damage caused by anticancer drugs [22–24], whereas indirectly, anticancer drugs may disturb the function of the hypothalamus–pituitary gland, resulting in growth hormone reduction [25]. During the follow-up, there were no patients with disturbed brain functions, including mental health. The standard systemic chemotherapy treatment for osteosarcoma patients is mainly composed of methotrexate, doxorubicin, cisplatin, and ifosfamide [1]. Among these key drugs, Leeuwen [22–24] reported that doxorubicin and methotrexate directly impaired increase in bone length in an in vivo animal model. Doxorubicin was reported to reduce plate height growth, affecting the proliferation zone, whereas methotrexate increased the height of the hypertrophic layer in the growth plate and disturbed the trabecular structure.

Our study has some limitations. This study was retrospective, and the small sample was comprised of patients of the same ethnicity (Japanese) from a single Japanese institution. Therefore, the results may not always be applicable to general osteosarcoma patients. The height was measured with a different type of instrument at the diagnosis and at the final follow-up; therefore, some errors were possible. The cumulative dose of the anticancer agents was not same, and the enrolled patients were being treated using two different protocols. Moreover, actual height values were compared with values predicted using Paley's multiplier method but not with values that could be predicted using other methods, such as those by Bayley [18] and Tanner [19]. The use of other prediction methods was not possible because of a lack of radiographs of skeletal age, nude height, occurrence of menarche, and mid-parent height at the time of osteosarcoma diagnosis, which are data we do not routinely collect. Therefore, our evaluation of predicted height was limited to chronological age instead of skeletal age. The average interval from the diagnosis to last follow-up was 89.6 months, and a longer follow-up of over 10 or 20 years might find different results.

5. Conclusions

Orthopedic oncologists should be convinced and be able to inform pediatric osteosarcoma patients that systemic chemotherapy does not affect skeletal growth as a treatment-related late adverse effect, unlike leukemia and brain tumors.

Author Contributions: Conceptualization, M.H.; methodology, M.H.; software, Y.B.; validation, M.H.; formal analysis, M.H.; writing—original draft preparation, M.H.; writing—review and editing, N.O. and T.I.; supervision, H.N. All authors have read and agreed to the published version of the manuscript.

Funding: This research received no external funding.

Institutional Review Board Statement: The study was conducted according to the guidelines of the Declaration of Helsinki and approved by the Institutional Review Board of Osaka Metropolitan University Graduate School of Medicine (approval no.: 4425).

Informed Consent Statement: Written informed consent was obtained from the patient and her family to publish this paper.

Data Availability Statement: All data are available from the corresponding author upon reasonable request.

Conflicts of Interest: The authors declare no conflict of interest.

References

1. Rosen, G.; Nirenberg, A. Neoadjuvant chemotherapy for osteogenic sarcoma: A five year follow-up (T-10) and preliminary report of new studies (T-12). *Prog. Clin. Biol. Res.* **1985**, *201*, 39–51. [PubMed]
2. Link, M.P.; Goorin, A.M.; Horowitz, M.; Meyer, W.H.; Belasco, J.; Baker, A.; Ayala, A.; Shuster, J. Adjuvant chemotherapy of high-grade osteosarcoma of the extremity. Updated results of the Multi-Institutional Osteosarcoma Study. *Clin. Orthop. Relat. Res.* **1991**, *270*, 8–14. [CrossRef]
3. Bielack, S.S.; Kempf-Bielack, B.; Delling, G.; Exner, G.U.; Flege, S.; Helmke, K.; Kotz, R.; Salzer-Kuntschik, M.; Werner, M.; Winkelmann, W.; et al. Prognostic factors in high-grade osteosarcoma of the extremities or trunk: An analysis of 1,702 patients treated on neoadjuvant cooperative osteosarcoma study group protocols. *J. Clin. Oncol.* **2002**, *20*, 776–790. [CrossRef] [PubMed]
4. Meyers, P.A.; Heller, G.; Healey, J.; Huvos, A.; Lane, J.; Marcove, R.; Applewhite, A.; Vlamis, V.; Rosen, G. Chemotherapy for nonmetastatic osteogenic sarcoma: The Memorial Sloan-Kettering experience. *J. Clin. Oncol.* **1992**, *10*, 5–15. [CrossRef] [PubMed]
5. Longhi, A.; Ferrari, S.; Tamburini, A.; Luksch, R.; Fagioli, F.; Bacci, G.; Ferrari, C. Late effects of chemotherapy and radiotherapy in osteosarcoma and Ewing sarcoma patients: The Italian Sarcoma Group Experience (1983–2006). *Cancer* **2012**, *118*, 5050–5059. [CrossRef]
6. Ottaviani, G.; Jaffe, N. The etiology of osteosarcoma. *Cancer Treat Res.* **2009**, *152*, 15–32. [PubMed]
7. Viana, M.B.; Vilela, M.I. Height deficit during and many years after treatment for acute lymphoblastic leukemia in children: A review. *Pediatr. Blood Cancer* **2008**, *50*, 509–516. [CrossRef]

8. Gurney, J.G.; Ness, K.K.; Stovall, M.; Wolden, S.; Punyko, J.A.; Neglia, J.P.; Mertens, A.C.; Packer, R.J.; Robison, L.L.; Sklar, C.A. Final Height and Body Mass Index Among Adult Survivors of Childhood Brain Cancer: Childhood Cancer Survivor Study. *J. Clin. Endocrinol. Metab.* **2003**, *88*, 4731–4739. [CrossRef] [PubMed]
9. Paley, J.; Talor, J.; Levin, A.; Bhave, A.; Paley, D.; Herzenberg, J.E. The multiplier method for prediction of adult height. *J. Pediatr. Orthop.* **2004**, *24*, 732–737. [CrossRef] [PubMed]
10. The Japanese Society for Pediatric Endocrinology. Cross-Sectional Growth Chart for Boys (0–18 yrs) and Cross-Sectional Growth Chart for Girls (0–18 yrs). Clinical Growth Charts. Available online: http://jspe.umin.jp/medical/chart_dl.html (accessed on 10 February 2022).
11. Kudawara, I.; Aoki, Y.; Ueda, T.; Araki, N.; Naka, N.; Nakanishi, H.; Matsumine, A.; Ieguchi, M.; Mori, S.; Myoui, A.; et al. Neoadjuvant and adjuvant chemotherapy with high-dose ifosfamide, doxorubicin, cisplatin and high-dose methotrexate in non-metastatic osteosarcoma of the extremities: A phase II trial in Japan. *J. Chemother.* **2013**, *25*, 41–48. [CrossRef]
12. Tsuchiya, H.; Tomita, K.; Mori, Y.; Asada, N.; Yamamoto, N. Marginal excision for osteosarcoma with caffeine assisted chemotherapy. *Clin. Orthop. Relat. Res.* **1999**, *358*, 27–35. [CrossRef]
13. Dalton, V.K.; Rue, M.; Silverman, L.B.; Gelber, R.D.; Asselin, B.L.; Barr, R.D.; Clavell, L.A.; Hurwitz, C.A.; Moghrabi, A.; Samson, Y.; et al. Height and weight in children treated for acute lymphoblastic leukemia: Relationship to CNS treatment. *J. Clin. Oncol.* **2003**, *21*, 2953–2960. [CrossRef] [PubMed]
14. Vilela, M.I.; Viana, M.B. Longitudinal growth and risk factors for growth deficiency in children treated for acute lymphoblastic leukemia. *Pediatr. Blood Cancer* **2007**, *48*, 86–92. [CrossRef]
15. Glasser, D.B.; Duane, K.; Lane, J.M.; Healey, J.H.; Caparros-Sison, B. The effect of chemotherapy on growth in the skeletally immature individual. *Clin. Orthop. Relat. Res.* **1991**, *262*, 93–100. [CrossRef]
16. Cool, W.P.; Grimer, R.J.; Carter, S.R.; Tillman, R.M.; Davies, A.M. Longitudinal growth following treatment for osteosarcoma. *Sarcoma* **1998**, *2*, 115–119. [CrossRef]
17. Gilg, M.M.; Wibmer, C.; Andreou, D.; Avian, A.; Sovinz, P.; Maurer-Ertl, W.; Tunn, P.U.; Leithner, A. Paley's multiplier method does not accurately predict adult height in children with bone sarcoma. *Clin. Orthop. Relat. Res.* **2014**, *472*, 2506–2513. [CrossRef]
18. Bayley, N.; Pinneau, S. Tables for predicting adult height from skeletal age. *J. Pediatr.* **1952**, *14*, 432.
19. Tanner, J.M.; Whitehouse, R.H.; Marshall, W.A. Prediction of adult height from height, bone age, and occurrence of menarche, at ages 4 to 16 with allowance for midparent height. *Arch. Dis. Child* **1975**, *50*, 14–26. [CrossRef]
20. Roche, A.F.; Wainer, H.; Thissen, D. The RWT method for the prediction of adult stature. *Pediatrics* **1975**, *56*, 1027–1033. [CrossRef]
21. Sklar, C.; Mertens, A.; Walter, A.; Mitchell, D.; Nesbit, M.; O'Leary, M.; Hutchinson, R.; Meadows, A.; Robison, L. Final height after treatment for childhood acute lymphoblastic leukemia: Comparison of no cranial irradiation with 1800 and 2400 centigrays of cranial irradiation. *J. Pediatr.* **1993**, *123*, 59–64. [CrossRef]
22. van Leeuwen, B.L.; Kamps, W.A.; Jansen, H.W.; Hoekstra, H.J. The effect of chemotherapy on the growing skeleton. *Cancer Treat Rev.* **2000**, *26*, 363–376. [CrossRef]
23. van Leeuwen, B.L.; Kamps, W.A.; Hartel, R.M.; Veth, R.P.; Sluiter, W.J.; Hoekstra, H.J. Effect of single chemotherapeutic agents on the growing skeleton of the rat. *Ann. Oncol.* **2000**, *11*, 1121–1126. [CrossRef]
24. van Leeuwen, B.L.; Hartel, R.M.; Jansen, H.W.; Kamps, W.A.; Hoekstra, H.J. The effect of chemotherapy on the morphology of the growth plate and metaphysis of the growing skeleton. *Eur. J. Surg. Oncol.* **2003**, *29*, 49–58. [CrossRef]
25. Roman, J.; Villaizán, C.J.; García-Foncillas, J.; Salvador, J.; Sierrasesúmaga, L. Growth and growth hormone secretion in children with cancer treated with chemotherapy. *J. Pediatr.* **1997**, *131*, 105–112. [CrossRef]

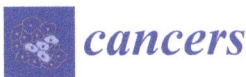

Systematic Review

Metastasectomy in Leiomyosarcoma: A Systematic Review and Pooled Survival Analysis

Megan Delisle [1], Bader Alshamsan [2,3], Kalki Nagaratnam [4], Denise Smith [5], Ying Wang [6,7] and Amirrtha Srikanthan [3,8,9,*]

1. Division of General Surgery, The Ottawa Hospital, University of Ottawa, Ottawa, ON K1N 6N5, Canada; megandelisle@gmail.com
2. Department of Medicine, College of Medicine, Qassim University, Buraydah 52571, Saudi Arabia; bshmsan@qu.edu.sa
3. Department of Medicine, University of Ottawa Faculty of Medicine, Ottawa, ON K1N 6N5, Canada
4. Interdisciplinary School of Health Sciences, Faculty of Health Sciences, University of Ottawa, Ottawa, ON K1N 6N5, Canada; knaga018@uottawa.ca
5. Health Sciences Library, McMaster University, Hamilton, ON L8S 4L8, Canada; dsmith@mcmaster.ca
6. Division of Medical Oncology, BC Cancer—Vancouver Cancer Centre, Vancouver, BC V5Z 4E6, Canada; ying.wang@bccancer.bc.ca
7. Department of Medicine, University of British Columbia, Vancouver, BC V6T 1Z4, Canada
8. Division of Medical Oncology, The Ottawa Hospital, Ottawa, ON K1H 8L6, Canada
9. Ottawa Hospital Research Institute, Ottawa, ON K1H 8L6, Canada
* Correspondence: asrikanthan@toh.ca

Simple Summary: Leiomyosarcoma (LMS) is an aggressive soft tissue sarcoma with a poor prognosis. Approximately 40% of patients will develop metastatic disease. The optimal treatment for patients with metastatic LMS is not well established, and there are no randomized controlled trials regarding metastasectomy. This systematic review and pooled survival analysis aims to assess the survival in patients undergoing a metastasectomy for LMS and compare the outcomes based on the site of metastasectomy. We identified that patients with LMS metastases in the lungs, liver, spine, and brain can undergo metastasectomy with acceptable survival. Two studies have compared survival outcomes between patients treated and not treated with metastasectomy; despite their low quality, these studies support a survival benefit associated with metastasectomy.

Abstract: This study assesses the survival in patients undergoing metastasectomy for leiomyosarcoma (LMS) and compares the outcomes by the site of metastasectomy. We conducted a systematic review and pooled survival analysis of patients undergoing metastasectomy for LMS. Survival was compared between sites of metastasectomy. We identified 23 studies including 573 patients undergoing metastasectomy for LMS. The pooled median survival was 59.6 months (95% CI 33.3 to 66.0). The pooled median survival was longest for lung metastasectomy (72.8 months 95% CI 63.0 to 82.5), followed by liver (34.8 months 95% CI 22.3 to 47.2), spine (14.1 months 95% CI 8.6 to 19.7), and brain (14 months 95% CI 6.7 to 21.3). Two studies compared the survival outcomes between patients who did, versus who did not undergo metastasectomy; both demonstrated a significantly improved survival with metastasectomy. We conclude that surgery is currently being utilized for LMS metastases to the lung, liver, spine, and brain with acceptable survival. Although low quality, comparative studies support a survival benefit with metastasectomy. In the absence of randomized studies, it is impossible to determine whether the survival benefit associated with metastasectomy is due to careful patient selection rather than a surgical advantage; limited data were included about patient selection.

Keywords: sarcoma; metastasis; leiomyosarcoma; metastasectomy; surgery; survival; systematic review

Citation: Delisle, M.; Alshamsan, B.; Nagaratnam, K.; Smith, D.; Wang, Y.; Srikanthan, A. Metastasectomy in Leiomyosarcoma: A Systematic Review and Pooled Survival Analysis. *Cancers* **2022**, *14*, 3055. https://doi.org/10.3390/cancers14133055

Academic Editors: Shinji Miwa, Po-Kuei Wu and Hiroyuki Tsuchiya

Received: 28 May 2022
Accepted: 20 June 2022
Published: 21 June 2022

Publisher's Note: MDPI stays neutral with regard to jurisdictional claims in published maps and institutional affiliations.

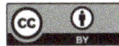

Copyright: © 2022 by the authors. Licensee MDPI, Basel, Switzerland. This article is an open access article distributed under the terms and conditions of the Creative Commons Attribution (CC BY) license (https://creativecommons.org/licenses/by/4.0/).

1. Introduction

Leiomyosarcoma (LMS) is a malignant mesenchymal tumor arising from smooth muscle cells that accounts for 10–20% of soft tissue sarcomas [1,2]. LMSs most commonly occur in the uterus, followed by the abdomen, the retroperitoneum, and larger blood vessels [3]. LMSs are principally tumors of adults and are more common in women [3]. Most LMSs are sporadic, but some may be associated with hereditary syndromes, such as retinoblastoma and Li-Fraumeni. Compared to other histologic types of soft tissue sarcomas (STS), LMSs are inherently aggressive, with 90% of patients diagnosed with grade two or three tumors [4,5]. LMSs have a poorer prognosis with a tendency for distant recurrence and a decreased disease-free survival [6,7].

Surgery to achieve negative margins remains the only curative treatment modality for patients presenting with localized LMS. Adjunctive therapies, such as radiotherapy and systemic treatment, are used in only specific cases [8–10]. Despite optimal local treatment, the risk of developing metastatic disease is approximately 40% [11]. The optimal treatment for patients with metastatic LMS is not well established, and there are no randomized controlled trials regarding metastasectomy. Many studies on this topic include multiple sarcoma histologies, limiting generalizability to distinct individual histologies, which can vary in clinical course, outcome, and sensitivity to radiotherapy and systemic therapy. Most patients with metastatic LMSs are not curable, and palliative systemic or radiotherapy is the mainstay of management. Retrospective studies have demonstrated an association with improved survival in carefully selected patients. The role of metastasectomy is most well accepted for patients with oligometastatic pulmonary metastases, but other sites of metastasectomy are increasingly reported in the literature [12–14]. This study aims to assess the survival in patients undergoing metastasectomy for LMS and compare the outcomes based on the site of metastasectomy.

2. Materials and Methods

This study is a part of a series systematically summarizing survival outcomes for patients with soft tissue and bone sarcoma undergoing metastasectomy. This study focuses on survival outcomes of patients who underwent metastasectomy for LMS. Details on information sources, search strategy, eligibility criteria, study screening and selection, data collection, and extraction can be found elsewhere [15]. The protocol is registered within the prospective international register of systematic reviews (PROSPERO) database (registration ID: CRD42019126906), and this study is reported in compliance with PRISMA 2020 statement [16].

2.1. Search Strategy

The literature search was developed by a research librarian (D.S.). The search included Medline, Embase, Cochrane Central Register of Controlled Trials, and ClinicalTrials.gov from inception to 28 May 2021, and a PubMed search for studies not yet indexed or not found in Medline. The search strategy was tailored to each database. Conference abstracts for the last three years from three major sarcoma conferences were also searched: the Connective Tissue Oncology Society, the American Society of Clinical Oncology, and the European Society of Clinical Oncology. Reference lists of all included studies and relevant systematic reviews were reviewed for additional references.

2.2. Selection Process

We included studies that evaluated metastasectomy for LMS with survival outcomes, were peer-reviewed in the English language, and had a minimum of five patients with LMS undergoing metastasectomy. Studies that included a broad range of cancer histologies (sarcoma and non-sarcoma histologies) and reported the survival outcomes for the subgroup of patients undergoing metastasectomy for LMS were included. These studies did not have to report the sociodemographic and clinical data for the subgroup of LMS patients to be included. Four reviewers (working in pairs—B.A., M.D., A.S., and Y.W.) screened titles and abstracts independently and in duplicate in the first stage, then reviewed the full texts of potentially eligible studies in a second stage to determine the final eligible studies. Disagreements were resolved by referring to a third reviewer if necessary.

2.3. Data Collection

Data were extracted by two individual members (B.A. and M.D.) and compared for accuracy. A third member (A.S.) reviewed the data extraction and resolved inconsistencies where necessary. When patients undergoing metastasectomy for LMS were a subgroup of the entire study population, two attempts at contacting primary authors were made to obtain LMS-specific patient and treatment data. If still unavailable, these data were extracted for the entire study population.

2.4. Data Synthesis and Analysis

The details of the included articles are presented in table format. The LMS-specific baseline data were included when studies reported the sociodemographic and clinical characteristics of patients diagnosed with LMS undergoing metastasectomy [17–24]. Among studies with a broad range of cancer types, of which LMS was included, the sociodemographic and clinical characteristics of patients with LMS undergoing metastasectomy were not consistently reported [11,13,14,25–36]. Thus, these characteristics are reported for the entire study population to provide details despite representing multiple cancer histologies. The LMS-specific survival outcomes were reported by all studies and are summarized in table format.

The yearly Kaplan–Meier estimated survival rates and numbers at risk for LMS patients were extracted from each study. For studies where these data were not reported, if the Kaplan–Meier curves indicated the time at which patients were censored or a risk table was provided, this was used to derive the patient-level data from the study. For studies reporting Kaplan–Meier curves of overall survival, WebPlotDigitizer v4.5 was used to identify the follow-up time and estimated survival rate at each "step" of the curve [37]. If censoring times were not available, then *IPDfromKM* web-based Shiny application was utilized to reconstruct individual patient data from published Kaplan–Meier curves [38]. The numbers of deaths and numbers at risk at each year of the follow-up period were then used to calculate standard errors for the yearly survival estimates and median overall survival. If only median overall survival was reported and Kaplan–Meier curves or risk tables were not available, the standard error was calculated using methods described by Hozo et al. [39]. Median overall survival and yearly survival estimates were then pooled across studies using inverse-variance weighted random-effects meta-analysis models [40].

2.5. Risk of Bias Assessment and Certainty of Evidence

Risk of bias assessments were completed by two individual members (B.A. and K.N.), with a third member (M.D.) resolving disagreements where necessary. First, the study design was determined using accepted definitions [41]. Studies reporting survival for both metastasectomy and non-metastasectomy patients were defined as cohort studies. Studies reporting survival for only metastasectomy patients were defined as case series. Patients who did not undergo metastasectomy may have received other treatments, such as chemotherapy or radiation.

The Joanna Briggs Institute (JBI) Critical Appraisal Checklist for Case Series and the Newcastle-Ottawa Quality Assessment Scale (NOS) were selected as the methodological quality assessment tools based on expert recommendations [42–44]. Specific decision trees were developed and agreed upon by all authors to adjudicate each criterion.

The constructs of the GRADE (Grading of Recommendation, Assessment, Development, and Evaluation) approach to assess the certainty of evidence were applied [45]. Although we did not perform a comparative meta-analysis, the components of GRADE can still be used to address evidence synthesis of quantitative estimates of effect (and thus summarized narratively) [46].

3. Results

3.1. Study Characteristics

Out of 37,241 articles, 23 studies published between 1998 and 2020 were included (Supplementary Figure S1, Table 1) [11,13,14,17–36]. Twenty-one studies were case series, [13,14,17–35] and two were cohort studies [11,36]. Collectively, the articles included 1970 patients diagnosed between 1976 and 2018, of which 656 (33%) were diagnosed with metastatic LMS and 573 (29%) underwent metastasectomy for LMS (Supplementary Table S1).

Table 1. Study details.

Study	Country	Center(s)/Registry	Inclusion Dates	Study Design	Inclusion Criteria
Anraku, 2004	Japan	Metastatic lung tumor study group of Japan	1984–2002	Case series	Pulmonary metastasectomy for uterine malignancies
Blackmon, 2009	USA	University of Texas M. D. Anderson Cancer Center	1998–2006	Case series	Pulmonary metastasectomy for STS and bone sarcoma
Burt, 2011	USA	The Brigham and Women's Hospital	1989–2004	Case series	Pulmonary metastasectomy for STS and bone sarcoma
Chen, 1998	USA	The Johns Hopkins Hospital	1984–1995	Case series	Hepatic metastasectomy for LMS
Chudgar, 2017	USA	Memorial Sloan Kettering Cancer Center	1991–2014	Case series	Pulmonary metastasectomy for STS
Deguchi, 2020	Japan	Six institutes in Japan	2002–2018	Case series	Brain metastasectomy for STS and bone sarcoma
Ercolani, 2005	Italy	University of Bologna	1990–2003	Case series	Hepatic metastasectomy for noncolorectal nonneuroendocrine tumors
Faraj, 2015	Lebanon	American University of Beirut Medical Center	1998–2009	Case series	Hepatic metastasectomy for colorectal LMS
Farid, 2013	Singapore	National University of Singapore	2002–2010	Cohort study	All LMS
Goumard, 2018	USA	University of Texas M. D. Anderson Cancer Center	1998–2015	Case series	Hepatic metastasectomy for non-GIST sarcoma
Kato, 2020	Japan	Kanazawa University	2005–2016	Case series	Spine metastasectomy for LMS
Kim, 2017	Korea	Asian Medical Center	2003–2015	Case series	Hepatic metastasectomy for intra-abdominal LMS
Lang, 2000	Germany	Hanover Medical School	1982–1996	Case series	Hepatic metastasectomy for LMS
Liebl, 2007	Germany	University Medical Centre	1990–2005	Case series	Pulmonary metastasectomy for STS
Lin, 2015	USA	University of California Los Angeles Medical Center	1990–2010	Case series	Pulmonary metastasectomy for STS and bone sarcoma
Marudanayagam, 2010	UK	Queen Elizabeth University Hospital	1997–2009	Case series	Hepatic metastasectomy for STS
Paramanathan, 2013	Australia	Peter MacCallum Cancer Center and St. Vincent's Health	2001–2011	Case Series	Pulmonary metastasectomy for sarcoma of gynecologic origin and STS
Rao, 2008	USA	University of Texas M. D. Anderson Cancer Center	1993–2005	Case series	Spine resection for primary or metastatic STS or bone sarcoma
Smith, 2009	USA	Roswell Park Cancer Institute	1976–2000	Case series	Pulmonary metastasectomy for STS surviving longer than five years
Van Cann, 2018	Belgium	University Hospitals Leuven	2000–2014	Cohort study	Metastatic LMS
Zacherl, 2011	Austria	Medical University of Vienna and Medical University of Graz	1987–2006	Case series	Hepatic metastasectomy for STS
Zhang, 2015	China	Central Hospital of PLA	2000–2009	Case series	Hepatic metastasectomy for extremity STS surviving longer than five years
Ziewacz, 2012	USA	University of Michigan	2005–2011	Case series	Spine metastasectomy for LMS

Eight studies reported the sociodemographic and clinical data for patients diagnosed with LMS undergoing metastasectomy (Table 2A) [17–24]. The other 15 studies included a broad range of cancer types, of which metastatic LMS was a subgroup and the survival outcomes for patients undergoing metastasectomy for LMS were explicitly reported (Table 2B) [11,13,14,25–36]. The proportion of patients undergoing metastasectomy for LMS in these studies ranged from 8% [25] to 60% [34].

Table 2. Sociodemographic and clinical characteristics of included patients from studies reporting (A) and not reporting (B) these details for patients with LMS undergoing metastasectomy.

A. Sociodemographic and Clinical Characteristics of Patients from Studies Reporting These Details for the LMS Patients Undergoing Metastasectomy

Study	Total # Undergoing Metastasectomy for LMS	Median Age Years (Range)	Male #	Primary Site Location #	Synchronous #/Metachronous #	DFI (Months) from Primary Tumor to Metastases	Site of Metastases #,[a]
Burt, 2011	31	Mean 52 (SD ± 9.3)	7	Uterus 13; extremity 10; retroperitoneum 4; trunk 2; other 2	NR	Mean 48 (SD ± 61)	Lung 31
Chen, 1998	11	57 (30–69)	2	Retroperitoneum 5; gastric 3; small intestine 2; uterine/adnexal 1	NR	Mean 16 (SD ± 4, range 0–40 months)	Liver 11
Faraj, 2015	5	47 (24–69)	2	Colon 4; rectum 1	3/2	NR	Liver 5; adrenal 1 Spine 10; liver 1; lymph nodes 1 peritoneum 3; lung 3
Kato, 2020	10	Mean 53 (24–69)	5	Retroperitoneum 3; uterus 2; stomach 2; extremity 2; maxillary sinus 1	1/9	Mean 50 (range 10–204)	
Kim, 2017	10	48 (38–69)	3	Retroperitoneum 5; pancreas 1; small bowel 2; colon 1; stomach 1	2/8	Median 15 (range 5–38)	Liver 10
Lang, 2000 [b]	26	Mean 54 (23–67)	18	Stomach 8; small bowel 4; vena cava 1; kidney 1; colon 1; upper abdomen/stomach 5; retroperitoneum 5; not specified 1	8/15 [c]	Median 33 (range 0–164)	Liver 23; peritoneum 4; bone 1; lymph nodes 4
Paramanathan, 2013 [d]	12	58 (44–76)	0	Uterus 12; broad ligament/adnexal 1	0/13	Median 26 (range 7–156)	Lung 13
Ziewacz, 2012	8	Mean 51 (25–66)	3	Uterus 4; chest wall 1; extremity 2; retroperitoneum 1	NR	NR	Spine 8

B. Sociodemographic and Clinical Characteristics of Metastatic Patients of Studies Not Reporting These Details for the LMS Patients Undergoing Metastasectomy[e]

Study	Total # Included	Median Age Years (Range)	Male #	Histology #	Primary Site Location #	Synchronous #/Metachronous #	DFI (Months) from Primary Tumor to Metastases	Site of Metastases #,[a]
Anraku, 2004	133	Mean 56 (26–80)	0	Squamous cell carcinoma 58; adenocarcinoma 13; endometrial adenocarcinoma 23; choriocarcinoma 16; LMS 11; other 12	Uterine 133	8/125	Range 0–243 months (0 months 8; 1–11 months 23; 12–35 months 38; ≥36 months 60)	Lung 133; extra-pulmonary 8

Table 2. Cont.

Study			Age		Histology	Site		Follow-up	Metastases
Blackmon, 2009	234	41	Mean 43 (8–83)	123	Osteosarcoma 46; MFH 33; SS 29; LMS 41; other 85	Extremity 136; NR 98	NR	NR	Lung only 197; lung + extra-pulmonary metastases 37
Chudgar, 2017	539	169	54 (15–90)	227	LMS 169; pleomorphic sarcoma/MFH 130; SS 81; other 81; fibrosarcoma 33; LPS 30; MPNST 15	Extremity 249; trunk 65; retroperitoneum/abdomen/pelvis 65; Visceral/GU/gynecologic 136; head and neck 24	71/468	Median 16 months (IQR 8–36)	Lung only 492; lung + extra-pulmonary metastases 47
Deguchi, 2020	22	5	45 (18–76)	11	ASPS 6; RMS 1; LMS 5; MPNST 1; osteosarcoma 1; epithelioid cell tumor 1; pleomorphic sarcoma 2 SS 2; undifferentiated sarcoma 1; UPS 2	NR	2/20	Median 20 months (range 0–267)	Brain 22; lung 19
Ercolani, 2005	83	10	Mean 55 (18–76)	35	NR	GI 18; breast 21; GU 15; soft tissue 10; other 19	11/72	≤1 year 34; >1 year 49	Liver 83
Farid, 2013 [f,g]	97	11	51 (28–87)	23	LMS 97	Uterine 51; extremity 16; retroperitoneum 9; pelvis 8; GI 6; GU 5; other 2	27/NR	NR	Uterine LMS [h]: liver 12.5%; lungs 81.3%; brain 6.3%; bones 12.5%; peritoneal 18.6%; lymph nodes 15.6%; others 25%. Extrauterine LMS [h]: liver 38.5%; lungs 50%; bones 11.5%; peritoneal 19.2%; lymph nodes 19.2%; others 26.9%
Goumard, 2018	126	62	54 (4–79)	56	LMS 62; LPS 14; hemangiopericytoma/SFT 9; vascular 7 (hemangioendothelioma 4; angiosarcoma 3); osteosarcoma 2; RMS 1; unclassified 26; NR 4	Abdominal 105; extra-abdominal 21	44/82	Median 12 months (range 0–298); >24 months 45	Liver 126; extra-hepatic metastases 26
Liebl, 2007	42	13	Mean 50 (17–73)	25	Alveolar sarcoma 2; extraskeletal chondrosarcoma 4; fibrosarcoma 4; LMS 13; MPNST 3; MFH 7; SS 4; spindle cell sarcoma 2; other 5	NR	10/32	Median 12 months; >18 months 16; ≤18 months 26	Lung 42

Table 2. Cont.

Study	#	Age	#	Histology	Primary site	NR/NR	Follow-up	Metastatic sites
Lin, 2015	155	Mean 47 (11–92)	87	LMS 26; osteosarcoma 21; SS 19; chondrosarcoma 14; LPS 10; undifferentiated sarcoma/MFH 7; Ewing's sarcoma 5; MPNST 5; alveolar soft part sarcoma 3; RMS 2; other 25; NR 18	Extremity 87; non-extremity 52; Visceral-gynecologic 16	23/132	Median 20 months (range 1–268)	Lung 155
Marudanayagam, 2010 [c]	36	58 (23–81)	13	Spindle cell sarcoma 1; angiosarcoma 1; osteosarcoma 1; carcinosarcoma 2; LPS 2; sarcomatoid renal cell tumor 4; GIST 5; LMS 20	Lung 1; vena cava 2; retroperitoneum 2; leg 3; skin 1; breast 1; ovary 1; uterus 3; kidney 4; colon 1; small bowel 5; mesentery 6; stomach 6	13/23	Median 17 months (range 0–322)	Liver 36; extra-hepatic metastases 11
Rao, 2008	80	53 (9–77)	NR	Chondrosarcoma 21; LMS 22; Osteosarcoma 10; LPS 9; RMS 1; SS 4; unclassified sarcoma 9; other 4	NR 51	NR/NR	Median 32 months (range 0–127)	Spine 51; active extraspinal disease 35
Smith, 2009	94	49 (9–75)	47	MFH 16; SS 18; LMS 22; LPS 12; other 26	Extremity 47; retroperitoneum 6; uterus 12; other 29	18/76	Median 15 months (range 0–176)	Lung 94; extra-pulmonary metastases 34
Van Cann, 2018 [c]	122	60 (19–84)	45	Pleiomorphic sarcoma 1; LMS 9; chondrosarcoma 1; GIST 2; malignant schwannoma 1; malignant GI autonomic nerve tumor 1	Extremity 43; uterine 24; abdominal 23; vascular 13; GI 12; thoracic 5; cutaneous 2	38/84	Median 14 months (range 1–140)	Lung 78; liver 33; bone 9; lung only 47; liver only 10; bone only 3
Zacherl, 2011	15	Mean 62 (SD ± 12)	5		Small intestine 4; bone 3; pancreas 1; stomach 1; kidney 1; uterus 1; retroperitoneum 1; unknown primary 3	5/10	Median 33 months (range 15–124)	Liver 15
Zhang, 2015	27	42 (16–64)	15	LMS 12; SS 4; LPS 5; MFH 3; spindle cell sarcoma 3	Extremity 27	3/24	Median 31 months (range 0–104)	Liver 27

[a] Patients may be included more than once; [b] Data for patients undergoing first liver metastasectomy; [c] Data only available for 23 patients; [d] One patient with endometrial stromal sarcoma included in the data presented; [e] Sociodemographic and clinical data listed in this table are for the entire metastatic cohort and includes patients diagnosed with LMS and other cancer histologies; [f] The entire study cohort included LMS patients of which only a subgroup underwent metastasectomy; [g] Sociodemographic and clinical characteristics reported are for both metastatic and non-metastatic patients at the time of diagnosis of the primary tumor; [h] Sites of metastatic disease were only reported as percentages stratified by uterine versus extrauterine sites of primary tumor. These include both synchronous and metachronous metastatic disease; NR: Not reported; #: Number of patients.

3.2. Sociodemographic and Clinical Characteristics of Patients Undergoing Metastasectomy for LMS

The sociodemographic and clinical data for patients with LMS undergoing metastasectomy were available for 113 patients from eight studies and will be discussed here (Table 2A) [17–24]. The mean or median age was between 47 and 58, with individual patient age ranges between 23 and 76. Fifty-eight (51%) patients were male. The most common site of origin of LMS was gastrointestinal ($n = 34$, 30%), uterine/adnexal ($n = 33$, 29%), retroperitoneal ($n = 23$, 20%), extremity/trunk ($n = 17$, 15%), other ($n = 6$, 5%), and vena cava ($n = 1$, 1%). The primary tumor in patients undergoing metastasectomy was reported to be well controlled (no additional details provided) in six studies [17–21,23].

Seven studies reported either the disease-free interval (DFI) or the proportion of patients presenting with synchronous versus metachronous metastatic disease [17–23]. Fourteen patients (23%) had synchronous disease and 47 (77%) had metachronous disease. The median DFI was between 15 and 50 months, with an individual patient range between zero and 204 months. The most common sites of metastases included liver ($n = 59$, 42%), lung ($n = 47$, 33%), spine ($n = 18$, 13%), peritoneum ($n = 7$, 5%), lymph nodes ($n = 5$, 4%), other ($n = 4$, 3%), bone ($n = 1$, 1%), and adrenal ($n = 1$, 1%).

3.3. Management of Patients Undergoing Metastasectomy for LMS

Out of 656 patients with metastatic LMS included in all 23 studies, 573 (87%) underwent at least one metastasectomy (Table 3). The most commonly reported site of metastasectomy for LMS was lung ($n = 353$, 62%) followed by liver ($n = 165$, 29%), spine ($n = 39$, 7%), and brain ($n = 5$, 1%). The site of metastasectomy was not specified for 11 (2%) patients. Nine studies reported the intent for metastasectomy, and the criteria used to select patients for metastasectomy were reported by ten studies (Table 4).

Six studies reported whether perioperative systemic therapy was used in patients undergoing metastasectomy for LMS, of which 48 (52%) received perioperative systemic treatment [11,17–20,24]. Only three studies reported the type of systemic therapy used [11,18,19]. Van Cann et al. reported that seven out of 28 patients received systemic treatment before their first metastasectomy, of which four received an anthracycline combined with an alkylating agent regimen, two received a single-agent anthracycline, and one received the oral tyrosine kinase inhibitor, pazopanib [11]. Chen et al. reported that four out of 11 patients received perioperative systemic therapy; one patient received adriamycin, dacarbazine, and etoposide preoperatively, and, postoperatively, one patient received doxorubicin, dacarbazine, ifosfamide, and mesna, another received doxorubicin, dacarbazine, and etoposide, and a third received cytoxan and vincristine [18]. Faraj et al. reported that two out of five patients with synchronous disease who underwent the simultaneous resection of all disease received postoperative chemotherapy [19]. One patient received doxorubicin and ifosfamide and another received doxorubicin alone [19].

Five studies reported whether perioperative radiotherapy was used in patients undergoing metastasectomy for LMS, of which 18 (20%) received perioperative radiotherapy [11,17,18,20,24]. The details of the radiotherapy's type, dose, and frequency were not consistently reported.

Table 3. Management of metastatic disease in studies reporting (A) and not reporting (B) these details for the LMS patients undergoing metastasectomy.

A. Management of Metastatic Disease in Studies Reporting These Details for the LMS Patients Undergoing Metastasectomy

Study	Site of Metastasectomy #, [a]	Number of Resected Metastases #	Size of Resected Metastases	Completeness of Metastasectomy #	Type of Resection #	Perioperative Systemic Therapy #	Perioperative Radiotherapy #
Burt, 2011	Lung 31	Mean 1.9 +/− 1.5 (range 1–8)	Size of largest resected metastases 2.9 cm ± 2.4	R0 28; R1 3	Wedge 22; segmentectomy 2; lobectomy 7	Perioperative chemotherapy 20	Perioperative 7
Chen, 1998	Liver 11	Mean 2.6 (range 1–6)	Size of largest lesion mean 3.8 cm (range 1.1–10)	R0 6; R1/2 5	Segmentectomy 5; lobectomy 4; complex resection 2	Preoperative chemotherapy 1; postoperative chemotherapy 3	Preoperative 1
Faraj, 2015	Liver 5; adrenal 1	Multiple 5	Size of largest metastases median 12 cm (range 6–16)	R0 3; unknown 2	Major hepatectomy 4; left adrenalectomy + right hepatectomy 1	Postoperative chemotherapy 2	NR
Kato, 2020	Spine 10	Solitary 10	NR	NR	Single vertebral resection 5; two or three consecutive vertebral resections 5	Preoperative chemotherapy 2; postoperative chemotherapy 6	Preoperative 2; postoperative 1
Kim, 2017	Liver 10	Solitary 6; multiple 4	Maximum size of metastasis median 2.6 cm (range 0.9–3)	R0 9; R1 1	Wedge 8; sectionectomy 1; right hepatectomy 1	NR	NR
Lang, 2000 [b]	Liver 23	Solitary 10; two metastases 3; three metastases 4; >three metastases 6	Largest tumor diameter median 8 cm (range 2–25 cm)	R0 15; R1 3; R2 5	Segmentectomies 12, major hepatectomies 7, extracorporeal resections 4	NR	NR
Paramanathan, 2013	Lung 13	One metastasis 6; > one metastasis 7	NR	R0 11; R1 1; unresectable at the time of surgery 1	Wedge 7; segmentectomy 1; lobectomy 5	Some patients had pre or postoperative chemotherapy [c]	NR
Ziewacz, 2012	Spine 8	NR	NR	NR	Intralesional 8	Perioperative chemotherapy 7	Perioperative 6

Table 3. Cont.

B. Management of Metastatic Disease in the Studies Not Reporting These Details for the LMS Patients Undergoing Metastasectomy. [d]

Study	Site of Metastasectomy #,[e]	Number of Resected Metastases	Size of Resected Metastases	Completeness of Metastasectomy #	Type of Resection	Perioperative Systemic Therapy #	Perioperative Radiotherapy #,[e]
Anraku, 2004	Lung 133	One metastasis resected 77; 2–3 metastases resected 31; ≥4 metastases resected 23; NR 2	<3 cm 71; ≥3 cm 52; NR 10	NR	Pneumonectomy 3; bilobectomy 3; lobectomy 61 [f]; wedge or segmentectomy 84 [f] Lung resection combined with mediastinal or hilar lymphadenectomy 45	NR	NR
Blackmon, 2009	Lung 234; abdomen 12; bone 16; brain 7; extra-pulmonary thoracic 3; pelvis 3; retroperitoneum 2; soft tissue/skin 7; scalp 5; spine 8	≤ Two 94; >2 132	NR	R0 184; R1 21; R2 29	For the first pulmonary resection only: Wedge 200; lobectomy, bilobectomy or sleeve 18; segmentectomy 15; pneumonectomy 1; Lung resection combined with lymph node dissection 7	NR	NR
Chudgar, 2017	Lung 539 One metastasis 229; 2 metastases 87; three metastases 57; four metastases 28; ≥5 metastases 138	NR	R0 490; R1 18; R2 31	Wedge 422; lobectomy 107; pneumonectomy 10	Preoperative chemotherapy 160; postoperative chemotherapy 53	NR	
Deguchi, 2020	Brain 22	Single brain metastases 14; multiple brain metastases 8	Maximum metastasis size median 39 mm (range 5–80)	GTR 21; STR 1	NR	Postoperative chemotherapy 3; Postoperative tyrosine kinase inhibitor 3	WBRT 10; Stereotactic 12
Ercolani, 2005	Liver 83	Single metastasis 58; multiple metastases 25	<5 cm 50; >5 cm 33	NR	Wedge resection 11; major hepatectomy 72	Postoperative chemotherapy 26	NR
Farid, 2013	NR	NR	NR	NR	NR	NR	NR
Goumard, 2018	Liver 126; resection of all extra-hepatic metastases 17	≥2 51	Maximum metastasis size 38 mm (range 3–330)	R0 107	Major liver resection 68; associated RFA 17; associated abdominal extrahepatic resection 37; associated thoracic extrahepatic resection 9	Preoperative chemotherapy 65; postoperative chemotherapy 33	Postoperative radiation 2

Table 3. Cont.

Liebl, 2007	Lung 42	Solitary 16; multiple 26	≤2 cm 22; >2 cm 20	NR	NR	Preoperative chemotherapy 12	NR
Lin, 2015	Lung 155	Average 4 +/− 4; range 1–29	Diameter of largest metastasis mean 2.9 cm +/− 3.0 (range 0.3–16)	R0 105; R1 13; R2 12; NR 25	Wedge 102; segmentectomy 20; lobectomy 27; pneumonectomy 6	Preoperative therapy not otherwise specified 93	NR
Marudanayagam, 2010	Liver 36; extra-hepatic metastases 11	Median 1 (range 1–6)	Maximum diameter of metastasis 11 cm (range 1–26)	NR	Segmentectomy 6; wedge 8; hemihepatectomy 17; trisectionectomy 5	NR	NR
Rao, 2008	Spine 51	NR	NR	NR	En bloc resection 6; intralesional resection 45	NR	NR
Smith, 2009	Lung 94; extra-pulmonary metastases 34	One pulmonary metastasis 34; >1 pulmonary metastasis 60	NR	R0 74; R1/2 20	Wedge resection 74; lobectomy 17; pneumonectomy 3	Postoperative chemotherapy 53	Perioperative radiation 7; intraoperative radiation 7
Van Cann, 2017	Lung 28	NR	NR	NR	NR	Perioperative systemic therapy 7	Postoperative radiotherapy 1
Zacherl, 2011	Liver 15	Solitary 5; multiple 10	Median tumor diameter 60 mm (range 20–200)	R0 10; R1 3; R2 2	Hemihepatectomy 9; Segmentectomy 4; wedge 3	Postoperative chemotherapy 4	NR
Zhang, 2015	Liver 27	<Two metastases 16; ≥2 metastases 11 Median 3 (range 1–13)	NR	R0 21; R1 6	Wedge 17; segmentectomy 8; Hemihepatectomy 2	Postoperative chemotherapy 22	NR

[a] Patients may be included more than once; [b] Data presented for patients undergoing first metastasectomy only; [c] The number of patients that preoperative and postoperative chemotherapy was not reported; [d] The management listed in this table are for the entire metastatic cohort and includes patients diagnosed with LMS and other types of cancers; [e] Patients may be included more than once; [f] Includes second resection of staged operation; NR: Not reported; R0: negative margins; R1: microscopically positive margin; R2: macroscopically/gross positive margin. NR: Not reported; #: Number of patients.

Table 4. Intent and criteria for metastasectomy reported by studies.

Study	Intent	Criteria
Anraku, 2004	NR	NR
Blackmon, 2009	Curative and palliative	Local control of the primary tumor. Immediate metastasectomy was recommended if there was a single or limited number of pulmonary metastases and a long DFI (minimum duration not specified) otherwise chemotherapy was recommended followed by metastasectomy if there was stable, responding, or slowly progressing disease.
Burt, 2011	Curative	Control of all extra-thoracic disease and lack of a better alternative systemic therapy.
Chen, 1998	NR	NR
Chudgar, 2017	NR	NR
Deguchi, 2020	Palliative	NR
Ercolani, 2005	Curative	Metastatic disease limited to the liver.
Faraj, 2015	Curative	NR
Farid, 2013	NR	NR
Goumard, 2018	NR	NR
Kato, 2020	NR	Solitary metastasis of the spine involving three or fewer consecutive spinal levels, an Eastern Cooperative Oncology Group Performance Status (ECOG) equal to or less than three, stable disease, and three or fewer metastases in other organs.
Kim, 2017	NR	NR
Lang, 2000	NR	NR
Liebl, 2007	NR	NR
Lin, 2015	NR	Chemotherapy followed by metastasectomy was preferred in patients with a short disease-free interval, multiple lesions involving both lungs, high-grade sarcoma, or when preoperative chemotherapy was recommended for the primary tumor in synchronous disease.
Marudanayagam, 2010	NR	Resectable with enough functional liver remanent, extrahepatic metastases a preclusion to hepatic resection.
Paramanathan, 2013	Curative	Control of the primary tumor and no extra-thoracic disease.
Rao, 2008	NR	NR
Smith, 2009	Curative	NR
Van Cann, 2018	Curative	NR
Zacherl, 2011	NR	Resectable with enough functional liver remanent.
Zhang, 2015	Curative	Metastatic disease limited to the liver.
Ziewacz, 2012	Palliative	Life expectancy of at least three years and neurological deficits, refractory pain, radiographic instability, or tumor progression despite chemotherapy and radiation.

NR: Not reported.

3.4. Post-Metastasectomy Outcomes

For the assessment of overall survival, the median follow-up time ranged from 14 to 60 months across the studies (Supplementary Table S2). All 23 studies reported either a median overall survival or a one-year, three-year, or five-year overall survival for patients with LMS undergoing metastasectomy (Supplementary Table S2).

Kaplan–Meier curves or risk tables were available in 14 studies, allowing for individual patient data to be extracted and pooled yearly survival estimates to be calculated [13,17–25,28,29,34,36]. Two additional studies reported the median overall survival and range, from which the standard error could be calculated, and were included in the pooled median overall survival analysis [11,14].

The pooled median survival was 59.6 (95% CI 33.3 to 66.0) months. The pooled median overall survival was longest for patients undergoing lung metastasectomy (72.8 months 95% CI 63.0 to 82.5), followed by liver (34.8 months 95% CI 22.3 to 47.2), spine (14.1 months 95% CI 8.6 to 19.7), and brain (14 months 95% CI 6.7 to 21.3). The yearly pooled overall survival estimates are available in Table 5, and the yearly pooled estimates by the site of metastasectomy are displayed in Figure 1. Patients undergoing lung and liver metastasectomy did better than those undergoing brain and spine metastasectomy (Figure 1).

Table 5. Pooled overall survival estimates.

Study	Site of Metastasectomy	Total #	1-Year Overall Survival		2-Year Overall Survival		3-Year Overall Survival		4-Year Overall Survival		5-Year Overall Survival	
			# At Risk	Rate (%)	# At Risk	Rate (%)	# At Risk	Rate (%)	# At Risk	Rate (%)	# At Risk	Rate (%)
Anraku, 2003	Lung	11	7	64	5	55	4	38	3	38	2	38
Burt, 2011	Lung	31	29	98	25	87	19	72	16	64	13	52
Chen, 1998	Liver	11	11	100	7	72	4	52	1	35	0	0
Deguchi, 2020	Brain	5	2	80	0	0	0	0	0	0	0	0
Ercolani, 2005	Liver	10	8	80	6	60	6	60	5	50	3	30
Faraj, 2015	Liver	5	3	60	2	40	1	20	0	0	0	0
Farid, 2013	Other	11	11	100	9	100	7	78	7	78	6	67
Goumard, 2018	Liver	55	52	98	36	89	26	69	19	58	17	52
Kato, 2020	Spine	10	9	90	7	70	6	60	5	50	4	40
Kim, 2017	Liver	10	8	100	2	58	2	58	1	58	1	58
Lang, 2000	Liver	23	17	74	13	57	8	35	4	17	3	13
Paramanathan, 2013	Lung	13	12	92	11	92	8	76	6	66	4	66
Zacherl, 2011	Liver	9	5	56	5	56	3	33	1	11	1	11
Ziewacz, 2012	Spine	8	3	57	0	0	0	0	0	0	0	0
Pooled overall survival (95% CI)				86 (78–94)		65 (52–79)		49 (36–62)		38 (24–53)		31 (18–44)

#: Number of patients.

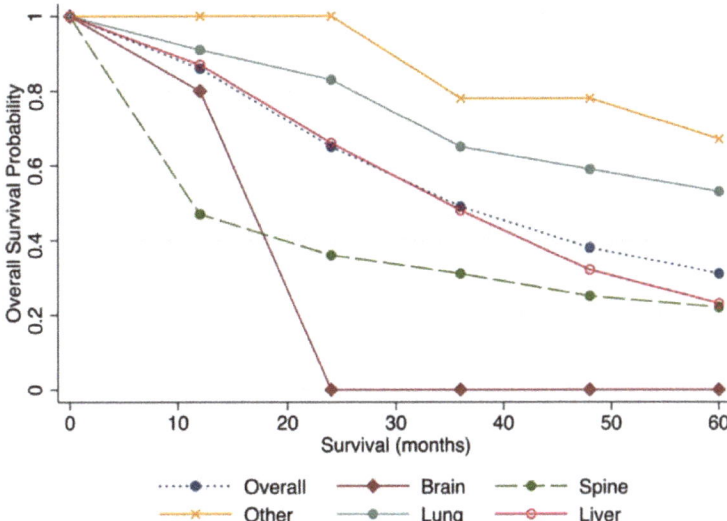

Figure 1. Pooled overall survival by site of metastasectomy.

Two studies compared survival outcomes for patients with metastatic LMS versus those who did not undergo metastasectomy [11,36]. Both these studies reported metastasectomy was for curative intent; however, neither presented the criteria used to select patients for metastasectomy. Van Cann et al. found that among patients who underwent metastasectomy, the median overall survival was 83 months (range 4–127) compared to 16 months (range 0–83) among those who did not undergo metastasectomy (multivariable analysis HR 0.4 95% CI 0.2–0.8 p = 0.01) [11]. Farid et al. found that among patients who underwent metastasectomy, the median overall survival was 205 months (range 45–205) compared to 40 months (range 5–140) among those who did not [36]. On univariable analysis, those who did not undergo metastasectomy were at a significantly higher risk of death compared to those who did (HR 5.30 95% CI 1.52–18.49 p = 0.004), and this risk was even higher in a subgroup analysis of patients with lung metastases (HR 9.09 95% CI 1.16–100 p = 0.012) [36].

3.5. Prognostic Factors Associated with Post-Metastasectomy Outcomes

3.5.1. Lung

Burt et al. identified that patients with a longer DFI had an improved overall survival on multivariable analysis (DFI included as a monthly continuous variable, HR 0.97 95% CI 0.94–0.99 p = 0.001) [17]. Paramanathan et al. identified that patients with a more favorable International Registry of Lung Metastases prognostic group (i.e., those with a completely resectable single metastasis with a DFI greater than 36 months) had improved survival (survival outcomes not reported quantitatively by authors) [47].

3.5.2. Liver

Chen et al. identified that patients undergoing an R0 resection had a significantly longer median overall survival (median overall survival not reached, range 19–55 months) than those undergoing an R1/2 resection (median overall survival 25 months range 18–39 p = 0.03) [18]. Chen et al. also found no difference in survival between high- versus low-grade LMS, the number of liver metastases, the size of liver metastases, or the extent of liver resection [18]. Lang et al. found a prolonged survival among those undergoing first liver resections for metastatic disease who achieved an R0 resection (median overall survival 32 months range 1–84, five-year overall survival 20%) compared to an R1/2 resection (median overall survival 21 months range 1–49 p = 0.31, five-year overall survival 0%) [22]. Lang et al. also identified that patients undergoing liver resection for synchronous disease had a lower median overall survival than those with metachronous disease (22 versus 32 months, respectively, p = 0.61) [22]. Lang et al. did not find the presence of an extra-hepatic tumor to be associated with worse survival if they were able to achieve an R0 resection [22].

3.5.3. Spine

Kato et al. assessed for various prognostic factors in univariable analyses and found postoperative Eastern Cooperative Oncology Group (ECOG) status was the only significant predictor of three-year overall survival after spine metastasectomy [20]. The three-year overall survival of patients with a postoperative ECOG status greater than three was 0% compared to 78% among those with an ECOG less than three (p = 0.003) [20].

3.6. Recurrence Post-Metastasectomy

Six studies reported recurrence post-metastasectomy for patients with LMS [17,19–21,23,24]. Of those, including patients who underwent lung metastasectomy, Burt et al. identified that 25 out of 31 patients recurred, of which 11 were managed with repeat metastasectomy [17]. Paramanthan et al. reported that eight out of 13 developed a recurrence [23]. Only one underwent repeat metastasectomy [23]. Of patients undergoing liver metastasectomy for LMS, Faraj et al. reported that all patients included in their study died of metastatic disease; the site of recurrence and management of recurrence was not specified [19]. Kim et al. reported that five out of 10 patients developed a recurrence. Two of these patients were managed with additional surgery. Among patients who underwent spine metastasectomy, Kato et al. reported that all patients included in their study died of metastatic disease, but the site of recurrence and the management of recurrence was not specified [20]. Ziewacz et al. reported that five out of eight patients recurred in their spine, of which, four underwent additional surgery and experienced improvement in their symptoms [24].

The outcomes of patients undergoing repeat metastasectomy were only reported by Lang et al.; the five-year overall survival was 0% and the median overall survival was

31 months (range 5–51) among the nine patients undergoing a second and third liver metastasectomy [22].

3.7. Risk of Bias and Certainty of Evidence

The risk of bias assessments are available in the supplementary material (Supplementary Tables S3 and S4). All included studies were at risk of bias. Based on the risk of bias assessments and review of the studies, the certainty of the bias was deemed very low (Supplementary Table S5).

4. Discussion

The role of metastasectomy in LMS is not currently well described in the literature. This study is the first to systematically synthesize and critique the available literature on this topic, thereby providing specific data that clinicians can generalize to LMS patients with metastases. We identified only two studies comparing the survival outcomes between patients who did, versus who did not undergo metastasectomy, which suggested an improved survival associated with surgery. In the absence of randomized studies, it is impossible to determine whether these findings are due to careful patient selection and favorable biology rather than a surgical advantage, as limited data was included in the publications about patient selection. However, most metastatic LMS are caused by high-grade tumors that are not indolent in their clinical behavior, and patients with metastatic LMS often have a poor prognosis without treatment.

Among patients undergoing metastasectomy for LMS, we found a pooled five-year overall survival of 31% (95% CI 18–44%) and a median overall survival of 59.6 months (95% CI 33.3 to 66.0). Before our study, the survival outcomes of patients undergoing metastasectomy for LMS were derived from large retrospective cohort studies with diverse histologies and were mostly limited to lung metastasectomy [27,48,49]. In these studies, the five-year overall survival post-lung metastasectomy ranged between 34 and 40%, with a median overall survival of 33 months. Compared to other histologic types of STSs, lung metastasectomy for LMS is suggested to be associated with a more favorable prognosis, and our results confirm this [27]. We estimated the pooled five-year overall survival among patients undergoing lung metastasectomy was 53% (95% CI 39–67%) and the median overall was 72.8 months (95% CI 63.0 to 82.5). Considerably less evidence exists describing the outcomes of patients undergoing metastasectomy for LMS at other sites. Our results suggest that patients with liver metastasectomy may also experience acceptable survival post-metastasectomy. In contrast, spine and brain metastasectomy may be more appropriately considered in palliative situations to improve quality of life.

We aimed to identify criteria that could be used to guide clinicians in the selection of patients with LMS appropriate for metastasectomy. The criteria used to select patients and the intent of metastasectomy were not uniformly reported by all studies. It was often not detailed enough to be used or replicated in clinical practice when reported. For example, the authors most commonly described selecting patients for metastasectomy if they had a long DFI, limited sites of metastatic disease, and demonstrated disease stability on chemotherapy. Additional considerations were noted to guide the selection of patients undergoing spine and brain metastasectomy, including their estimated prognosis, current performance status, and symptom burden. However, the specific details of how these criteria were evaluated or defined were not available, limiting the ability of clinicians to use these meaningfully in their clinical practice.

We identified that some patients undergoing liver (13, 34%), spine (1, 10%), and brain (2, 40%) metastasectomy had synchronous disease compared to none undergoing lung metastasectomy. In addition, patients undergoing liver (DFI range 16–50 months) and brain (DFI range 9–89 months) metastasectomy had a shorter median DFI compared to those undergoing lung (DFI range 26–48 months) and spine (DFI range 32–50 months) metastasectomies. Patients with brain and spine metastases are more prone to experience symptoms that impair their quality of life and could be eased by metastasectomy. For these reasons, patients with unfavorable prognostic characteristics, such as a short DFI and a synchronous presentation, may be more likely to be evaluated for metastasectomy if the treatment can improve their quality of life. However, it is unclear why there are more patients with synchronous disease and a shorter DFI undergoing liver compared to lung metastasectomies. It may be to decrease the systemic tumor burden, which may be associated with improved survival when resection of the primary tumor site is also performed. This difference in patient characteristics for those undergoing liver versus lung metastasectomy may partly explain why patients with lung metastasectomy had the most prolonged survival on pooled analysis. Developing more rigorous criteria for selecting patients who can benefit from metastasectomy is a priority for future research.

We found that few prognostic factors were evaluated quantitatively. Metachronous disease, a longer DFI, and R0 metastasectomy were favorable prognostic factors among lung and liver metastasectomy patients. The study by Paramanathan et al. was the only one to define a long DFI (i.e., 36 months) based on the International Registry of Lung Metastases prognostic group [23]. Patients undergoing lung metastasectomy were less likely to have additional sites of metastases compared to those undergoing liver metastasectomy. Interestingly, patients undergoing liver metastasectomy with extrahepatic disease who achieved complete resection of all disease had comparable survival to those without extrahepatic disease. This is an important finding, as patients with multiple sites of metastatic disease are often less likely to be considered for metastasectomy. For patients undergoing spine metastasectomy, post-metastasectomy performance status was the only significant prognostic factor. This has limited clinical utility as it is often difficult to predict how patients will respond to surgery. Additional research is required to determine which patients should be selected and who are most likely to benefit from metastasectomy.

We found that perioperative systemic and radiotherapy were infrequently utilized among patients undergoing metastasectomy for LMS. There is currently no evidence to support these treatment modalities in the perioperative metastatic setting. On the other hand, in the context of unresectable, metastatic STS, there is evidence to support cytotoxic chemotherapy. Anthracyclines, with or without ifosfamide, are regarded as an acceptable first-line treatment in this setting [50–53]. Many of the patients included in this systematic review were treated when our understanding of the various histologic types of STS was limited and before the practice of histology-driven treatment [10,53,54]. LMS has moderate sensitivity to ifosfamide-based regimens. As single therapies, doxorubicin and ifosfamide have demonstrated response rates of between 10% and 25% in LMS [10]. Dacarbazine had an overall response rate of 16% as a single agent, and retrospective data indicate overall response rates of nearly 37% when used in combination with doxorubicin [55,56]. In addition, gemcitabine and docetaxel also have demonstrated activity in LMS and this combination is used as a first-line therapy in the metastatic setting in some jurisdictions [57,58]. Newer treatments, including trabectedin, pazopanib and eribulin, have shown promising results in metastatic, unresectable LMS in later line settings [59–71]. It is imperative to evaluate the role of metastasectomy in the era of these modern systemic therapy regimens, even for all STS. Furthermore, because the majority of patients undergoing metastasectomy for LMS experience disease recurrence within a short interval, it is imperative to apply new treatment modalities for these metastases.

There is increasing evidence to support the feasibility and effectiveness of local interventional treatments, such as radiofrequency ablation, cryoablation, and stereotactic body radiation therapy [72–76]. Hepatic artery embolization with or without chemotherapy and radioembolization are further interventional treatments for liver metastases that can now be used in conjunction with other treatments. None of the studies included in this systematic review compared these local treatments to metastasectomy. As with many other rare diseases, retrospective data constitute the strongest available evidence, and decision-making around the management of these complex patients should be based on patient preferences in the context of multidisciplinary management.

Despite the promising survival outcomes, our results show that patients undergoing metastasectomy for LMS experienced high recurrence rates. For example, the five-year disease-free survival of patients undergoing lung metastasectomy was 9%, and the median disease-free survival was reported to be between 6 and 40 months. The five-year disease-free survival of patients undergoing liver metastasectomy was 22%, with a median disease-free survival between 13 and 16 months. The disease-free survival was not reported for patients undergoing spine and brain metastasectomies. Some patients who experienced recurrences underwent additional metastasectomies; this was performed for patients with lung, liver, and spine metastases. Currently, repeat metastasectomy is most well described and accepted for patients with lung metastases from various STS histologies, with the median overall survival after repeat metastasectomy reported to range between 25 and 65 months [77–80]. Prognostic factors associated with an improved median overall survival after repeat lung metastasectomy in these studies include achieving R0 margins, low-grade tumors, one or two sites of metastatic nodules, and the largest size of metastases less than 2 cm. Our results suggest that repeat liver metastasectomy results in comparable survival to repeat lung metastasectomy, and repeat spine metastasectomy may be warranted to improve symptoms [22]. Additional information on the criteria used to select patients for repeat metastasectomy and more data on survival outcomes are required to understand the feasibility.

Limitations

Limitations of the evidence in this review include the retrospective nature of the existing case series and cohort studies. These non-randomized studies introduce potential biases due to careful patient selection. Most of the survival outcomes reported were not stratified or adjusted based on important prognostic factors. Given the small sample size of many included, it is unlikely such a stratified analysis would have been possible. Being limited to small study samples also increases the risk of the "small-study effects," where smaller studies are more likely to be published if they report larger or more significant effects [81]. This is particularly important if unadjusted or unstratified estimates are reported. Another important limitation is that some studies included patients before the widespread use of the c-kit receptor for differentiation of gastrointestinal stromal tumors (GIST) versus LMS, which can otherwise have similarities on histopathology [82,83]. This is important as the outcomes for patients with GISTs are much better compared to LMS, which may have biased the results, particularly for the cohort of LMS arising from the gastrointestinal tract undergoing liver metastasectomy, as this is commonly the presentation of GISTs [84].

5. Conclusions

Surgery is currently being utilized to manage LMS metastases to the lung, liver, spine, and brain. Although low quality, comparative studies support a survival benefit, but patient selection and tumor biology are likely to have influenced these results. Recommendations regarding which patients should be considered for metastasectomy are limited by the variability in the criteria used to select patients for metastasectomy across studies and the sites of metastases. The majority of patients undergoing metastasectomy experience disease recurrence within a short interval. Additional research is required to establish the role of metastasectomy in the era of modern systemic therapy regimens and local ablative techniques. Leveraging international collaborations and registry data is one way to move forward with more robust and nuanced patient assessments in this rare disease [85].

Supplementary Materials: The following supporting information can be downloaded at: https://www.mdpi.com/article/10.3390/cancers14133055/s1, Figure S1: PRISMA Flow Diagram, Table S1: Total Patients Included in Each Study, Table S2: Post-Metastasectomy LMS-Specific Outcomes, Table S3: JBI Critical Appraisal Checklist for Case Series, Table S4: NOS for Cohort Studies, Table S5:

Components of GRADE (Grading of Recommendation, Assessment, Development and Evaluation) to Assess the Certainty of Evidence.

Author Contributions: Conceptualization, M.D., Y.W., D.S. and A.S.; methodology, M.D., Y.W., D.S. and A.S.; validation, M.D., B.A., K.N. and A.S.; formal analysis, M.D., K.N. and B.A.; resources, Y.W. and A.S.; data curation, M.D., B.A., K.N. and A.S.; writing—original draft preparation, M.D.; writing—review and editing, M.D., B.A. and A.S.; visualization, M.D., B.A., K.N. and A.S.; supervision, Y.W. and A.S.; project administration, M.D., Y.W. and A.S. All authors have read and agreed to the published version of the manuscript.

Funding: This research received no external funding.

Institutional Review Board Statement: Not applicable.

Informed Consent Statement: Not applicable.

Data Availability Statement: Data sharing is not applicable to this article as no new data were created or analyzed in this study.

Acknowledgments: The authors would like to acknowledge Ranjeeta Mallick and the Ottawa Methods Center for the expert advice regarding the statistical analysis. The researchers would like to thank the Deanship of Scientific Research, Qassim University for funding the publication of this project.

Conflicts of Interest: The authors declare no conflict of interest.

Abbreviations

ASPS	Alveolar soft part sarcoma
CI	Confidence interval
CSS	Cancer specific survival
DFI	Disease free interval
ECOG	Eastern Cooperative Oncology Group
GI	Gastrointestinal
GIST	Gastrointestinal stromal tumor
GTR	Gross total removal
GU	Genitourinary
IQR	Interquartile range
JBI	Joanna Briggs Institute
LMS	Leiomyosarcoma
LPS	Liposarcoma
MFH	Malignant fibrous histiocytoma
MPNST	Malignant peripheral nerve sheath tumor
NOS	Newcastle-Ottawa Quality Assessment Scale
NR	Not reported
OS	Overall survival
RMS	Rhabdomyosarcoma
SD	Standard deviation
SFT	Solitary fibrous tumor
SS	Synovial sarcoma
STR	Subtotal removal
STS	Soft tissue sarcoma
UPS	Undifferentiated pleomorphic sarcoma
WBRT	Whole brain radiation therapy

References

1. George, S.; Serrano, C.; Hensley, M.L.; Ray-Coquard, I. Soft Tissue and Uterine Leiomyosarcoma. *J. Clin. Oncol.* **2017**, *36*, 144–150. [CrossRef] [PubMed]
2. Bathan, A.J.; Constantinidou, A.; Pollack, S.M.; Jones, R.L. Diagnosis, Prognosis, and Management of Leiomyosarcoma: Recognition of Anatomic Variants. *Curr. Opin. Oncol.* **2013**, *25*, 384–389. [CrossRef] [PubMed]
3. Goldblum, J.; Volpe, A.; Weiss, S. Leiomyosarcoma. In *Enzinger & Weiss's Soft Tissue Tumors*; Goldblum, J., Folpe, A., Weiss, S., Eds.; Elsevier: Philadelphia, PA, USA, 2020; pp. 591–613.

4. Brennan, M.F.; Antonescu, C.R.; Moraco, N.; Singer, S. Lessons Learned from the Study of 10,000 Patients with Soft Tissue Sarcoma. *Ann. Surg.* **2014**, *260*, 416–422. [CrossRef] [PubMed]
5. Yadav, U.; Mangla, A. Leiomyosarcoma. Available online: https://www.ncbi.nlm.nih.gov/books/NBK551667/ (accessed on 19 February 2022).
6. Pisters, P.W.; Leung, D.H.; Woodruff, J.; Shi, W.; Brennan, M.F. Analysis of Prognostic Factors in 1,041 Patients with Localized Soft Tissue Sarcomas of the Extremities. *J. Clin. Oncol.* **1996**, *14*, 1679–1689. [CrossRef]
7. Gronchi, A.; Strauss, D.C.; Miceli, R.; Bonvalot, S.; Swallow, C.J.; Hohenberger, P.; van Coevorden, F.; Rutkowski, P.; Callegaro, D.; Hayes, A.J.; et al. Variability in Patterns of Recurrence after Resection of Primary Retroperitoneal Sarcoma (RPS). A Report on 1007 Patients from the Multi-Institutional Collaborative RPS Working Group. *Ann. Surg.* **2016**, *263*, 1002–1009. [CrossRef]
8. Yang, J.C.; Chang, A.E.; Baker, A.R.; Sindelar, W.F.; Danforth, D.N.; Topalian, S.L.; DeLaney, T.; Glatstein, E.; Steinberg, S.M.; Merino, M.J.; et al. Randomized Prospective Study of the Benefit of Adjuvant Radiation Therapy in the Treatment of Soft Tissue Sarcomas of the Extremity. *J. Clin. Oncol.* **1998**, *16*, 197–203. [CrossRef]
9. Bonvalot, S.; Gronchi, A.; le Péchoux, C.; Swallow, C.J.; Strauss, D.; Meeus, P.; van Coevorden, F.; Stoldt, S.; Stoeckle, E.; Rutkowski, P.; et al. Preoperative Radiotherapy plus Surgery versus Surgery Alone for Patients with Primary Retroperitoneal Sarcoma (EORTC-62092: STRASS): A Multicentre, Open-Label, Randomised, Phase 3 Trial. *Lancet Oncol.* **2020**, *21*, 1366–1377. [CrossRef]
10. Gamboa, A.C.; Gronchi, A.; Cardona, K. Soft-tissue Sarcoma in Adults: An Update on the Current State of Histiotype-specific Management in an Era of Personalized Medicine. *CA Cancer J. Clin.* **2020**, *70*, 200–229. [CrossRef]
11. Van Cann, T.; Cornillie, J.; Wozniak, A.; Debiec-Rychter, M.; Sciot, R.; Hompes, D.; Vergote, I.; Schöffski, P. Retrospective Analysis of Outcome of Patients with Metastatic Leiomyosarcoma in a Tertiary Referral Center. *Oncol. Res. Treat.* **2018**, *41*, 206–213. [CrossRef]
12. Tirotta, F.; Hodson, J.; Parente, A.; Pasquali, S.; Sutcliffe, R.; Desai, A.; Muiesan, P.; Ford, S.J.; Fiore, M.; Gronchi, A.; et al. Liver Resection for Sarcoma Metastases: A Systematic Review and Experience from Two European Centres. *Eur. J. Surg. Oncol.* **2020**, *46*, 1807–1813. [CrossRef]
13. Deguchi, S.; Nakasu, Y.; Sakaida, T.; Akimoto, J.; Tanahashi, K.; Natsume, A.; Takahashi, M.; Okuda, T.; Asakura, H.; Mitsuya, K.; et al. Surgical Outcome and Graded Prognostic Assessment of Patients with Brain Metastasis from Adult Sarcoma: Multi-Institutional Retrospective Study in Japan. *Int. J. Clin. Oncol.* **2020**, *25*, 1995–2005. [CrossRef] [PubMed]
14. Rao, G.; Suki, D.; Chakrabarti, I.; Feiz-Erfan, I.; Mody, M.G.; McCutcheon, I.E.; Gokaslan, Z.; Patel, S.; Rhines, L.D. Surgical Management of Primary and Metastatic Sarcoma of the Mobile Spine. *J. Neurosurg. Spine* **2008**, *9*, 120–128. [CrossRef] [PubMed]
15. Wang, Y.; Delisle, M.; Smith, D.; Srikanthan, A. Survival by Histology among Patients with Bone and Soft Tissue Sarcoma Who Undergo Metastasectomy: Protocol for a Systematic Review and Meta-Analysis. *Syst. Rev.* **2020**, *9*, 189. [CrossRef]
16. Page, M.J.; McKenzie, J.E.; Bossuyt, P.M.; Boutron, I.; Hoffmann, T.C.; Mulrow, C.D.; Shamseer, L.; Tetzlaff, J.M.; Akl, E.A.; Brennan, S.E.; et al. The PRISMA 2020 Statement: An Updated Guideline for Reporting Systematic Reviews. *BMJ* **2021**, *372*, n160. [CrossRef] [PubMed]
17. Burt, B.M.; Ocejo, S.; Mery, C.M.; Dasilva, M.; Bueno, R.; Sugarbaker, D.J.; Jaklitsch, M.T. Repeated and Aggressive Pulmonary Resections for Leiomyosarcoma Metastases Extends Survival. *Ann. Thorac. Surg.* **2011**, *92*, 1202–1207. [CrossRef] [PubMed]
18. Chen, H. Complete Hepatic Resection of Metastases from Leiomyosarcoma Prolongs Survival. *J. Gastrointest. Surg.* **1998**, *2*, 151–155. [CrossRef]
19. Faraj, W.; El-Kehdy, J.; el Nounou, G.; Deeba, S.; Fakih, H.; Jabbour, M.; Haydar, A.; el Naaj, A.A.; Abou-Alfa, G.K.; O'Reilly, E.M.; et al. Liver Resection for Metastatic Colorectal Leiomyosarcoma: A Single Center Experience. *J. Gastrointest. Oncol.* **2015**, *6*, E70–E76. [CrossRef]
20. Kato, S.; Demura, S.; Shinmura, K.; Yokogawa, N.; Yonezawa, N.; Shimizu, T.; Oku, N.; Kitagawa, R.; Murakami, H.; Kawahara, N.; et al. Clinical Outcomes and Survivals after Total En Bloc Spondylectomy for Metastatic Leiomyosarcoma in the Spine. *Eur. Spine J.* **2020**, *29*, 3237–3244. [CrossRef]
21. Kim, Y.W.; Lee, J.H.; Kim, J.E.; Kang, J. Surgical Resection of Liver Metastasis of Leiomyosarcoma. *Korean J. Clin. Oncol.* **2017**, *13*, 143–146. [CrossRef]
22. Lang, H.; Nußbaum, K.-T.; Kaudel, P.; Frü Hauf, N.; Flemming, P.; Raab, R. Hepatic Metastases from Leiomyosarcoma A Single-Center Experience with 34 Liver Resections During a 15-Year Period. *Ann. Surg.* **2000**, *231*, 500–505. [CrossRef]
23. Paramanathan, A.; Wright, G. Pulmonary Metastasectomy for Sarcoma of Gynaecologic Origin. *Heart Lung Circ.* **2013**, *22*, 270–275. [CrossRef]
24. Ziewacz, J.E.; Lau, D.; la Marca, F.; Park, P. Outcomes after Surgery for Spinal Metastatic Leiomyosarcoma. *J. Neurosurg. Spine* **2012**, *17*, 432–437. [CrossRef] [PubMed]
25. Anraku, M.; Yokoi, K.; Nakagawa, K.; Fujisawa, T.; Nakajima, J.; Akiyama, H.; Nishimura, Y.; Kobayashi, K. Pulmonary Metastases from Uterine Malignancies: Results of Surgical Resection in 133 Patients. *J. Thorac. Cardiovasc. Surg.* **2004**, *127*, 1107–1112. [CrossRef] [PubMed]
26. Blackmon, S.H.; Shah, N.; Roth, J.A.; Correa, A.M.; Vaporciyan, A.A.; Rice, D.C.; Hofstetter, W.; Walsh, G.L.; Benjamin, R.; Pollock, R.; et al. Resection of Pulmonary and Extrapulmonary Sarcomatous Metastases Is Associated with Long-Term Survival. *Ann. Thorac. Surg.* **2009**, *88*, 877–885. [CrossRef] [PubMed]

27. Chudgar, N.P.; Brennan, M.F.; Munhoz, R.R.; Bucciarelli, P.R.; Tan, K.S.; D'Angelo, S.P.; Bains, M.S.; Bott, M.; Huang, J.; Park, B.J.; et al. Pulmonary Metastasectomy with Therapeutic Intent for Soft-Tissue Sarcoma. *J. Thorac. Cardiovasc. Surg.* **2017**, *154*, 319–330.e1. [CrossRef]
28. Ercolani, G.; Grazi, G.L.; Ravaioli, M.; Ramacciato, G.; Cescon, M.; Varotti, G.; del Gaudio, M.; Vetrone, G.; Pinna, A.D. The Role of Liver Resections for Noncolorectal, Nonneuroendocrine Metastases: Experience with 142 Observed Cases. *Ann. Surg. Oncol.* **2005**, *12*, 459–466. [CrossRef]
29. Goumard, C.; Marcal, L.P.; Wang, W.L.; Somaiah, N.; Okuno, M.; Roland, C.L.; Tzeng, C.W.D.; Chun, Y.S.; Feig, B.W.; Vauthey, J.N.; et al. Long-Term Survival According to Histology and Radiologic Response to Preoperative Chemotherapy in 126 Patients Undergoing Resection of Non-GIST Sarcoma Liver Metastases. *Ann. Surg. Oncol.* **2018**, *25*, 107–116. [CrossRef]
30. Liebl, L.S.; Elson, F.; Quaas, A.; Gawad, K.A.; Izbicki, J.R. Value of Repeat Resection for Survival in Pulmonary Metastases from Soft Tissue Sarcoma. *Anticancer Res.* **2007**, *27*, 2897–2902.
31. Lin, A.Y.; Kotova, S.; Yanagawa, J.; Elbuluk, O.; Wang, G.; Kar, N.; Elashoff, D.; Grogan, T.; Cameron, R.B.; Singh, A.; et al. Risk Stratification of Patients Undergoing Pulmonary Metastasectomy for Soft Tissue and Bone Sarcomas. *J. Thorac. Cardiovasc. Surg.* **2015**, *149*, 85–92. [CrossRef]
32. Marudanayagam, R.; Sandhu, B.; Perera, M.T.P.R.; Bramhall, S.R.; Mayer, D.; Buckels, J.A.C.; Mirza, D.F. Liver Resection for Metastatic Soft Tissue Sarcoma: An Analysis of Prognostic Factors. *Eur. J. Surg. Oncol.* **2010**, *37*, 87–92. [CrossRef]
33. Smith, R.; Pak, Y.; Kraybill, W.; Kane, J.M. Factors Associated with Actual Long-Term Survival Following Soft Tissue Sarcoma Pulmonary Metastasectomy. *Eur. J. Surg. Oncol.* **2009**, *35*, 356–361. [CrossRef] [PubMed]
34. Zacherl, M.; Bernhardt, G.A.; Zacherl, J.; Gruber, G.; Kornprat, P.; Bacher, H.; Mischinger, H.J.; Windhager, R.; Jakesz, R.; Grünberger, T. Surgery for Liver Metastases Originating from Sarcoma-Case Series. *Langenbeck's Arch. Surg.* **2011**, *396*, 1083–1091. [CrossRef]
35. Zhang, F.; Wang, J. Clinical Features of Surgical Resection for Liver Metastasis from Extremity Soft Tissue Sarcoma. *Hepatogastroenterology* **2015**, *62*, 677–682.
36. Farid, M.; Ong, W.S.; Tan, M.H.; Foo, L.S.S.; Lim, Y.K.; Chia, W.K.; Soh, L.T.; Poon, D.; Lee, M.J.F.; Ho, Z.C.; et al. The Influence of Primary Site on Outcomes in Leiomyosarcoma. *Am. J. Clin. Oncol.* **2013**, *36*, 368–374. [CrossRef] [PubMed]
37. Rohatgi, A. *WebPlotDigitizer*; Version 4.5; 2021.
38. Liu, N.; Zhou, Y.; Lee, J.J. IPDfromKM: Reconstruct Individual Patient Data from Published Kaplan-Meier Survival Curves. *BMC Med. Res. Methodol.* **2021**, *21*, 111. [CrossRef]
39. Hozo, S.P.; Djulbegovic, B.; Hozo, I. Estimating the Mean and Variance from the Median, Range, and the Size of a Sample. *BMC Med. Res. Methodol.* **2005**, *5*, 13. [CrossRef]
40. Deeks, J.; Higgins, J.; Altman, D. Random-Effects Methods for Meta-Analysis. In *Cochrane Handbook for Systematic Reviews of Interventions*; Thomas, J., Higgins, J., Eds.; Wiley-Blackwell: Chicester, UK, 2022.
41. Mathes, T.; Pieper, D. Study Design Classification of Registry-Based Studies in Systematic Reviews. *J. Clin. Epidemiol.* **2018**, *93*, 84–87. [CrossRef] [PubMed]
42. Moola, S.; Munn, Z.; Tufanaru, C.; Aromataris, E.; Sears, K.; Sfetcu, R.; Currie, M.; Qureshi, R.; Mattis, P.; Lisy, K.; et al. Systematic Reviews of Etiology and Risk. In *Joanna Briggs Institute Reviewer's Manual*; Aromataris, E., Munn, Z., Eds.; 2017. Available online: https://synthesismanual.jbi.global (accessed on 20 February 2022).
43. The Newcastle-Ottawa Scale (NOS) for Assessing the Quality of Nonrandomised Studies in Meta-Analyses. Available online: http://www.ohri.ca/programs/clinical_epidemiology/oxford.asp (accessed on 20 February 2022).
44. Ma, L.-L.; Wang, Y.-Y.; Yang, Z.-H.; Huang, D.; Weng, H.; Zeng, X.-T. Methodological Quality (Risk of Bias) Assessment Tools for Primary and Secondary Medical Studies: What Are They and Which Is Better? *Mil. Med. Res.* **2020**, *7*, 7. [CrossRef]
45. Santesso, N.; Glenton, C.; Dahm, P.; Garner, P.; Akl, E.A.; Alper, B.; Brignardello-Petersen, R.; Carrasco-Labra, A.; de Beer, H.; Hultcrantz, M.; et al. GRADE Guidelines 26: Informative Statements to Communicate the Findings of Systematic Reviews of Interventions. *J. Clin. Epidemiol.* **2020**, *119*, 126–135. [CrossRef]
46. Murad, M.H.; Mustafa, R.A.; Schünemann, H.J.; Sultan, S.; Santesso, N. Rating the Certainty in Evidence in the Absence of a Single Estimate of Effect. *Evid.-Based Med.* **2017**, *22*, 85–87. [CrossRef]
47. Pastorino, U.; Buyse, M.; Friedel, S.G.; Ginsberg, R.J.; Girard, P.; Goldstraw, P.; Johnston, M.; Mccormack, P.; Pass, H.; Putnam, J.B. Long-Term Results of Lung Metastasectomy: Prognostic Analyses Based on 5206 Cases. *J. Thorac. Cardiovasc. Surg.* **1997**, *113*, 37–49. [CrossRef]
48. Van Geel, A.N.; Pastorino, U.; Jauch, K.; Judson, I.R.; van Coevorden, F.; Buesa, J.M.; Niesien, S.; Boudinet, A.; Tursz, T.; Schmitz, P.I.M.; et al. Surgical Treatment of Lung Metastases the European Organization for Research and Treatment of Cancer-Soft Tissue and Bone Sarcoma Group Study of 255 Patients. *Cancer* **1996**, *77*, 675–682. [CrossRef]
49. Choong, P.F.M.; Pritchard, D.J.; Rock, M.G.; Sim, F.H.; Frassica, F.J. Survival after Pulmonary Metastasectomy in Soft Tissue Sarcoma: Prognostic Factors in 214 Patients. *Acta Orthop. Scand.* **1995**, *66*, 561–568. [CrossRef]
50. Maurel, J.; López-Pousa, A.; de Las Peñas, R.; Fra, J.; Martín, J.; Cruz, J.; Casado, A.; Poveda, A.; Martínez-Trufero, J.; Balañá, C.; et al. Efficacy of Sequential High-Dose Doxorubicin and Ifosfamide Compared with Standard-Dose Doxorubicin in Patients with Advanced Soft Tissue Sarcoma: An Open-Label Randomized Phase II Study of the Spanish Group for Research on Sarcomas. *J. Clin. Oncol.* **2009**, *27*, 1893–1898. [CrossRef] [PubMed]

51. Tap, W.D.; Papai, Z.; van Tine, B.A.; Attia, S.; Ganjoo, K.N.; Jones, R.L.; Schuetze, S.; Reed, D.; Chawla, S.P.; Riedel, R.F.; et al. Doxorubicin plus Evofosfamide versus Doxorubicin Alone in Locally Advanced, Unresectable or Metastatic Soft-Tissue Sarcoma (TH CR-406/SARC021): An International, Multicentre, Open-Label, Randomised Phase 3 Trial. *Lancet Oncol.* **2017**, *18*, 1089–1103. [CrossRef]
52. Judson, I.; Verweij, J.; Gelderblom, H.; Hartmann, J.T.; Schöffski, P.; Blay, J.-Y.; Kerst, J.M.; Sufliarsky, J.; Whelan, J.; Hohenberger, P.; et al. Doxorubicin Alone versus Intensified Doxorubicin plus Ifosfamide for First-Line Treatment of Advanced or Metastatic Soft-Tissue Sarcoma: A Randomised Controlled Phase 3 Trial. *Lancet Oncol.* **2014**, *15*, 415–423. [CrossRef]
53. Edmonson, J.H.; Ryan, L.M.; Blum, R.H.; Brooks, J.S.; Shiraki, M.; Frytak, S.; Parkinson, D.R. Randomized Comparison of Doxorubicin Alone versus Ifosfamide plus Doxorubicin or Mitomycin, Doxorubicin, and Cisplatin against Advanced Soft Tissue Sarcomas. *J. Clin. Oncol.* **1993**, *11*, 1269–1275. [CrossRef]
54. Oosten, A.W.; Seynaeve, C.; Schmitz, P.I.M.; den Bakker, M.A.; Verweij, J.; Sleijfer, S. Outcomes of First-Line Chemotherapy in Patients with Advanced or Metastatic Leiomyosarcoma of Uterine and Non-Uterine Origin. *Sarcoma* **2009**, *2009*, 348910. [CrossRef]
55. Talbot, S.M.; Keohan, M.L.; Hesdorffer, M.; Orrico, R.; Bagiella, E.; Troxel, A.B.; Taub, R.N. A Phase II Trial of Temozolomide in Patients with Unresectable or Metastatic Soft Tissue Sarcoma. *Cancer* **2003**, *98*, 1942–1946. [CrossRef]
56. D'Ambrosio, L.; Touati, N.; Blay, J.; Grignani, G.; Flippot, R.; Czarnecka, A.M.; Piperno-Neumann, S.; Martin-Broto, J.; Sanfilippo, R.; Katz, D.; et al. Doxorubicin plus Dacarbazine, Doxorubicin plus Ifosfamide, or Doxorubicin Alone as a First-line Treatment for Advanced Leiomyosarcoma: A Propensity Score Matching Analysis from the European Organization for Research and Treatment of Cancer Soft Tissue and Bone Sarcoma Group. *Cancer* **2020**, *126*, 2637–2647. [CrossRef]
57. Hensley, M.L.; Blessing, J.A.; Mannel, R.; Rose, P.G. Fixed-Dose Rate Gemcitabine plus Docetaxel as First-Line Therapy for Metastatic Uterine Leiomyosarcoma: A Gynecologic Oncology Group Phase II Trial. *Gynecol. Oncol.* **2008**, *109*, 329–334. [CrossRef] [PubMed]
58. Hensley, M.L.; Blessing, J.A.; DeGeest, K.; Abulafia, O.; Rose, P.G.; Homesley, H.D. Fixed-Dose Rate Gemcitabine plus Docetaxel as Second-Line Therapy for Metastatic Uterine Leiomyosarcoma: A Gynecologic Oncology Group Phase II Study. *Gynecol. Oncol.* **2008**, *109*, 323–328. [CrossRef] [PubMed]
59. Schöffski, P.; Chawla, S.; Maki, R.G.; Italiano, A.; Gelderblom, H.; Choy, E.; Grignani, G.; Camargo, V.; Bauer, S.; Rha, S.Y.; et al. Eribulin versus Dacarbazine in Previously Treated Patients with Advanced Liposarcoma or Leiomyosarcoma: A Randomised, Open-Label, Multicentre, Phase 3 Trial. *Lancet* **2016**, *387*, 1629–1637. [CrossRef]
60. Blay, J.-Y.; Schöffski, P.; Bauer, S.; Krarup-Hansen, A.; Benson, C.; D'Adamo, D.R.; Jia, Y.; Maki, R.G. Eribulin versus Dacarbazine in Patients with Leiomyosarcoma: Subgroup Analysis from a Phase 3, Open-Label, Randomised Study. *Br. J. Cancer* **2019**, *120*, 1026–1032. [CrossRef]
61. Hirbe, A.C.; Eulo, V.; Moon, C.I.; Luo, J.; Myles, S.; Seetharam, M.; Toeniskoetter, J.; Kershner, T.; Haarberg, S.; Agulnik, M.; et al. A Phase II Study of Pazopanib as Front-Line Therapy in Patients with Non-Resectable or Metastatic Soft-Tissue Sarcomas Who Are Not Candidates for Chemotherapy. *Eur. J. Cancer* **2020**, *137*, P1–P9. [CrossRef] [PubMed]
62. Grünwald, V.; Karch, A.; Schuler, M.; Schöffski, P.; Kopp, H.-G.; Bauer, S.; Kasper, B.; Lindner, L.H.; Chemnitz, J.-M.; Crysandt, M.; et al. Randomized Comparison of Pazopanib and Doxorubicin as First-Line Treatment in Patients with Metastatic Soft Tissue Sarcoma Age 60 Years or Older: Results of a German Intergroup Study. *J. Clin. Oncol.* **2020**, *38*, 3555–3564. [CrossRef] [PubMed]
63. Grosso, F.; D'Ambrosio, L.; Zucchetti, M.; Ibrahim, T.; Tamberi, S.; Matteo, C.; Rulli, E.; Comandini, D.; Palmerini, E.; Baldi, G.G.; et al. Pharmacokinetics, Safety, and Activity of Trabectedin as First-Line Treatment in Elderly Patients Who Are Affected by Advanced Sarcoma and Are Unfit to Receive Standard Chemotherapy: A Phase 2 Study (TR1US Study) from the Italian Sarcoma Group. *Cancer* **2020**, *126*, 4726–4734. [CrossRef]
64. Kawai, A.; Araki, N.; Sugiura, H.; Ueda, T.; Yonemoto, T.; Takahashi, M.; Morioka, H.; Hiraga, H.; Hiruma, T.; Kunisada, T.; et al. Trabectedin Monotherapy after Standard Chemotherapy versus Best Supportive Care in Patients with Advanced, Translocation-Related Sarcoma: A Randomised, Open-Label, Phase 2 Study. *Lancet Oncol.* **2015**, *16*, 406–416. [CrossRef]
65. Garcia-Carbonero, R.; Supko, J.G.; Maki, R.G.; Manola, J.; Ryan, D.P.; Harmon, D.; Puchalski, T.A.; Goss, G.; Seiden, M.V.; Waxman, A.; et al. Ecteinascidin-743 (ET-743) for Chemotherapy-Naive Patients with Advanced Soft Tissue Sarcomas: Multicenter Phase II and Pharmacokinetic Study. *J. Clin. Oncol.* **2005**, *23*, 5484–5492. [CrossRef]
66. Garcia-Carbonero, R.; Supko, J.G.; Manola, J.; Seiden, M.V.; Harmon, D.; Ryan, D.P.; Quigley, M.T.; Merriam, P.; Canniff, J.; Goss, G.; et al. Phase II and Pharmacokinetic Study of Ecteinascidin 743 in Patients with Progressive Sarcomas of Soft Tissues Refractory to Chemotherapy. *J. Clin. Oncol.* **2004**, *22*, 1480–1490. [CrossRef]
67. Le Cesne, A.; Blay, J.Y.; Judson, I.; van Oosterom, A.; Verweij, J.; Radford, J.; Lorigan, P.; Rodenhuis, S.; Ray-Coquard, I.; Bonvalot, S.; et al. Phase II Study of ET-743 in Advanced Soft Tissue Sarcomas: A European Organisation for the Research and Treatment of Cancer (EORTC) Soft Tissue and Bone Sarcoma Group Trial. *J. Clin. Oncol* **2005**, *23*, 576–584. [CrossRef] [PubMed]
68. Yovine, A.; Riofrio, M.; Blay, J.Y.; Brain, E.; Alexandre, J.; Kahatt, C.; Taamma, A.; Jimeno, J.; Martin, C.; Salhi, Y.; et al. Phase II Study of Ecteinascidin-743 in Advanced Pretreated Soft Tissue Sarcoma Patients. *J. Clin. Oncol.* **2004**, *22*, 890–899. [CrossRef] [PubMed]
69. Martin-Broto, J.; Pousa, A.L.; de Las Peñas, R.; García Del Muro, X.; Gutierrez, A.; Martinez-Trufero, J.; Cruz, J.; Alvarez, R.; Cubedo, R.; Redondo, A.; et al. Randomized Phase II Study of Trabectedin and Doxorubicin Compared with Doxorubicin Alone

as First-Line Treatment in Patients with Advanced Soft Tissue Sarcomas: A Spanish Group for Research on Sarcoma Study. *J. Clin. Oncol.* **2016**, *34*, 2294–2302. [CrossRef]
70. Patel, S.; von Mehren, M.; Reed, D.R.; Kaiser, P.; Charlson, J.; Ryan, C.W.; Rushing, D.; Livingston, M.; Singh, A.; Seth, R.; et al. Overall Survival and Histology-Specific Subgroup Analyses from a Phase 3, Randomized Controlled Study of Trabectedin or Dacarbazine in Patients with Advanced Liposarcoma or Leiomyosarcoma. *Cancer* **2019**, *125*, 2610–2620. [CrossRef] [PubMed]
71. Demetri, G.D.; von Mehren, M.; Jones, R.L.; Hensley, M.L.; Schuetze, S.M.; Staddon, A.; Milhem, M.; Elias, A.; Ganjoo, K.; Tawbi, H.; et al. Efficacy and Safety of Trabectedin or Dacarbazine for Metastatic Liposarcoma or Leiomyosarcoma After Failure of Conventional Chemotherapy: Results of a Phase III Randomized Multicenter Clinical Trial. *J. Clin. Oncol.* **2016**, *34*, 786–793. [CrossRef] [PubMed]
72. Jones, R.L.; McCall, J.; Adam, A.; O'Donnell, D.; Ashley, S.; Al-Muderis, O.; Thway, K.; Fisher, C.; Judson, I.R. Radiofrequency Ablation Is a Feasible Therapeutic Option in the Multi Modality Management of Sarcoma. *Eur. J. Surg. Oncol.* **2010**, *36*, 477–482. [CrossRef] [PubMed]
73. Berber, E.; Ari, E.; Herceg, N.; Siperstein, A. Laparoscopic Radiofrequency Thermal Ablation for Unusual Hepatic Tumors: Operative Indications and Outcomes. *Surg. Endosc.* **2005**, *19*, 1613–1617. [CrossRef]
74. Dhakal, S.; Corbin, K.S.; Milano, M.T.; Philip, A.; Sahasrabudhe, D.; Jones, C.; Constine, L.S. Stereotactic Body Radiotherapy for Pulmonary Metastases from Soft-Tissue Sarcomas: Excellent Local Lesion Control and Improved Patient Survival. *Int. J. Radiat. Oncol. Biol. Phys.* **2012**, *82*, 940–945. [CrossRef]
75. Navarria, P.; Ascolese, A.M.; Cozzi, L.; Tomatis, S.; D'Agostino, G.R.; de Rose, F.; de Sanctis, R.; Marrari, A.; Santoro, A.; Fogliata, A.; et al. Stereotactic Body Radiation Therapy for Lung Metastases from Soft Tissue Sarcoma. *Eur. J. Cancer* **2015**, *51*, 668–674. [CrossRef]
76. Nakamura, T.; Matsumine, A.; Yamakado, K.; Matsubara, T.; Takaki, H.; Nakatsuka, A.; Takeda, K.; Abo, D.; Shimizu, T.; Uchida, A. Lung Radiofrequency Ablation in Patients with Pulmonary Metastases from Musculoskeletal Sarcomas. *Cancer* **2009**, *115*, 3774–3781. [CrossRef]
77. Wigge, S.; Heißner, K.; Steger, V.; Ladurner, R.; Traub, F.; Sipos, B.; Bösmüller, H.; Kanz, L.; Mayer, F.; Kopp, H.-G. Impact of Surgery in Patients with Metastatic Soft Tissue Sarcoma: A Monocentric Retrospective Analysis. *J. Surg. Oncol.* **2018**, *118*, 167–176. [CrossRef] [PubMed]
78. Weiser, M.R.; Downey, R.J.; Leung, D.H.; Brennan, M.F. Repeat Resection of Pulmonary Metastases in Patients with Soft-Tissue Sarcoma. *J. Am. Coll. Surg.* **2000**, *191*, 184–190. [CrossRef]
79. Casson, A.G.; Putnam, J.B.; Natarajan, G.; Johnston, D.A.; Mountain, C.; McMurtrey, M.; Roth, J.A. Efficacy of Pulmonary Metastasectomy for Recurrent Soft Tissue Sarcoma. *J. Surg. Oncol.* **1991**, *47*, 1–4. [CrossRef] [PubMed]
80. Pogrebniak, H.W.; Roth, J.A.; Steinberg, S.M.; Rosenberg, S.A.; Pass, H.I. Reoperative Pulmonary Resection in Patients with Metastatic Soft Tissue Sarcoma. *Ann. Thorac. Surg.* **1991**, *52*, 197–203. [CrossRef]
81. Sterne, J.A.C.; Sutton, A.J.; Ioannidis, J.P.A.; Terrin, N.; Jones, D.R.; Lau, J.; Carpenter, J.; Rucker, G.; Harbord, R.M.; Schmid, C.H.; et al. Recommendations for Examining and Interpreting Funnel Plot Asymmetry in Meta-Analyses of Randomised Controlled Trials. *BMJ* **2011**, *343*, d4002. [CrossRef] [PubMed]
82. Hirota, S.; Isozaki, K.; Moriyama, Y.; Hashimoto, K.; Nishida, T.; Ishiguro, S.; Kawano, K.; Hanada, M.; Kurata, A.; Takeda, M.; et al. Gain-of-Function Mutations of c-*Kit* in Human Gastrointestinal Stromal Tumors. *Science* **1998**, *279*, 577–580. [CrossRef]
83. Newman, P.L.; Wadden, C.; Fletcher, C.D. Gastrointestinal Stromal Tumours: Correlation of Immunophenotype with Clinicopathological Features. *J. Pathol.* **1991**, *164*, 107–117. [CrossRef]
84. Van Glabbeke, M.; van Oosterom, A.T.; Oosterhuis, J.W.; Mouridsen, H.; Crowther, D.; Somers, R.; Verweij, J.; Santoro, A.; Buesa, J.; Tursz, T. Prognostic Factors for the Outcome of Chemotherapy in Advanced Soft Tissue Sarcoma: An Analysis of 2,185 Patients Treated with Anthracycline-Containing First-Line Regimens—A European Organization for Research and Treatment of Cancer Soft Tissue and Bone Sarcoma Group Study. *J. Clin. Oncol.* **1999**, *17*, 150–157. [CrossRef]
85. Van Houdt, W.J.; Raut, C.P.; Bonvalot, S.; Swallow, C.J.; Haas, R.; Gronchi, A. New Research Strategies in Retroperitoneal Sarcoma. The Case of TARPSWG, STRASS and RESAR: Making Progress through Collaboration. *Curr. Opin. Oncol.* **2019**, *31*, 310–316. [CrossRef]

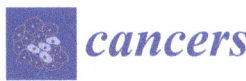

Systematic Review

Radiotherapy in the Management of Gastrointestinal Stromal Tumors: A Systematic Review

Haidong Zhang [1,†], Tianxiang Jiang [1,†], Mingchun Mu [1], Zhou Zhao [1], Xiaonan Yin [1], Zhaolun Cai [1], Bo Zhang [1,2,*] and Yuan Yin [1,*]

[1] Department of Gastrointestinal Surgery, West China Hospital, Sichuan University, Chengdu 610041, China; zhd3287332910@163.com (H.Z.); jiangtx98@163.com (T.J.); mmcmmcmmc163@163.com (M.M.); zhaozhou_med@163.com (Z.Z.); yxnyinxiaonan@163.com (X.Y.); caizhaolun@foxmail.com (Z.C.)

[2] Department of Gastrointestinal Surgery, Sanya People's Hospital, West China Sanya Hospital, Sichuan University, Sanya 572000, China

* Correspondence: zhangbo7310@126.com (B.Z.); yinyuan10@wchscu.cn (Y.Y.)

† These authors contributed equally to this work.

Simple Summary: Gastrointestinal stromal tumors are considered to be insensitive to radiotherapy. However, with the development of radiation techniques and the accumulation of cases, some studies have indicated that radiotherapy could help achieve objective response in advanced or metastatic gastrointestinal stromal tumors. Therefore, it is necessary to conduct a systematic review to reassess the role of radiotherapy in gastrointestinal stromal tumors. The purpose of this study was to draw the attention of scholars and clinicians to radiotherapy and promote further research on radiotherapy in gastrointestinal stromal tumors.

Abstract: Gastrointestinal stromal tumors (GISTs) are considered insensitive to radiotherapy. However, a growing number of case reports and case series have shown that some lesions treated by radiotherapy achieved an objective response. The aim of the study was to perform a systematic review of all reported cases, case series, and clinical studies of GISTs treated with radiotherapy to reevaluate the role of radiotherapy in GISTs. A systematic search of the English-written literature was conducted using PubMed, Web of Science, and Embase databases. Overall, 41 articles describing 112 patients were retrieved. The included articles were of low to moderate quality. Bone was the most common site treated by radiotherapy, followed by the abdomen. In order to exclude the influence of effective tyrosine kinase inhibitors (TKIs), a subgroup analysis was conducted on whether and which TKIs were concurrently applied with radiotherapy. Results showed that radiotherapy alone or combined with resistant TKIs could help achieve objective response in selected patients with advanced or metastatic GISTs; however, survival benefits were not observed in the included studies. Pain was the most common symptom in symptomatic GISTs, followed by neurological dysfunction and bleeding. The symptom palliation rate was 78.6% after excluding the influence of effective TKIs. The adverse reactions were mainly graded 1–2. Radiotherapy was generally well-tolerated. Overall, radiotherapy may relieve symptoms for GIST patients with advanced or metastatic lesions and even help achieve objective response in selected patients without significantly reducing the quality of life. In addition to bone metastases, fixed abdominal lesions may be treated by radiotherapy. Publication bias and insufficient quality of included studies were the main limitations in this review. Further clinical studies are needed and justified.

Keywords: gastrointestinal stromal tumor; GIST; management; radiotherapy; radiation therapy; symptom palliation; adverse events

Citation: Zhang, H.; Jiang, T.; Mu, M.; Zhao, Z.; Yin, X.; Cai, Z.; Zhang, B.; Yin, Y. Radiotherapy in the Management of Gastrointestinal Stromal Tumors: A Systematic Review. *Cancers* 2022, *14*, 3169. https://doi.org/10.3390/cancers14133169

Academic Editors: Shinji Miwa, Po-Kuei Wu and Hiroyuki Tsuchiya

Received: 31 May 2022
Accepted: 26 June 2022
Published: 28 June 2022

Publisher's Note: MDPI stays neutral with regard to jurisdictional claims in published maps and institutional affiliations.

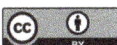

Copyright: © 2022 by the authors. Licensee MDPI, Basel, Switzerland. This article is an open access article distributed under the terms and conditions of the Creative Commons Attribution (CC BY) license (https://creativecommons.org/licenses/by/4.0/).

1. Introduction

Gastrointestinal stromal tumor (GIST) is the most common mesenchymal tumor in the gastrointestinal tract [1], with significant variations in reported incidence (from 0.4 to 2 cases per 100,000 per year [2,3]. The most common site of GISTs is the stomach, followed by the small intestine, which is now thought to originate from interstitial cells of Cajal (ICC) [4]. Functional mutations in the *KIT* gene and *PDGFRA* gene drive approximately 90% of GISTs [5]. At present, complete surgical resection is the standard treatment for locoregional lesions. Adjuvant 3-year imatinib therapy is given after surgery for GISTs, with significant recurrence risk. In contrast, the standard treatment for advanced, inoperable, and metastatic disease is tyrosine kinase inhibitors (TKIs) [2]. Although the use of molecularly targeted drugs such as imatinib significantly prolonged the overall survival of patients with GISTs [6,7], local treatment, such as surgery, radiofrequency ablation, and hepatic artery embolization, may be recommended for selected patients with advanced or metastatic GISTs [8]. In the past, GISTs were considered insensitive to radiotherapy [9], which is recommended for palliative intent in patients with advanced lesions or metastatic disease [2]. However, with the development of radiotherapy technology, some published cases and case series have shown that radiotherapy may be used for therapeutic purposes [10,11]. Radiotherapy is rarely used in GISTs, and the literature is limited to case reports and a few clinical studies with a limited number of cases. Therefore, a systematic review of the literature synthesizing these reports helps physicians by providing the best evidence for reassessing radiotherapy in the management of GISTs. The aim of the present study was to perform a systematic review of all reported radiation-treated cases.

2. Methods and Data Management

2.1. Protocol

This systematic review was reported according to the Preferred Reporting Items for Systematic Reviews and Meta-Analyses (PRISMA) checklist [12] (Table S1). This protocol was prospectively registered in the Open Science Framework Registry (https://osf.io/qba6j, accessed on 22 June 2022).

2.2. Study Design

A systematic review was performed that analyzed radiotherapy in the management of GISTs to answer the following question: "What is the potential value of radiotherapy in GISTs"?

2.3. Eligibility Criteria

2.3.1. Inclusion Criteria

Articles in which patients with confirmed GISTs were treated with radiotherapy combined with/without TKIs and/or surgery were included, irrespective of what type of treatment the patients previously had. Case series were defined as reports on treatment outcomes in more than 2 patients. In addition, at least one of the following was obtained from the included articles: (1) patient response to radiotherapy; (2) duration of disease control (time to progression, time to recurrence, and survival); (3) symptom palliation; (4) adverse events.

2.3.2. Exclusion Criteria

Studies written in non-English languages, cases with synchronous or heterochronous tumors, case series with other types of tumors and reviews, and unavailable full texts were excluded.

2.4. Information Sources and Search Strategy

A systematic review of the English-written literature was conducted using PubMed, Web of Science, and Embase databases, with individual search strategies for each database.

A comprehensive search was undertaken to retrieve original studies using the keywords gastrointestinal stromal tumor, GIST, radiotherapy, and their variations. No time limit was imposed on publication dates. The last search was performed on 18 May 2022. The reference lists of all relevant articles were scanned to identify any possible related studies to be included [13].

2.5. Study Selection

The selection was completed in two phases. In phase one, all retrieved abstracts were screened by two authors (H.Z. and T.J.). For each one that met the inclusion criteria, the full text was obtained. In phase two, full-text reading was performed independently by the same two authors. They had discussions to reach a consensus when disagreements arose. When a consensus was not reached, a third author (Y.Y.) was involved in making a final decision.

2.6. Methodological Quality Assessment of Included Studies

The Joanna Briggs Institute (JBI) Critical Appraisal Checklist for Case Reports and Case series and the CARE Checklist were adapted and applied for the methodological quality assessment [14,15]. Regarding JBI quality appraisal, two reviewers (H.Z. and T.J.) scored 9 items, including whether to report according to the CARE Checklist, as "yes", "no", "unclear", and "not applicable" for case reports, and 10 items for case series. Any disagreement was resolved by consensus or the decision of a third author (Y.Y.). The quality evaluation results were divided into three grades: low, moderate, and high. In case reports, we attached more importance to the details of diagnosis, treatment procedures, and effects. Therefore, "low quality" was defined as not all of items 4, 5, and 6 receiving a "yes" response. "Moderate quality" was defined as all items 4, 5, and 6 receiving "yes" while not all other nine items receiving a "yes" score. "High quality" was defined as all nine items receiving "yes". For item 1, we gave "yes" to case reports in which the age and sex could at least be obtained. In addition, the histological results—namely, immunohistochemical analysis for item 4; radiation dose and fractions for item 5; and symptom palliation, response to radiotherapy, or recurrence for item 6—could also at least be retrieved. In addition, in case series, we attached more importance to inclusion criteria, diagnosis, consistent inclusion, treatment procedure, and outcomes or follow-up. Therefore, "low quality" was defined as not all items 1, 3, 4, 7, and 8 receiving a "yes" response. "Moderate quality" was defined as all items 1, 3, 4, 7, and 8 receiving a "yes" score while not 10 items receiving "yes". "High quality" was defined as all 10 items receiving a "yes" response (Table S2).

2.7. Data Collection Process and Data Items

Age, sex, sites treated by radiotherapy, dose and fractions, previous and concomitant TKIs, symptom palliation, adverse events, disease response, time to progression, time to recurrence, and survival time were recorded by one author (H.Z.). A second author (T.J.) cross-checked all the collected information. Again, any disagreement was resolved by consensus or the decision of a third author (Y.Y.). The results of response to radiotherapy and recurrence should be supported by objective images (pre- and post-treatment images) or based on definite criteria that were presented in articles. Regarding response, we defined articles in which definite criteria and objective images were not presented as "not available". When the authors evaluated a response according to specific criteria or images presented in studies, we accepted it. When the articles presented images and did not evaluate responses to radiotherapy, we evaluated the responses based on the images according to Response Evaluation Criteria in Solid Tumors (RECIST criteria).

2.8. Outcomes of Interest

The included studies were synthesized in qualitative and quantitative descriptions. Response and symptom palliation after radiotherapy were the primary outcomes. In addition, we defined the initiation of radiotherapy as the starting point for follow-up. Overall survival (OS) was calculated from the date of radiotherapy initiation to the date of death. Time to progression and recurrence were calculated from radiotherapy initiation to progression and recurrence, respectively. Local progression and recurrence were defined as any clinical or radiographic evidence of tumor growth. Local progression-free survival (PFS), local recurrence-free survival (RFS), and OS were estimated using the Kaplan–Meier method. OS, PFS, RFS, and adverse events related to radiotherapy were the secondary outcomes.

3. Results

3.1. Study Selection

Finally, 412 studies were retrieved from the 3 electronic databases, and 2 were obtained from reference lists. Then, duplicate articles were removed, resulting in 315 remaining studies. Then, a comprehensive evaluation of the abstracts was conducted, and 265 articles were excluded. Therefore, 50 manuscripts were selected for full-text review. Later, four case reports were excluded due to reporting GISTs with synchronous or heterochronous tumors, and five case series were excluded due to reporting GISTs with other types of tumors. There were a total of 41 retrieved articles describing 112 patients [10,11,16–54] for qualitative analysis (Figure 1). Among them, 35 articles were case reports (Table 1), and 6 were case series (Table 2). According to the quality assessment, there were 20 low-quality and 15 moderate-quality case reports. There were five low-quality and one moderate-quality case series. There were no high-quality studies in either case reports or case series (Table S2). These patients consisted of 36 females (32.1%) and 76 males (67.9%), with ages ranging from 19.7 to 86.5 years.

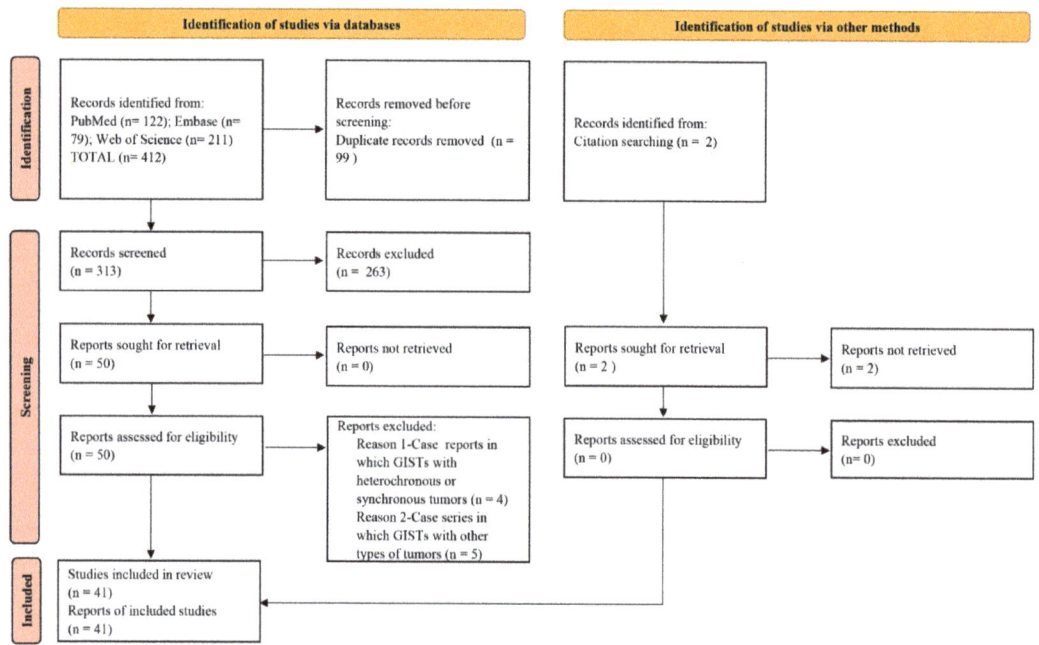

Figure 1. Flow diagram of the literature search and selection criteria.

Table 1. Description of the cases treated by radiotherapy.

References	Age/Gender	Location	Previous TKIs	Means/Total Dose*Fractions #	Concomitant TKIs	Palliation	Response	Side Effects	Follow-Up (Recurrence or Progression/TTR or TTP (mo)/A or D/OS (mo)
Shioyama et al., 2001 [50]	75/female	retroperitoneum	None	R + C + I/51Gy*34	None	Yes	PR	NA	No/72/A/72
Pollock et al., 2001 [25]	77/female	rectum	None	S + R/50.4Gy*NA	None	Yes	-	desquamation of perineum/grade 2	No/18/A/18
Akiyama et al., 2004 [37]	60/male	around the left optic nerve	None	R/54Gy*18	None	Yes	NA	NA	NA/NA/D/4.5
Puri et al., 2006 [44]	42/male	right parietal lobe	None	S + R + C/60Gy*NA	None	Yes	-	NA	No/20/D/20
Boruban et al., 2007 [23]	55/male	pelvic	None	S(I) + R + T/54Gy*27	imatinib	Yes	CR	NA	No/37/A/37
Barrière et al., 2009 [41]	57/male	clivus/lumbar spine	imatinib/sunitinib (R)	R + T/NA	sunitinib/nilotinib	No	NA	NA	NA/NA/D/5
Ciresa et al., 2009 [52]	54/male	rectum	None	R + T/37.8Gy*21	imatinib	Yes	PR	neutropenia/grade 3/proctitis/grade 2	NA/NA/NA/NA
Hamada et al., 2010 [27]	54/female	left frontal lobe	imatinib(W)	S + R/NA	None	NA	-	NA	No/6/A/6
Tezcan et al., 2011 [30]	83/male	right femur head	None	R + T/30Gy*10	imatinib	Yes	NA	NA	NA/NA/A/NA
Knowlton et al., 2011 [16]	37/male	stomach	None	S + R/36Gy*24	None	Yes	-	No	No/240/D/240
Naoe et al., 2011 [19]	77/female	right cerebral peduncle/left occipital lobe	None	R + T/NA/S + R + T/NA	Imatinib (I)	NA	NA/-	NA	No/2/D/2
Lolli et al., 2011 [10]	48/female	left supraclavicular	imatinib/sunitinib/nilotinib/sorafenib (R)	R + T/50Gy*25	sorafenib	Yes	SD	well tolerated	No/NA/A/NA
Di Scioscio et al., 2011 [29]	62/male	spine	None	R + T/30Gy*NA	imatinib	Yes	NA	NA	Yes/24/D/34
Abuzakhm et al., 2011 [34]	57/female	left humerus	imatinib/sunitinib (R)	R + T/NA	sunitinib	NA	NA	NA	NA/NA/A/NA
Wong et al., 2011 [38]	26/male	left frontal temporal	imatinib/sunitinib (R)	S + R/NA	None	Yes	-	NA	No/4/A/4
Slimack et al., 2012 [36]	37/male	spine	imatinib (R)	S + R + C/NA	None	Yes	-	NA	No/24/A/24

Table 1. Cont.

References	Age/Gender	Location	Previous TKIs	Means/Total Dose*Fractions #	Concomitant TKIs	Palliation	Response	Side Effects	Follow-Up (Recurrence or Progression/TTR or TTP (mo)/A or D/OS (mo)
Halpern et al., 2012 [28]	62/male	right upper quadrant/retroperitoneum	imatinib (I)	R/63.4Gy*NA	None	Yes	PR	well tolerated	No/3/A/3
Feki et al., 2012 [35]	58/male	sternoclavicular joint	None	R + T/30Gy*NA	imatinib	Yes	PR	NA	No/10/A/19
Drazin et al., 2013 [39]	60/male	left frontal lobe/left cerebellum	None	R/18Gy*1/S + R/NA	None	Yes	NA/-	NA	No/15/A/15
Takeuchi et al., 2014 [26]	74/male	right lateral ventricle	imatinib/sunitinib (R)	R + T/NA	sunitinib	-	CR	NA	No/4/A/4
Sato et al., 2014 [40]	80/male	vermis	None	S + R/22Gy*11	None	Yes	-	NA	Yes/1/D/3
Aktan et al., 2015 [31]	56/male	right femur/L1–3 vertebrae	Imatinib (R)	R + T/30Gy*10	imatinib	Yes	NA	NA	NA/NA/D/2
	70/male	L2 vertebra	Imatinib (R)	R + T/30Gy*NA	imatinib	Yes	NA	NA	NA/NA/D/1.5
Gupta et al., 2016 [24]	64/female	right frontal skull	Imatinib (R)	S + R + T/35Gy*14	imatinib/sunitinib	Yes	-	NA	Yes/21/A/24
Gatto et al., 2017 [22]	62/male	paracaval lesion	imatinib/sunitinib (R)	R + T/35Gy*14	regorafenib	Yes	PR	No	No/36/A/36
	44/male	pararenal/supraclavicular	imatinib/sunitinib (R)	R/85Gy*9/R + T/32Gy*5	sunitinib	Yes	SD	nausea/NA	No/5/A/5
Loaiza-Bonilla et al., 2017 [46]	35/male	liver/right retropharyngeal	imatinib (R)	R + T/NA	regorafenib	-	SD	NA	NA/NA/A/3
Badri et al., 2018 [42]	66/male	right cerebellum	None	S + R/NA	NA	NA	-	NA	No/12/A/12
Jang et al., 2018 [43]	70/male	liver	Imatinib (R)	E + R + T/40Gy*16	Imatinib	Yes	NA	NA	No/6/A/6
Yang et al., 2018 [51]	74/male	duodenal bulb	imatinib/sunitinib (R)	R/32.5Gy*13	None	Yes	PR	NA	Yes/9/D/16
Katayanagi et al., 2019 [32]	56/male	T8 vertebra/right ilium	imatinib/sunitinib (R)	R + T/37.5Gy*15	sunitinib/imatinib	NA	NA	NA	NA/NA/D/19
Yilmaz et al., 2020 [17]	31/male	right iliac bone	imatinib (R)	R + T/24Gy*3	sunitinib	Yes	CR	No	No/16/A/16
Carvalho et al., 2020 [18]	76/female	left frontal lobe/right cerebellar	imatinib (R)	S + R + T/NA/R + T/NA	imatinib	No	-/NA	NA	NA/NA/D/6

Table 1. Cont.

References	Age/Gender	Location	Previous TKIs	Means/Total Dose*Fractions #	Concomitant TKIs	Palliation Response	Side Effects	Follow-Up (Recurrence or Progression/TTR or TTP (mo)/A or D/OS (mo)
Andruska et al., 2020 [21]	29/female	caudate lobe of liver	imatinib/sunitinib/sorafenib/regorafenib (R)	R + T/30Gy*10	regorafenib/sunitinib	NA	NA	NA/NA/D/NA
Lo et al., 2020 [33]	63/male	T9 vertebra	imatinib/sunitinib/regorafenib/dasatinib (R)	S + R/30Gy*10	None	NA	NA	NA/NA/D/2
Maria et al., 2022 [20]	77/male	left maxillary	imatinib/2 additional lines (R)	R/35Gy*10	None	Yes	mucositis/grade2/dermatitis/grade1	NA/NA/D/8
Al-Jarani et al., 2022 [54]	52/female	liver/xiphoid	NA	NA	NA	NA	change in skin, dermatitis, sclerosis, fistula/NA	NA/NA/A/48

Total dose and fractions; Abbreviations: T, tyrosine kinase inhibitors (TKIs); S, surgery; R, radiotherapy; C, chemotherapy; E, embolization; I, immunotherapy; NA, not available; CR, complete response; PR, partial response; SD, stable disease; PD, progressive disease; (R), resistance; (I), intolerance; (W), withdrawal; Gy, gray; TTP, time to progression; TTR, time to recurrence; (mo), month; A, alive; D, dead.

Table 2. Description of the case series treated by radiotherapy.

References	Sex, Total No. (Male/Female)	Age, Median (Range),y	Sites	Previous TKIs, Patients No.	Means/Dose Range	Concomitant TKIs, Patients No.	Symptom Palliation, Patients No.	Response	Follow-Up, Range (mo)/Outcome
Baik et al., 2007 [45]	4 (1/3)	53 (41–68)	Rectum	None	R/45–54 Gy	None	NA	-	21–75/No recurrence and all alive
Cuaron et al., 2013 [11]	15 (8/7)	68 (41–86)	Bone/Abdomen/Pelvis	11	R/15–50 Gy	5	12	PR in 5 patients, SD in 9	1.4–28.3/12 deaths
Joensuu et al., 2015 [47]	25 (17/8)	61.4 (19.7–86.5)	Abdomen	25	R/30–40 Gy	19	NA	PR in 2 patients, SD in 20	2–74/20 patients progressed and 18 deaths
Rathmann et al., 2015 [49]	9 (7/2)	55 (34–74)	Liver	9	RE/0.55–1.88 Gbq	9	NA	CR in 3 patients, PR in 5, SD in 1	10–72/8 progressed and 4 deaths
Omari et al., 2019 [48]	10 (9/1)	58.5 (37–68)	Liver/Peritoneum	10	iBT/6.7–22.0 Gy	7	NA	LTC 97.5%	2.3–92.9/one relapse and 6 deaths
Patterson et al., 2022 [53]	12 (7/5)	69 (36–79)	NA	NA	R/20–50 Gy	12	9	SD in 1 patient, PD in 1	NA

Abbreviations: T, tyrosine kinase inhibitors (TKIs); mo, month; S, surgery; R, radiotherapy; RE, radioembolization; iBT, interstitial brachytherapy; Gy, gray; NA, not available; LTC, local tumor control; CR, complete response; PR, partial response; SD, stable disease.

3.2. Patient Response to Radiation and Follow-Up

There were 34 case reports and 2 case series, covering 70 lesions in 55 patients, which clearly described the patients' responses to radiotherapy and the specific scenarios of radiotherapy combined with TKIs [10,11,16–46,50–52]. The total doses of radiation ranged from 15 Gy to 85 Gy. The most common pattern was 30 Gy in 10 fractions. We divided the 70 lesions into 2 parts: 53 defined irradiated lesions in 41 patients (specific lesions in images or macroscopic incompletely resected lesions) and 17 undefined lesions in 17 patients (macroscopic completely resected lesions; radiotherapy was used as adjuvant therapy after complete resection).

We divided the 53 defined irradiated lesions into 4 groups according to radiotherapy with/without concomitant TKIs: radiotherapy (R), radiotherapy with new TKIs (R + nT, radiotherapy with further lines of TKIs after resistance), radiotherapy with resistant TKIs (R + rT, radiotherapy with previous resistant TKIs), and radiotherapy with sensitive TKIs (R + sT, radiotherapy with imatinib in cases in which no TKIs have been used before). The responses of the lesions are presented in Table 3. There were a total of 32 evaluable lesions. In particular, in the "R" group, partial response (PR) was observed in six lesions, and stable disease (SD) was observed in six lesions. In addition, in the "R + rT" group, complete response (CR) was seen in one lesion, PR in four, and SD in five. We further analyzed the locations of these 53 lesions, and the results are presented in Table 4. Bone and joints (26/53) were the most common sites treated by radiotherapy, followed by the abdomen (14/53).

Table 3. Response to radiotherapy with/without concomitant TKIs in the definite irradiated lesions.

Response	R	R + nT	R + rT	R + sT
CR	0	1	1	1
PR	6	1	4	2
SD	6	3	5	0
PD	2	0	0	0
NA	5	1	12	3
N	19	6	22	6

Abbreviations: CR, complete response; PR, partial response; SD, stable disease; PD, progressive disease; NA, not available; N, number; R, radiotherapy; R + nT, radiotherapy with new TKIs (radiotherapy with further lines of TKIs after resistance); R + rT, radiotherapy with resistant TKIs (radiotherapy with previously resistant TKIs); R + sT, radiotherapy with sensitive TKIs (radiotherapy with imatinib in cases in which no TKIs have been used before).

Table 4. Response of GIST at different locations to radiotherapy.

Response	Brain	Neck	Chest	Abdomen	Pelvis	Bone and Joint	N
CR	1				1	1	3
PR			1	6	1	5	13
SD		3	1	5	1	4	14
PD						2	2
NA	4			3		14	21
N	5	3	2	14	3	26	53

Abbreviations: GISTs, gastrointestinal stromal tumors; CR, complete response; PR, partial response; SD, stable disease; PD, progressive disease; N, number.

Among the 41 patients who had defined lesions treated by radiotherapy, Cuaron et al. reported 15 patients with locally advanced or metastatic GISTs [11]. There were 12 deaths, with a median follow-up of 5.1 months (range, 1.4–28.3). The estimated 6-month local progression-free survival was 57.0%. The median survival was 6.6 months, and the estimated 6-month overall survival was 57.8%. Among the remaining 26 patients who were from 24 case reports [10,17–23,26,28–32,34,35,37,39,41,43,46,50–52], 22 patients had clear follow-up information (progressive or dead outcomes and duration). Among the 22 patients, 8 patients were not resistant to TKIs before radiotherapy, 6 patients were resistant to 1 line of TKIs (all were imatinib-resistant), 7 patients were resistant to 2 lines of TKIs (all were imatinib- and sunitinib-resistant) and 1 patient was resistant to 3 lines. Since the role of radiotherapy in GISTs should be discussed after excluding the influence of effective TKIs, we analyzed the cases in which radiotherapy was used alone, as well as those in which radiotherapy was used with previously resistant TKIs. There were six patients treated by radiotherapy without any continued TKIs and eight patients treated by radiotherapy with previously resistant TKIs (Table 5). For the six patients with advanced or metastatic GISTs in the abdomen (three), brain (two), and bone (one), there were four patients not resistant to TKIs, one patient resistant to imatinib and sunitinib, and one patient resistant to three lines of TKIs. The median follow-up was 11.5 months (range, 3–72), and there were three deaths (one of the three deaths had a definite progression of irradiated lesions during follow-up). The estimated median PFS was 9 months (Figure 2A). Regarding the eight patients with advanced or metastatic GISTs in the bone (five), brain (one), liver (one), and pararenal and supraclavicular regions (one) treated by radiotherapy with previously resistant TKIs, four patients were imatinib-resistant, and four patients were imatinib- and sunitinib-resistant. There were five deaths, with a median follow-up of 4.5 months (range, 1.5–19). The estimated PFS was 5 months (Figure 2B).

Table 5. Application of TKIs in 22 patients with defined lesions before and after radiotherapy.

Continued TKIs	Resistant to 0 TKIs	Resistant to 1 TKI	Resistant to 2 TKIs	Resistant to ≥3TKIs
None	4		1	1
rTKI	-	4	4	
nTKI	-	2	2	
sTKI	4	-	-	-
NA				
N	8	6	7	1

Abbreviations: TKIs: tyrosine kinase Inhibitors; rTKI, previously resistant TKIs; nTKI, further lines of TKIs after resistance; sTKI, imatinib in cases in which no TKIs were previously used; NA, not available; N, number.

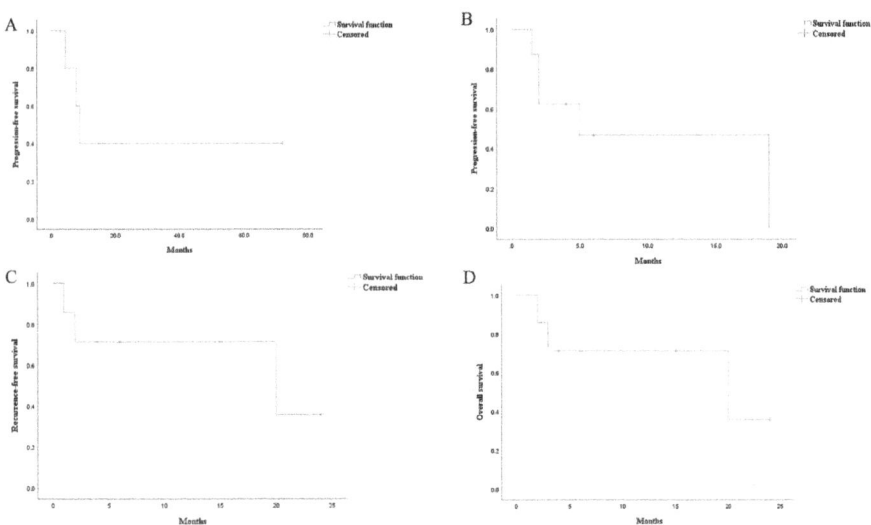

Figure 2. Kaplan–Meier estimates of survival: (A) progression-free survival in the 6 patients treated by radiotherapy without any continued TKIs; (B) progression-free survival in the 8 patients treated by radiotherapy with previously resistant TKIs; (C) recurrence-free survival in the 7 patients treated by radiotherapy without continued TKIs after surgery; (D) overall survival in the 7 patients treated by radiotherapy without continued TKIs after surgery.

Regarding the 17 undefined irradiated lesions in 17 patients, 13 patients were from 13 case reports [16,18,19,24,25,27,33,36,38–40,42,44], and the other 4 patients were from one case series [45]. The four patients with rectal GISTs treated by adjuvant radiotherapy without TKIs after surgery were all alive and had no recurrence during a follow-up of 21–75 months. The remaining 13 lesions in 13 patients included 1 lesion in the rectum, 1 in the stomach, 3 in the bone (1 in the skull and the other 2 in the spine), and 8 in the brain. Among the 13 patients, 8 patients were not resistant to TKIs before radiotherapy, 3 were resistant to 1 line of TKIs (all were imatinib-resistant), 1 was resistant to 2 lines of TKIs (imatinib- and sunitinib-resistant), and 1 was resistant to 4 lines of TKIs. There were 9 patients treated by radiotherapy without continued TKIs after surgery in these 13 patients (Table 6). Two of the nine patients received radiotherapy for the primary lesion areas (rectum and stomach), while the other seven patients received radiotherapy for the brain (five) and spine (two) metastases. Given that metastatic GISTs had a profound impact on prognosis, we performed survival analysis on the seven patients. Among the seven patients, there were four patients not resistant to TKIs, one patient resistant to imatinib, one patient resistant to imatinib and sunitinib, and one patient resistant to imatinib, sunitinib, regorafenib, and dasatinib. There were three deaths (one of the three deaths had definite recurrence during follow-up), with a median follow-up of 6 months (range, 2–24). The estimated median RFS was 20 months (Figure 2C), and the estimated OS was 20 months (Figure 2D).

Table 6. Application of TKIs in 13 patients with undefined lesions before and after radiotherapy.

Continued TKIs	Resistant to 0 TKIs	Resistant to 1 TKI	Resistant to 2 TKIs	Resistant to ≥3 TKIs
None	6	1	1	1
rTKI	-	2		
nTKI	-			
sTKI	1	-	-	
NA	1			
N	8	3	1	1

Abbreviations: TKIs: tyrosine kinase Inhibitors; rTKI, previously resistant TKIs; nTKI, further lines of TKIs after resistance; sTKI, imatinib in cases in which no TKIs were previously used; NA, not available; N, number.

In addition, there were three other case series, which did not clearly describe the specific scenarios of radiotherapy combined with TKIs [47–49]. Joensuu et al. reported 25 patients with advanced or metastatic GISTs receiving radiotherapy, which was a prospective clinical study [47]. PR was seen in 2 patients, and SD was seen in 20. In total, 20 patients progressed, and 18 died, with a median follow-up of 9 months (range, 2–74). The estimated median time to target lesion progression was 16 months, and the median OS was 19 months.

Both interstitial brachytherapy (iBT) and radioembolization are internal irradiation. Omari et al. reported that among 10 imatinib-resistant metastatic GISTs treated with iBT (TKIs continued in 7 patients), 1 recurred, and 6 died during follow-up (range, 2.3–92.9 months), with a median PFS of 6.8 months (range, 3.0–20.2) and a median OS of 37.3 months (range, 11.4–89.7); local tumor control was 97.5% [48]. Rathmann et al. reported nine patients who received radioembolization for liver metastases [49]. CR was seen in three patients, PR in five patients, and SD in one. Eight patients progressed at the end of the study, with a median progression time of 15.9 months (range, 4–29). There were four deaths, and the median OS was 29.8 months (range, 10–72).

3.3. Symptom Palliation

We considered symptom palliation in defined lesions treated by radiotherapy alone or radiotherapy with previously resistant TKIs. Among the 41 patients who had defined lesions, 30 patients received radiotherapy alone or radiotherapy with previously resistant TKIs. There were 28 patients with symptomatic GISTs. Local pain, which occurred in

17 patients, was the most common symptom, followed by neurological dysfunction (4) and bleeding (3). There were 22 patients achieving partial or complete palliation. Two patients did not achieve palliation, and the other four patients were not available. The symptom palliation rate was 78.6% (22/28).In addition, the other case series reported symptom palliation in 12 patients with advanced or metastatic GISTs treated by radiotherapy with concomitant TKIs [53]. Pain, spinal cord compression, and bleeding were the main symptoms. There were nine patients who had at least partial palliation.

3.4. Adverse Events

There were five case reports and four case series reporting adverse events [11,20,22,25, 47–49,52,54]. Adverse reactions were reported in 14 patients from 5 case reports and 1 case series with nausea in 3 patients (grade 1), diarrhea in 3 (grade 1–3), fatigue in 3 (grade 1–2), esophagitis in 2 (grade 2), proctitis in 1 (grade 2), chest pain in 1 (grade 1), urinary urgency in 1 (grade 1), dysgeusia in 1 (grade 1), mucositis in 1 (grade 2), dermatitis in 2 (grade 1), and moist desquamation in 1 (grade 2) [11,20,22,25,52,54]. Al-Jarani et al. first reported pericardial cutaneous fistula after radiotherapy in a metastatic GIST patient [54]. In addition, Rathmann et al. reported that among nine GIST patients who received radioembolization for liver metastasis, laboratory findings increased from grade 0 to grade 1 toxicity in seven cases, and stomach ulceration was grade E in one patient according to the Society of Interventional Radiology (SIR) guidelines [49]. Joensuu et al. reported that transient diarrhea was the most common adverse event (52%), followed by pain (44%), nausea (36%), and fatigue (32%) in 25 patients. The adverse events were mainly mild to moderate (grade 1 or 2), and only a few were severe (grade 3). Only one patient developed grade 4 biliary tract necrosis [47]. Omari et al. reported that of 10 patients with imatinib-resistant metastatic GISTs who received iBT, 3 had elevated inflammatory parameters (grade 1), and 2 had local hepatic hemorrhage and pneumothorax (grade 3) [48].

4. Discussion

In the era of TKIs, the management of GISTs has undergone revolutionary changes [55,56]. The effectiveness and safety of TKIs have been demonstrated in basic and clinical studies and benefit most GIST patients [57–59]. However, we still have to address the problems of secondary resistant mutations. The accurately molecular analysis is the gold standard of GIST diagnosis and also helps patients choose the optimal treatment [60]. wild-type *KIT/PDGFRA* and some special mutation sites in GISTs such as *PDGFRA D842 V* result in a limited response to imatinib [61–63]. According to the guidelines, the standard treatment for multiple systemic metastases is TKIs [2]. However, there are a considerable number of patients with advanced or metastatic GISTs who need further effective treatment. Therefore, multimodal management of GIST patients (including surgery, radiotherapy, radiofrequency ablation, etc.) has been examined in advanced GISTs [22,64–66]. In the past, GISTs were thought to be resistant to radiation therapy [10]. However, some studies have shown that radiotherapy may have some effect on selected GIST patients. Therefore, the effectiveness and role of radiotherapy should be reevaluated.

According to the current systematic review, the quality of most case reports and case series included was low. High-quality research on radiotherapy in GISTs is needed in the future. Compared with many other malignant tumors, GISTs have a better prognosis, and patients are expected to live longer. In many published clinical studies, outcome events often require an extended follow-up [67,68], but most of the patients included in this study had advanced GISTs. Therefore, it is possible to observe the outcome events in a relatively short follow-up period.

We analyzed the defined irradiated lesions, which are presented in Table 3. We divided the lesions into four groups. Two of the four groups were "R" and "R + rT", in which some lesions achieved objective response when treated by radiotherapy. This may indicate that radiotherapy had some effect on selected patients. The previous view that GISTs were insensitive to radiotherapy may need to be reevaluated.

The latest NCCN guidelines recommend radiotherapy for the palliative treatment of bone metastases [69]. We further analyzed the sites of these defined irradiated lesions and found that bone was the most common site, followed by the abdomen. There were some lesions in the abdomen that achieved objective response and disease stabilization. This indicated that, in addition to bone, abdominal lesions may be treated by radiotherapy, especially if the tumor is relatively fixed in the abdominal cavity [51]. Even in the past, there were concerns about the adverse effects of radiation on the abdominal organs. Furthermore, radiotherapy combined with imatinib should be considered, especially for GISTs at high risk of local recurrence, where surgery is often demolitive, such as rectal and esophageal GISTs [11,22].

According to our study, there were six patients (four patients not resistant to TKIs) with advanced or metastatic GISTs treated by radiotherapy alone. PR was seen in three patients, with an estimated median PFS of 9 months in the six patients. Compared with patients with advanced GISTs treated initially with imatinib [70], radiotherapy may not benefit the survival of patients with advanced GISTs. In addition, eight patients (four patients were imatinib-resistant and four were imatinib- and sunitinib-resistant) received radiotherapy with previously resistant TKIs. CR was seen in one patient, and SD was seen in one patient, with an estimated median PFS of 5 months in the eight patients. Compared with patients treated by further lines of TKIs after imatinib or imatinib and sunitinib failure [71,72], radiotherapy with continuous use of previously resistant TKIs may not benefit survival for patients with advanced GISTs. Thus, TKIs are still the mainstay for advanced or metastatic GISTs. However, radiotherapy may help achieve objective response in selected patients. Therefore, when TKIs are not available, radiotherapy may be an option for some patients. Nevertheless, it may not benefit survival in patients with systematic metastases. In addition, the survival of the "R + rT" group was inferior to that of the "R" group, which may be because all eight patients were drug-resistant. Joensuu et al. reported that 25 patients who were progressive during or after TKIs were treated by radiotherapy. There were 19 patients treated with concomitant TKIs. The study did not further analyze the efficacy of radiotherapy alone or radiotherapy with concomitant previously resistant TKIs. Therefore, the results of the study failed to demonstrate the effectiveness of radiotherapy in GISTs.

There were seven patients with undefined irradiated lesions mainly located in the brain treated by radiotherapy alone. The estimated median RFS was 20 months. Sym et al. reported that compared with imatinib-resistant patients after surgery, patients responsive to imatinib had better survival after surgery [73]. The results should be interpreted with caution. Among the seven patients in our study, four patients were not resistant to TKIs and may benefit from the surgery. In addition, some patients might have been contaminated by TKIs after surgery, which was not reported. Meanwhile, previous studies have indicated that surgery should be chosen with greater caution in patients with multiple systemic metastases [48]. In cases of limited disease progression after TKIs, a more aggressive approach can be chosen [74,75], but the risks of surgical complications and potential benefits cannot be quantified [76,77]. Some studies have also pointed out that complete surgical resection has a significant impact on the survival of GIST patients. In contrast, adjuvant radiotherapy has no apparent benefit except for controlling the target area [78,79]. For locally advanced GISTs, previous studies have evaluated the effectiveness of TKIs in neoadjuvant settings [80]. However, there have been a few case reports about neoadjuvant radiotherapy in GISTs, which may need further investigation.

In addition, relatively high disease control has been achieved in radioembolization and iBT [48,49], which suggests that the two special radiation means may be superior to others for local tumor control. However, hepatopulmonary shunt and radiation pneumonia may limit the use of radioembolization [81].

Through the analysis of symptomatic GISTs, we found that the symptom palliation rate of radiotherapy alone and radiotherapy with concomitant previously resistant TKIs reached 78.6% (22/28), which supports the application of radiotherapy in GISTs for palliative purposes recommended by the guidelines [2]. In addition to pain, radiotherapy may also be used to relieve the symptoms of bleeding and spinal cord compression [51,53]. Patterson et al. reported that among 12 patients with advanced or metastatic GISTs treated by radiotherapy, 9 had improvement in symptoms to varying degrees [53]. However, all 12 patients received TKIs during radiotherapy. It was not clear whether further lines of TKIs after resistance or sensitive or resistant TKIs were used. Thus, the role of radiotherapy in symptom palliation was not clearly explained.

Radiotherapy with concomitant TKIs was well-tolerated. Most adverse events were grade 1–2. However, some adverse reactions suggested that we need to be cautious in simultaneous treatment. TKIs that inhibit *VEGF* receptors may be associated with local dermal toxicity and hepatotoxicity at irradiated sites [82–85].

Regarding the modes of radiotherapy, Joensuu et al. reported radiotherapy for liver and abdominal tumors, for which three-dimensional (3D) conformational radiotherapy and intensity-modulated radiotherapy (IMRT) were mainly used [47]. These methods belong to the category of stereotactic radiotherapy. Stereotactic radiotherapy has the advantages of precise localization, the concentration of dose, minor impact on the surrounding tissue of tumors, and a high ablative dose. Radioembolization and iBT have also shown good efficacy and safety in treating liver metastases [48,49]. These radiotherapy methods can deliver a relatively high dose to target lesions and can protect the important surrounding structures, ultimately achieving a better response [11,86–88].

5. Limitations

We must acknowledge that this study has several limitations.

Most importantly, publication bias was present in the current study. Because GISTs were considered insensitive to radiotherapy in the past, positive results of radiotherapy treatment had a tendency to be published, which may overstate our findings. Furthermore, with the wide application of TKIs, radiotherapy was rarely considered in GISTs, resulting in few publications reporting radiotherapy in GISTs. However, to discuss the application of radiotherapy in GISTs more comprehensively, we conducted an extensive literature search and included almost all the positive and negative cases of radiotherapy that could be retrieved. A considerable number of patients were not responsive to radiotherapy in our study. However, there were still many negative cases that could not be obtained through the literature search. Further research is, therefore, necessary on radiotherapy in GISTs.

Second, the articles included were low- to moderate-quality case reports and case series. In addition, there was data heterogeneity in these studies. Thus, in the future, we need to design high-quality randomized controlled studies to evaluate the efficacy and safety of radiotherapy in GISTs.

Third, in the era of TKIs, radiotherapy with concomitant TKIs has been more common, which may mean that the effects of radiotherapy cannot be effectively evaluated. Thus, it is necessary to strictly design research to assess the value of radiotherapy in GISTs from an ethical point of view.

6. Conclusions

Overall, radiotherapy may relieve symptoms for some GIST patients with advanced or metastatic lesions and even help achieve objective response in selected patients without significantly reducing the quality of life. In addition to bone metastases, fixed abdominal lesions may be treated by radiotherapy.

Nevertheless, the efficacy and safety of radiotherapy in GIST patients warrant further investigation.

Supplementary Materials: The following supporting information can be downloaded at: https://www.mdpi.com/article/10.3390/cancers14133169/s1, Table S1: PRISMA 2020 item checklist [12], Table S2: Methodological quality of included studies (adapted from the Joanna Briggs Institute (JBI) Critical Appraisal Checklist for Case Reports and Case series).

Author Contributions: Conceptualization, Y.Y. and B.Z.; methodology, Y.Y. and H.Z.; formal analysis, H.Z. and T.J.; investigation, H.Z. and T.J.; data curation, H.Z. and M.M.; writing—original draft preparation, H.Z.; writing—review and editing, H.Z., T.J., Y.Y. and M.M.; visualization, H.Z., Z.Z. and X.Y.; supervision, Y.Y. and Z.C.; project administration, Y.Y.; funding acquisition, Y.Y. All authors have read and agreed to the published version of the manuscript.

Funding: This research was supported by the Sichuan Provincial Health and Family Planning Commission Key Research Project, project number 20ZD007.

Institutional Review Board Statement: The research did not require ethical approval.

Informed Consent Statement: Not applicable.

Data Availability Statement: The paper has already contained all date sets.

Acknowledgments: We wish to thank the West China Hospital who set up the cooperation platform for research and kind help from the author's roommates.

Conflicts of Interest: The authors declare no conflict of interest.

References

1. Miettinen, M.; Lasota, J. Gastrointestinal stromal tumors—Definition, clinical, histological, immunohistochemical, and molecular genetic features and differential diagnosis. *Virchows Arch.* **2001**, *438*, 3–12. [CrossRef] [PubMed]
2. Casali, P.G.; Blay, J.Y.; Abecassis, N.; Bajpai, J.; Bauer, S.; Biagini, R.; Bielack, S.; Bonvalot, S.; Boukovinas, I.; Bovee, J.; et al. Gastrointestinal stromal tumours: ESMO-EURACAN-GENTURIS Clinical Practice Guidelines for diagnosis, treatment and follow-up. *Ann. Oncol.* **2022**, *33*, 20–33. [CrossRef] [PubMed]
3. Cai, Z.; Chen, X.; Zhang, B.; Cao, D. Apatinib Treatment in Metastatic Gastrointestinal Stromal Tumor. *Front. Oncol.* **2019**, *9*, 470. [CrossRef]
4. Mantese, G. Gastrointestinal stromal tumor: Epidemiology, diagnosis, and treatment. *Curr. Opin. Gastroenterol.* **2019**, *35*, 555–559. [CrossRef]
5. Joensuu, H. Gastrointestinal stromal tumor (GIST). *Ann. Oncol.* **2006**, *17* (Suppl. S10), x280–x286. [CrossRef]
6. Balachandran, V.P.; DeMatteo, R.P. Gastrointestinal stromal tumors: Who should get imatinib and for how long? *Adv. Surg.* **2014**, *48*, 165–183. [CrossRef]
7. Cai, Z.; Yin, Y.; Shen, C.; Tang, S.; Yin, X.; Chen, Z.; Zhang, B. Role of surgical resection for patients with recurrent or metastatic gastrointestinal stromal tumors: A systematic review and meta-analysis. *Int. J. Surg.* **2018**, *56*, 108–114. [CrossRef]
8. Ahmed, M. Recent advances in the management of gastrointestinal stromal tumor. *World J. Clin. Cases* **2020**, *8*, 3142–3155. [CrossRef]
9. Ahmed, K.A.; Caudell, J.J.; El-Haddad, G.; Berglund, A.E.; Welsh, E.A.; Yue, B.; Hoffe, S.E.; Naghavi, A.O.; Abuodeh, Y.A.; Frakes, J.M.; et al. Radiosensitivity Differences between Liver Metastases Based on Primary Histology Suggest Implications for Clinical Outcomes after Stereotactic Body Radiation Therapy. *Int. J. Radiat. Oncol. Biol. Phys.* **2016**, *95*, 1399–1404. [CrossRef]
10. Lolli, C.; Pantaleo, M.A.; Nannini, M.; Saponara, M.; Pallotti, M.C.; Scioscio, V.D.; Barbieri, E.; Mandrioli, A.; Biasco, G. Successful radiotherapy for local control of progressively increasing metastasis of gastrointestinal stromal tumor. *Rare Tumors* **2011**, *3*, e49. [CrossRef]
11. Cuaron, J.J.; Goodman, K.A.; Lee, N.; Wu, A.J. External beam radiation therapy for locally advanced and metastatic gastrointestinal stromal tumors. *Radiat. Oncol.* **2013**, *8*, 274. [CrossRef] [PubMed]
12. Page, M.J.; McKenzie, J.E.; Bossuyt, P.M.; Boutron, I.; Hoffmann, T.C.; Mulrow, C.D.; Shamseer, L.; Tetzlaff, J.M.; Akl, E.A.; Brennan, S.E.; et al. The PRISMA 2020 statement: An updated guideline for reporting systematic reviews. *Syst. Rev.* **2021**, *10*, 89. [CrossRef]
13. Cai, Z.; Liu, C.; Chang, C.; Shen, C.; Yin, Y.; Yin, X.; Jiang, Z.; Zhao, Z.; Mu, M.; Cao, D.; et al. Comparative safety and tolerability of approved PARP inhibitors in cancer: A systematic review and network meta-analysis. *Pharmacol. Res.* **2021**, *172*, 105808. [CrossRef] [PubMed]
14. Moola, S.; Munn, Z.; Tufanaru, C.; Aromataris, E.; Mu, P.F. Chapter 7: *Systematic Reviews of Etiology and Risk*; JBI Reviewer's Manual; The Joanna Briggs Institute: Adelaide, Australia, 2019.
15. Riley, D.S.; Barber, M.S.; Kienle, G.S.; Aronson, J.K.; von Schoen-Angerer, T.; Tugwell, P.; Kiene, H.; Helfand, M.; Altman, D.G.; Sox, H.; et al. CARE guidelines for case reports: Explanation and elaboration document. *J. Clin. Epidemiol.* **2017**, *89*, 218–235. [CrossRef] [PubMed]
16. Knowlton, C.A.; Brady, L.W.; Heintzelman, R.C. Radiotherapy in the treatment of gastrointestinal stromal tumor. *Rare Tumors* **2011**, *3*, e35. [CrossRef]
17. Yilmaz, M.T.; Gultekin, M.; Yalcin, S.; Tuncel, M.; Gedikoglu, G.; Yildiz, F.; Cengiz, M. Stereotactic ablative radiotherapy for bone metastasis of gastrointestinal stromal tumor: Case report and review of the literature. *Rep. Pract. Oncol. Radiother.* **2020**, *25*, 331–335. [CrossRef]

18. Carvalho, J.; Teixeira, M.; Silva, F.T.; Esteves, A.; Ribeiro, C.; Guerra, D. Esophageal Gastrointestinal Stromal Tumor with Rare Intracranial Metastasis. *Case Rep. Gastrointest Med.* **2020**, *2020*, 8842006. [CrossRef]
19. Naoe, H.; Kaku, E.; Ido, Y.; Gushima, R.; Maki, Y.; Saito, H.; Yokote, S.; Gushima, R.; Nonaka, K.; Hoshida, Y.; et al. Brain metastasis from gastrointestinal stromal tumor: A case report and review of the literature. *Case Rep. Gastroenterol.* **2011**, *5*, 583–589. [CrossRef]
20. Maria, O.M.; Alghamdi, O.; Baabdullah, R.; El-Hakim, M.; Al-Halabi, H.; Makhoul, N.M. Gastrointestinal stromal tumor with maxillary metastasis: A case report and literature review. *Oral Surg. Oral Med. Oral Pathol. Oral Radiol.* **2022**, *133*, e1–e5. [CrossRef]
21. Andruska, N.; Mahapatra, L.; Brenneman, R.; MacArthur, K.M.; Oppelt, P.; Baumann, B.C. False-positive pregnancy test secondary to ectopic expression of human chorionic gonadotropin by a gastrointestinal stromal tumor. *J. Surg. Oncol.* **2020**, online ahead of print. [CrossRef]
22. Gatto, L.; Nannini, M.; Saponara, M.; Di Scioscio, V.; Beltramo, G.; Frezza, G.P.; Ercolani, G.; Pinna, A.D.; Astolfi, A.; Urbini, M.; et al. Radiotherapy in the management of gist: State of the art and new potential scenarios. *Clin. Sarcoma Res.* **2017**, *7*, 1. [CrossRef]
23. Boruban, C.; Sencan, O.; Akmansu, M.; Atik, E.T.; Ozbek, S. Metastatic gastrointestinal stromal tumor with long-term response after treatment with concomitant radiotherapy and imatinib mesylate. *Anticancer Drugs* **2007**, *18*, 969–972. [CrossRef] [PubMed]
24. Gupta, S.; Bi, W.L.; Dunn, I.F. Metastatic Gastrointestinal Stromal Tumor to the Skull. *World Neurosurg.* **2016**, *89*, 725.e11-6. [CrossRef] [PubMed]
25. Pollock, J.; Morgan, D.; Denobile, J.; Williams, J. Adjuvant radiotherapy for gastrointestinal stromal tumor of the rectum. *Dig. Dis. Sci.* **2001**, *46*, 268–272. [CrossRef] [PubMed]
26. Takeuchi, H.; Koike, H.; Fujita, T.; Tsujino, H.; Iwamoto, Y. Sunitinib treatment for multiple brain metastases from jejunal gastrointestinal stromal tumor: Case report. *Neurol. Med. Chir.* **2014**, *54*, 664–669. [CrossRef]
27. Hamada, S.; Itami, A.; Watanabe, G.; Nakayama, S.; Tanaka, E.; Hojo, M.; Yoshizawa, A.; Hirota, S.; Sakai, Y. Intracranial metastasis from an esophageal gastrointestinal stromal tumor. *Intern. Med.* **2010**, *49*, 781–785. [CrossRef]
28. Halpern, J.; Kim, Y.J.; Sultana, R.; Villani, G. Effectiveness of radiation therapy in GIST: A case report. *J. Gastrointest Oncol.* **2012**, *3*, 143–146. [CrossRef] [PubMed]
29. Di Scioscio, V.; Greco, L.; Pallotti, M.C.; Pantaleo, M.A.; Maleddu, A.; Nannini, M.; Bazzocchi, A.; Di Battista, M.; Mandrioli, A.; Lolli, C.; et al. Three cases of bone metastases in patients with gastrointestinal stromal tumors. *Rare Tumors* **2011**, *3*, e17. [CrossRef]
30. Tezcan, Y.; Koç, M. Gastrointestinal stromal tumor of the rectum with bone and liver metastasis: A case study. *Med. Oncol.* **2011**, *28* (Suppl. S1), S204–S206. [CrossRef]
31. Aktan, M.; Koc, M.; Yavuz, B.B.; Kanyilmaz, G. Two cases of gastrointestinal stromal tumor of the small intestine with liver and bone metastasis. *Ann. Transl. Med.* **2015**, *3*, 259. [CrossRef]
32. Katayanagi, S.; Yokoyama, T.; Makuuchi, Y.; Osakabe, H.; Iwamoto, H.; Sumi, T.; Hirano, H.; Katsumata, K.; Tsuchida, A.; Hirota, S.; et al. Long-Term Survival after Multidisciplinary Treatment Including Surgery for Metachronous Metastases of Small Intestinal Gastrointestinal Stromal Tumors after Curative Resection: A Case Report. *Am. J. Case Rep.* **2019**, *20*, 1942–1948. [CrossRef]
33. Lo, Y.T.; Mak, D.S.K.; Nolan, C.P. Surgical management of vertebral metastatic gastrointestinal stromal tumor: Case illustration, literature review, and pooled analysis. *Surg. Neurol. Int.* **2020**, *11*, 343. [CrossRef] [PubMed]
34. Abuzakhm, S.M.; Acre-Lara, C.E.; Zhao, W.; Hitchcock, C.; Mohamed, N.; Arbogast, D.; Shah, M.H. Unusual metastases of gastrointestinal stromal tumor and genotypic correlates: Case report and review of the literature. *J. Gastrointest Oncol.* **2011**, *2*, 45–49. [CrossRef] [PubMed]
35. Feki, J.; Bouzguenda, R.; Ayedi, L.; Bradi, M.; Boudawara, T.; Daoud, J.; Frikha, M. Bone metastases from gastrointestinal stromal tumor: A case report. *Case Rep. Oncol. Med.* **2012**, *2012*, 509845. [CrossRef] [PubMed]
36. Slimack, N.P.; Liu, J.C.; Koski, T.; McClendon, J., Jr.; O'Shaughnessy, B.A. Metastatic gastrointestinal stromal tumor to the thoracic and lumbar spine: First reported case and surgical treatment. *Spine J.* **2012**, *12*, e7–e12. [CrossRef] [PubMed]
37. Akiyama, K.; Numaga, J.; Kagaya, F.; Takazawa, Y.; Suzuki, S.; Koseki, N.; Kato, S.; Kaburaki, T.; Kawashima, H. Case of optic nerve involvement in metastasis of a gastrointestinal stromal tumor. *Jpn. J. Ophthalmol.* **2004**, *48*, 166–168. [CrossRef]
38. Wong, C.S.; Chu, Y.C. Intra-cranial metastasis of gastrointestinal stromal tumor. *Chin. Med. J.* **2011**, *124*, 3595–3597.
39. Drazin, D.; Spitler, K.; Jeswani, S.; Shirzadi, A.; Bannykh, S.; Patil, C. Multiple intracranial metastases from a gastric gastrointestinal stromal tumor. *J. Clin. Neurosci.* **2013**, *20*, 471–473. [CrossRef]
40. Sato, K.; Tanaka, T.; Kato, N.; Ishii, T.; Terao, T.; Murayama, Y. Metastatic cerebellar gastrointestinal stromal tumor with obstructive hydrocephalus arising from the small intestine: A case report and review of the literature. *Case Rep. Oncol. Med.* **2014**, *2014*, 343178. [CrossRef]
41. Barrière, J.; Thariat, J.; Vandenbos, F.; Bondiau, P.Y.; Peyrottes, I.; Peyrade, F. Diplopia as the first symptom of an aggressive metastatic rectal stromal tumor. *Onkologie* **2009**, *32*, 345–347. [CrossRef]
42. Badri, M.; Chabaane, M.; Gader, G.; Bahri, K.; Zammel, I. Cerebellar metastasis of gastrointestinal stromal tumor: A case report and review of the literature. *Int. J. Surg. Case Rep.* **2018**, *42*, 165–168. [CrossRef]
43. Jang, S.J.; Kwon, J.H.; Han, Y. A Ruptured Metastatic Hepatic Gastrointestinal Stromal Tumor Treated by Angiographic Embolization. *Korean J. Gastroenterol.* **2018**, *72*, 205–208. [CrossRef] [PubMed]

44. Puri, T.; Gunabushanam, G.; Malik, M.; Goyal, S.; Das, A.K.; Julka, P.K.; Rath, G.K. Mesenteric gastrointestinal stromal tumour presenting as intracranial space occupying lesion. *World J. Surg. Oncol.* **2006**, *4*, 78. [CrossRef] [PubMed]
45. Baik, S.H.; Kim, N.K.; Lee, C.H.; Lee, K.Y.; Sohn, S.K.; Cho, C.H.; Kim, H.; Pyo, H.R.; Rha, S.Y.; Chung, H.C. Gastrointestinal stromal tumor of the rectum: An analysis of seven cases. *Surg. Today* **2007**, *37*, 455–459. [CrossRef] [PubMed]
46. Loaiza-Bonilla, A.; Bonilla-Reyes, P.A. Somatostatin Receptor Avidity in Gastrointestinal Stromal Tumors: Theranostic Implications of Gallium-68 Scan and Eligibility for Peptide Receptor Radionuclide Therapy. *Cureus* **2017**, *9*, e1710. [CrossRef]
47. Joensuu, H.; Eriksson, M.; Collan, J.; Balk, M.H.; Leyvraz, S.; Montemurro, M. Radiotherapy for GIST progressing during or after tyrosine kinase inhibitor therapy: A prospective study. *Radiother. Oncol.* **2015**, *116*, 233–238. [CrossRef]
48. Omari, J.; Drewes, R.; Matthias, M.; Mohnike, K.; Seidensticker, M.; Seidensticker, R.; Streitparth, T.; Ricke, J.; Powerski, M.; Pech, M. Treatment of metastatic, imatinib refractory, gastrointestinal stroma tumor with image-guided high-dose-rate interstitial brachytherapy. *Brachytherapy* **2019**, *18*, 63–70. [CrossRef]
49. Rathmann, N.; Diehl, S.J.; Dinter, D.; Schütte, J.; Pink, D.; Schoenberg, S.O.; Hohenberger, P. Radioembolization in patients with progressive gastrointestinal stromal tumor liver metastases undergoing treatment with tyrosine kinase inhibitors. *J. Vasc. Interv. Radiol.* **2015**, *26*, 231–238. [CrossRef]
50. Shioyama, Y.; Yakeishi, Y.; Watanabe, T.; Nakamura, K.; Kunitake, N.; Kimura, M.; Sasaki, M.; Honda, H.; Terashima, H.; Masuda, K. Long-term control for a retroperitoneal metastasis of malignant gastrointestinal stromal tumor after chemoradiotherapy and immunotherapy. *Acta Oncol.* **2001**, *40*, 102–104. [CrossRef]
51. Yang, P.C.; Guo, J.C. Radiotherapy as salvage treatment after failure of tyrosine kinase inhibitors for a patient with advanced gastrointestinal stromal tumor. *J. Cancer Res. Pract.* **2018**, *5*, 156–160. [CrossRef]
52. Ciresa, M.; D'Angelillo, R.M.; Ramella, S.; Cellini, F.; Gaudino, D.; Stimato, G.; Fiore, M.; Greco, C.; Nudo, R.; Trodella, L. Molecularly targeted therapy and radiotherapy in the management of localized gastrointestinal stromal tumor (GIST) of the rectum: A case report. *Tumori* **2009**, *95*, 236–239. [CrossRef]
53. Patterson, T.; Li, H.; Chai, J.; Debruyns, A.; Simmons, C.; Hart, J.; Pollock, P.; Holloway, C.L.; Truong, P.T.; Feng, X. Locoregional Treatments for Metastatic Gastrointestinal Stromal Tumor in British Columbia: A Retrospective Cohort Study from January 2008 to December 2017. *Cancers* **2022**, *14*, 1477. [CrossRef] [PubMed]
54. Al-Jarani, B.; Soon Chan, W.; Dulu, A.; Nahass, T.; Pastores, S. Radiation-induced pericardial cutaneous fistula. *Crit. Care Med.* **2022**, *50*, 163. [CrossRef]
55. Kelly, C.M.; Gutierrez Sainz, L.; Chi, P. The management of metastatic GIST: Current standard and investigational therapeutics. *J. Hematol. Oncol.* **2021**, *14*, 2. [CrossRef] [PubMed]
56. Nishida, T.; Blay, J.Y.; Hirota, S.; Kitagawa, Y.; Kang, Y.K. The standard diagnosis, treatment, and follow-up of gastrointestinal stromal tumors based on guidelines. *Gastric Cancer* **2016**, *19*, 3–14. [CrossRef] [PubMed]
57. Demetri, G.D.; von Mehren, M.; Blanke, C.D.; Van den Abbeele, A.D.; Eisenberg, B.; Roberts, P.J.; Heinrich, M.C.; Tuveson, D.A.; Singer, S.; Janicek, M.; et al. Efficacy and safety of imatinib mesylate in advanced gastrointestinal stromal tumors. *N. Engl. J. Med.* **2002**, *347*, 472–480. [CrossRef]
58. Cavnar, M.J.; Seier, K.; Curtin, C.; Balachandran, V.P.; Coit, D.G.; Yoon, S.S.; Crago, A.M.; Strong, V.E.; Tap, W.D.; Gönen, M.; et al. Outcome of 1000 Patients with Gastrointestinal Stromal Tumor (GIST) Treated by Surgery in the Pre- and Post-imatinib Eras. *Ann. Surg.* **2021**, *273*, 128–138. [CrossRef]
59. Joensuu, H.; Eriksson, M.; Sundby Hall, K.; Hartmann, J.T.; Pink, D.; Schütte, J.; Ramadori, G.; Hohenberger, P.; Duyster, J.; Al-Batran, S.E.; et al. One vs three years of adjuvant imatinib for operable gastrointestinal stromal tumor: A randomized trial. *JAMA* **2012**, *307*, 1265–1272. [CrossRef]
60. Wu, C.E.; Tzen, C.Y.; Wang, S.Y.; Yeh, C.N. Clinical Diagnosis of Gastrointestinal Stromal Tumor (GIST): From the Molecular Genetic Point of View. *Cancers* **2019**, *11*, 679. [CrossRef]
61. Grunewald, S.; Klug, L.R.; Mühlenberg, T.; Lategahn, J.; Falkenhorst, J.; Town, A.; Ehrt, C.; Wardelmann, E.; Hartmann, W.; Schildhaus, H.U.; et al. Resistance to Avapritinib in PDGFRA-Driven GIST Is Caused by Secondary Mutations in the PDGFRA Kinase Domain. *Cancer Discov.* **2021**, *11*, 108–125. [CrossRef]
62. von Mehren, M.; Joensuu, H. Gastrointestinal Stromal Tumors. *J. Clin. Oncol.* **2018**, *36*, 136–143. [CrossRef]
63. Fletcher, J.A.; Rubin, B.P. KIT mutations in GIST. *Curr. Opin. Genet Dev.* **2007**, *17*, 3–7. [CrossRef] [PubMed]
64. Saponara, M.; Pantaleo, M.A.; Nannini, M.; Biasco, G. Treatments for gastrointestinal stromal tumors that are resistant to standard therapies. *Future Oncol.* **2014**, *10*, 2045–2059. [CrossRef] [PubMed]
65. Raut, C.P.; Posner, M.; Desai, J.; Morgan, J.A.; George, S.; Zahrieh, D.; Fletcher, C.D.; Demetri, G.D.; Bertagnolli, M.M. Surgical management of advanced gastrointestinal stromal tumors after treatment with targeted systemic therapy using kinase inhibitors. *J. Clin. Oncol.* **2006**, *24*, 2325–2331. [CrossRef] [PubMed]
66. Jones, R.L.; McCall, J.; Adam, A.; O'Donnell, D.; Ashley, S.; Al-Muderis, O.; Thway, K.; Fisher, C.; Judson, I.R. Radiofrequency ablation is a feasible therapeutic option in the multi modality management of sarcoma. *Eur. J. Surg. Oncol.* **2010**, *36*, 477–482. [CrossRef]
67. Joensuu, H.; Eriksson, M.; Sundby Hall, K.; Reichardt, A.; Hermes, B.; Schütte, J.; Cameron, S.; Hohenberger, P.; Jost, P.J.; Al-Batran, S.E.; et al. Survival Outcomes Associated with 3 Years vs. 1 Year of Adjuvant Imatinib for Patients with High-Risk Gastrointestinal Stromal Tumors: An Analysis of a Randomized Clinical Trial after 10-Year Follow-Up. *JAMA Oncol.* **2020**, *6*, 1241–1246. [CrossRef]

68. Casali, P.G.; Zalcberg, J.; Le Cesne, A.; Reichardt, P.; Blay, J.Y.; Lindner, L.H.; Judson, I.R.; Schöffski, P.; Leyvraz, S.; Italiano, A.; et al. Ten-Year Progression-Free and Overall Survival in Patients with Unresectable or Metastatic GI Stromal Tumors: Long-Term Analysis of the European Organisation for Research and Treatment of Cancer, Italian Sarcoma Group, and Australasian Gastrointestinal Trials Group Intergroup Phase III Randomized Trial on Imatinib at Two Dose Levels. *J. Clin. Oncol.* **2017**, *35*, 1713–1720. [CrossRef]
69. Mehren, M.v.; Kane, J.M.; Agulnik, M.; Bui, M.M.; Carr-Ascher, J.; Choy, E.; Connelly, M.; Dry, S. National Comprehensive Cancer Network. NCCN Clinical Practice Guidelines in Oncology: Gastrointestinal Stromal Tumors (GISTs), Version 1. 2022. Available online: https://www.nccn.org/professionals/physician_gls/pdf/gist.pdf (accessed on 21 January 2022).
70. Rutkowski, P.; Bylina, E.; Lugowska, I.; Teterycz, P.; Klimczak, A.; Streb, J.; Czarnecka, A.M.; Osuch, C. Treatment outcomes in older patients with advanced gastrointestinal stromal tumor (GIST). *J. Geriatr. Oncol.* **2018**, *9*, 520–525. [CrossRef]
71. Shirao, K.; Nishida, T.; Doi, T.; Komatsu, Y.; Muro, K.; Li, Y.; Ueda, E.; Ohtsu, A. Phase I/II study of sunitinib malate in Japanese patients with gastrointestinal stromal tumor after failure of prior treatment with imatinib mesylate. *Investig. New Drugs* **2010**, *28*, 866–875. [CrossRef]
72. Komatsu, Y.; Doi, T.; Sawaki, A.; Kanda, T.; Yamada, Y.; Kuss, I.; Demetri, G.D.; Nishida, T. Regorafenib for advanced gastrointestinal stromal tumors following imatinib and sunitinib treatment: A subgroup analysis evaluating Japanese patients in the phase III GRID trial. *Int. J. Clin. Oncol.* **2015**, *20*, 905–912. [CrossRef]
73. Sym, S.J.; Ryu, M.H.; Lee, J.L.; Chang, H.M.; Kim, T.W.; Kim, H.C.; Kim, K.H.; Yook, J.H.; Kim, B.S.; Kang, Y.K. Surgical intervention following imatinib treatment in patients with advanced gastrointestinal stromal tumors (GISTs). *J. Surg. Oncol.* **2008**, *98*, 27–33. [CrossRef]
74. Yeh, C.N.; Hu, C.H.; Wang, S.Y.; Wu, C.E.; Chen, J.S.; Tsai, C.Y.; Hsu, J.T.; Yeh, T.S. Cytoreductive Surgery may be beneficial for highly selected patients with Metastatic Gastrointestinal Stromal Tumors receiving Regorafenib facing Local Progression: A Case Controlled Study. *J. Cancer* **2021**, *12*, 3335–3343. [CrossRef] [PubMed]
75. Fairweather, M.; Balachandran, V.P.; Li, G.Z.; Bertagnolli, M.M.; Antonescu, C.; Tap, W.; Singer, S.; DeMatteo, R.P.; Raut, C.P. Cytoreductive Surgery for Metastatic Gastrointestinal Stromal Tumors Treated with Tyrosine Kinase Inhibitors: A 2-institutional Analysis. *Ann. Surg.* **2018**, *268*, 296–302. [CrossRef] [PubMed]
76. von Mehren, M.; Randall, R.L.; Benjamin, R.S.; Boles, S.; Bui, M.M.; Ganjoo, K.N.; George, S.; Gonzalez, R.J.; Heslin, M.J.; Kane, J.M.; et al. Soft Tissue Sarcoma, Version 2.2018, NCCN Clinical Practice Guidelines in Oncology. *J. Natl. Compr. Canc Netw.* **2018**, *16*, 536–563. [CrossRef] [PubMed]
77. Casali, P.G.; Abecassis, N.; Aro, H.T.; Bauer, S.; Biagini, R.; Bielack, S.; Bonvalot, S.; Boukovinas, I.; Bovee, J.; Brodowicz, T.; et al. Gastrointestinal stromal tumours: ESMO-EURACAN Clinical Practice Guidelines for diagnosis, treatment and follow-up. *Ann. Oncol.* **2018**, *29*, iv267. [CrossRef] [PubMed]
78. Pierie, J.P.; Choudry, U.; Muzikansky, A.; Yeap, B.Y.; Souba, W.W.; Ott, M.J. The effect of surgery and grade on outcome of gastrointestinal stromal tumors. *Arch. Surg.* **2001**, *136*, 383–389. [CrossRef]
79. Crosby, J.A.; Catton, C.N.; Davis, A.; Couture, J.; O'Sullivan, B.; Kandel, R.; Swallow, C.J. Malignant gastrointestinal stromal tumors of the small intestine: A review of 50 cases from a prospective database. *Ann. Surg. Oncol.* **2001**, *8*, 50–59. [CrossRef] [PubMed]
80. Wang, S.Y.; Wu, C.E.; Lai, C.C.; Chen, J.S.; Tsai, C.Y.; Cheng, C.T.; Yeh, T.S.; Yeh, C.N. Prospective Evaluation of Neoadjuvant Imatinib Use in Locally Advanced Gastrointestinal Stromal Tumors: Emphasis on the Optimal Duration of Neoadjuvant Imatinib Use, Safety, and Oncological Outcome. *Cancers* **2019**, *11*, 424. [CrossRef]
81. Wright, C.L.; Werner, J.D.; Tran, J.M.; Gates, V.L.; Rikabi, A.A.; Shah, M.H.; Salem, R. Radiation pneumonitis following yttrium-90 radioembolization: Case report and literature review. *J. Vasc. Interv. Radiol.* **2012**, *23*, 669–674. [CrossRef]
82. Tejwani, A.; Wu, S.; Jia, Y.; Agulnik, M.; Millender, L.; Lacouture, M.E. Increased risk of high-grade dermatologic toxicities with radiation plus epidermal growth factor receptor inhibitor therapy. *Cancer* **2009**, *115*, 1286–1299. [CrossRef]
83. Tong, C.C.; Ko, E.C.; Sung, M.W.; Cesaretti, J.A.; Stock, R.G.; Packer, S.H.; Forsythe, K.; Genden, E.M.; Schwartz, M.; Lau, K.H.; et al. Phase II trial of concurrent sunitinib and image-guided radiotherapy for oligometastases. *PLoS ONE* **2012**, *7*, e36979. [CrossRef]
84. Kao, J.; Packer, S.; Vu, H.L.; Schwartz, M.E.; Sung, M.W.; Stock, R.G.; Lo, Y.C.; Huang, D.; Chen, S.H.; Cesaretti, J.A. Phase 1 study of concurrent sunitinib and image-guided radiotherapy followed by maintenance sunitinib for patients with oligometastases: Acute toxicity and preliminary response. *Cancer* **2009**, *115*, 3571–3580. [CrossRef]
85. Chen, S.W.; Lin, L.C.; Kuo, Y.C.; Liang, J.A.; Kuo, C.C.; Chiou, J.F. Phase 2 study of combined sorafenib and radiation therapy in patients with advanced hepatocellular carcinoma. *Int. J. Radiat. Oncol. Biol. Phys.* **2014**, *88*, 1041–1047. [CrossRef] [PubMed]
86. Zeng, K.L.; Tseng, C.L.; Soliman, H.; Weiss, Y.; Sahgal, A.; Myrehaug, S. Stereotactic Body Radiotherapy (SBRT) for Oligometastatic Spine Metastases: An Overview. *Front. Oncol.* **2019**, *9*, 337. [CrossRef] [PubMed]
87. De Rose, F.; Franceschini, D.; Reggiori, G.; Stravato, A.; Navarria, P.; Ascolese, A.M.; Tomatis, S.; Mancosu, P.; Scorsetti, M. Organs at risk in lung SBRT. *Phys. Med.* **2017**, *44*, 131–138. [CrossRef] [PubMed]
88. Ma, L.; Wang, L.; Tseng, C.L.; Sahgal, A. Emerging technologies in stereotactic body radiotherapy. *Chin. Clin. Oncol.* **2017**, *6*, S12. [CrossRef]

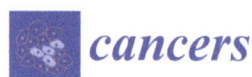

Article

Preoperative Planning Using Three-Dimensional Multimodality Imaging for Soft Tissue Sarcoma of the Axilla: A Pilot Study

Xiang Fang [1,†], Yan Xiong [1,†], Fang Yuan [2], Senlin Lei [1], Dechao Yuan [1], Yi Luo [1], Yong Zhou [1], Li Min [1], Wenli Zhang [1,*], Chongqi Tu [1] and Hong Duan [1]

1. Department of Orthopedics, Orthopedic Research Institute, West China Hospital, Sichuan University, Chengdu 610041, China; xiangfang@stu.scu.edu.cn (X.F.); luyibingli@163.com (Y.X.); lsl867172079@126.com (S.L.); lzyxyncszxyyydc@163.com (D.Y.); orthop_luoyi@163.com (Y.L.); changfshn@163.com (Y.Z.); jacky-min@163.com (L.M.); tcqbonetumor@163.com (C.T.); duanhong1970@126.com (H.D.)
2. Department of Radiology, West China Hospital, Sichuan University, Chengdu 610041, China; yuanfang@wchscu.cn
* Correspondence: zwlbox@163.com; Tel.: +86-18980606875
† These authors contributed equally to this work.

Simple Summary: Soft tissue sarcoma (STS) of the axilla, with its proximity to vital neurovascular bundles and occasional involvement, is a challenge for surgeons. Conventionally, surgeons need to build the whole tumour model with its adjacent anatomical structures by absorbing necessary information from each separate preoperative 2D and 3D image, which is very experience-demanding and potentially inaccurate. Therefore, a computer-generated 3D tumour model revealing tumour and adjacent key anatomical structures from multimodal images was developed, and we attempted to explore whether this digital model could facilitate surgical planning and outcomes for axillary STS. This study suggested significantly better performance in reducing surgical blood loss, operative time, and length of hospital stay. Considering that the surgeries were performed by two specialists with 15 years of experience, the real-world benefit might be even greater, especially for less-experienced STS surgeons. Therefore, this technology might change how preoperative planning is performed for complex STS in the future.

Abstract: Axillary soft tissue sarcoma (STS) is challenging due to its proximity to vital neurovascular bundles. We conducted a prospective observational pilot study to explore whether 3D multimodality imaging (3DMMI) can improve preoperative planning for and surgical outcomes of patients with axillary STS. Twenty-one patients with STS (diameter > 5 cm) of the axilla were allocated, at their discretion, to either a control group undergoing traditional preoperative planning with separate computed tomography angiography, magnetic resonance imaging, and magnetic resonance neurography, or an intervention group where 3DMMI, digitally created based on these images, revealed the tumour and adjacent skeletomuscular and neurovascular structures in three dimensions. Primary outcome measures were surgical margins and surgical complications. Secondary outcomes included operative time, blood loss, serum C-reactive protein and interleukin-6, length of hospital stay, and limb function. The 3DMMI group had a lower, although not significantly different, inadvertent positive margin rate (1/12 vs. 3/9, $p = 0.272$), a significantly shorter operative time ($p = 0.048$), reduced blood loss ($p = 0.038$), and reduced length of hospital stay ($p = 0.046$). This endorses larger trials to improve complex surgical procedures and study how preoperative planning could be performed in the future.

Keywords: axilla; soft tissue sarcoma; magnetic resonance neurography; surgical margin

Citation: Fang, X.; Xiong, Y.; Yuan, F.; Lei, S.; Yuan, D.; Luo, Y.; Zhou, Y.; Min, L.; Zhang, W.; Tu, C.; et al. Preoperative Planning Using Three-Dimensional Multimodality Imaging for Soft Tissue Sarcoma of the Axilla: A Pilot Study. *Cancers* 2022, 14, 3185. https://doi.org/10.3390/cancers14133185

Academic Editor: Robert J. Canter

Received: 4 June 2022
Accepted: 12 June 2022
Published: 29 June 2022

Publisher's Note: MDPI stays neutral with regard to jurisdictional claims in published maps and institutional affiliations.

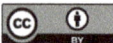

Copyright: © 2022 by the authors. Licensee MDPI, Basel, Switzerland. This article is an open access article distributed under the terms and conditions of the Creative Commons Attribution (CC BY) license (https://creativecommons.org/licenses/by/4.0/).

1. Introduction

Soft tissue sarcomas (STS) encompass over 100 histologic subtypes, accounting for 1% of all adult malignancies [1]. In 2018, approximately 13,040 individuals were diagnosed with STS in the USA, with an estimated 5150 deaths [2]. The most common subtypes are leiomyosarcoma, liposarcoma, and undifferentiated pleomorphic sarcoma, whereas the most common primary sites are extremities (43%), trunk (13%), and retroperitoneum (7%) [3]. Despite a multidisciplinary approach, the cornerstone treatment is surgical resection, in which en bloc resection with wide surgical margins is standard procedure [4,5].

Axillary STS has unique management challenges due to its proximity to important neurovascular structures. This makes wide surgical margins almost impossible and increases the risk of functional morbidity. Appropriate preoperative planning by experienced surgeons may reduce the risk of margin contamination and neurovascular injury. However, only a few studies have reported surgical improvement from the perspective of preoperative planning through imaging modalities [6–9]. Magnetic resonance imaging (MRI) and magnetic resonance neurography (MRN) are used for local staging and preoperative planning, especially regarding tumour location and its adjacent neural structures, usually in two dimensions (2D), whereas computed tomography (CT) plays a role in revealing vascular structures and calcified lesions in three dimensions (3D). In conventional surgical planning, the surgeon relies on these mixed 2D and 3D images to construct the tumour and its adjacent anatomical structures in the brain, which might be inaccurate, requires a high cognitive load, and demands very high experience.

3D multimodality imaging (3DMMI) is generated by radiologists using image registration and segmentation algorithms based on each imaging modality, where different images synergistically contribute to a more reliable computer-generated objective tumour building. Currently, 3DMMI is applied in neurosurgery, radiation therapy, and bone oncology surgery, where is demonstrates promising efficacy in clinical practice [10–13]. However, no relevant STS studies have been performed. This study aimed to report a pilot real-world experience with 3DMMI for the surgical treatment of axillary STS.

2. Materials and Methods

2.1. Study Design and Eligibility

This prospective observational study compared preoperative planning based on 3DMMI to traditional images for the surgical treatment of axillary STS. The ethical committee of our institution approved the study protocol (No. 2019-1062). This study followed the Strengthening the Reporting of Observational Studies in Epidemiology reporting guidelines (Figure 1) and was conducted in compliance with the ethical standards of our hospital and the Helsinki Declaration.

Eligibility requirements included biopsy-proven, resectable axillary STS, tumour diameter > 5 cm, age > 14 years, and a clinical course aimed at curative limb salvage surgery. The exclusion criteria were severe systemic disease and intolerance to surgery. Informed consent was obtained from all participants or their guardians.

2.2. Allocation and Management

The patients were allocated to two cohorts (3DMMI and non-3DMMI groups) at their own discretion. Each patient was evaluated by a multidisciplinary team of pathologists, radiologists, orthopaedic oncologists, radiation oncologists, and medical oncologists. Based on the biopsy histotypes, preoperative chemotherapy was administered in selected cases. Preoperative radiation therapy was indicated if an oncologically appropriate surgical margin was difficult to obtain [14].

Preoperative local imaging, including contrast-enhanced CT angiography and MRI, and MRN, was performed for all patients. For contrast-enhanced CT angiography, a multi-slice helical CT (SOMATOM Definition Flash, Siemens Healthcare, Erlangen, Germany) scan was performed with a slice thickness of 1 mm to generate plain scan images and artery and venous phase images. For contrast-enhanced MRI, using a 3.0-T MR scanner (MAGNETOM Skyra, Siemens Healthcare, Erlangen, Germany) with an 8-channel receive coil, a conventional T1 VIBE enhanced sequence was performed to generate T1 enhanced images to assist the registration process. Then, a T2W turbo spin echo (TSE) sampling perfection with application-optimised contrasts using different flip angle evolution (SPACE) sequences in the same MR device was prescribed for MRN in a coronal plane with the following parameters: echo time (TE) 195 ms; repetition time (TR) 3500 ms; inversion time 220 ms; flip angle 120; matrix size 512 × 512; field of view (FOV) 384 mm; slice thickness 1 mm.

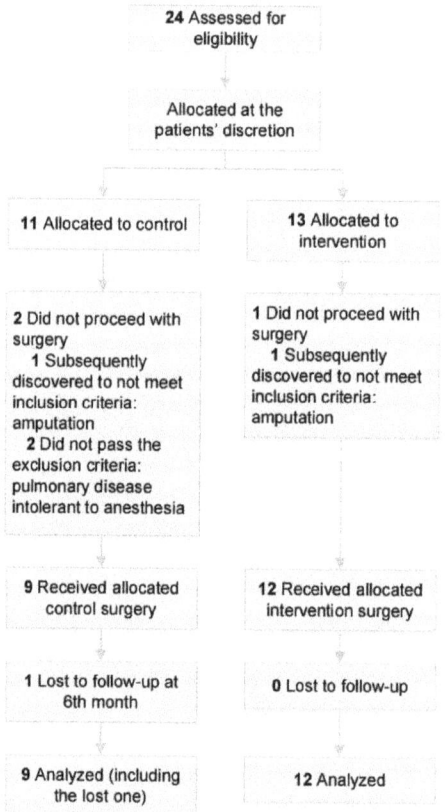

Figure 1. Flow of participants in the study of preoperative planning using 3D-multimodality imaging for soft tissue sarcoma of the axilla.

Preoperative planning and the definitive surgery were conducted by one of two surgeons (H.D. and C.T.) with over 15 years of experience in STS. In the 3DMMI group, the planning was conducted based on 3DMMI, whereas in the non-3DMMI group, it was conducted based on conventional planning using separate 2D or 3D images.

The intra- and postoperative treatment protocols were similar between groups. Gross dissection was conducted through normal tissue planes without tumour contamination, with reference to the preoperative planning. For tumours adjacent to bone, the periosteum was removed. For cortical or medullary invasion, the affected bone segment was resected or reimplanted after sterilisation. For tumours close to major vessels, the vessels were not resected if the underlying structures were grossly intact after adventitia removal [14]. Otherwise, major vessels were replaced with a great saphenous vein graft or artificial vessels. The major nerves were always retained, and the perineurium was removed if the nerves were immediately adjacent to the tumour.

Postoperative radiation therapy was indicated and recommended for patients with all positive surgical margins and stage II, IIIA, and IIIB extremity STS, according to the American Joint Committee on Cancer (AJCC) [14]. Chemotherapy was also considered for specific STS histotypes. The patients were followed up at two weeks and 1, 3, 6, and every 3 to 6 months thereafter in the outpatient department. Chest CT and axillary MRI were performed to detect lung metastasis and local recurrence, respectively.

2.3. Model Preparation and Use

In the 3DMMI group, MRI and MRN were mapped to CT in register using affine and diffeomorphic registration algorithms in advanced normalisation tools [11]. The tumour and adjacent critical structures were segmented with level-set, region-grow, and threshold control in 3D Slicer 4.11 (www.slicer.org, accessed on 20 March 2022) [15]. Quality assurance and manual correction were performed to achieve registration accuracy > 95% and a maximum segmentation error < 2 mm compared with the original DICOM data. The time spent on model preparation was recorded.

The model included the bones (scapula, clavicle, humerus, and ribs), tumour, major neurovascular structures (at least those adjacent to the tumour), muscles (segmented as much as possible), enlarged lymph nodes (if any), and bone oedema (if any), which were reviewed by surgeons using smartphones or computers (Figures 2 and 3).

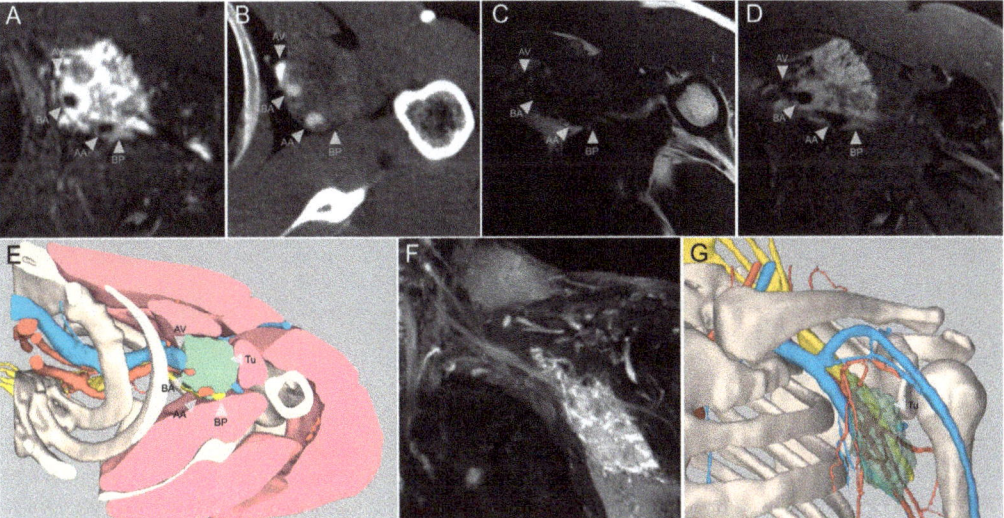

Figure 2. Classic images and their 3D reconstructions in a patient with axillary Ewing's sarcoma. (**A**) MR hydrography image; (**B**) CT angiography image; (**C**) T1-weighted MRI; (**D**) T2-weighted MRI; (**E**) multimodality 3D reconstruction image with similar axial views as (**A–D**); (**F**) coronary view of MR hydrography image; (**G**) anterior view image of multimodality 3D reconstruction. Traditional surgical planning (control group) relies on classic images (**A–D, F**) alone, whereas the 3D multimodality image group has additional 3D reconstructions based on these classic images. Abbreviations: AV, axillary vein; BA, brachial artery; AA, axillary artery; BP, brachial plexus; Tu, tumour.

2.4. Data Collection and End-Point Selection

The patient enrolment period was between November 2019 and December 2020, whereas data collection was from November 2019 to June 2021. Clinical baseline data included sex, age, tumour size, histology type, Fédération Nationale des Centres de Lutte

Contre le Cancer (FNCLCC) grading, stage, and neurovascular involvement [16]. Tumour size was recorded as the maximum diameter according to the preoperative cross-sectional images. Neurovascular involvement was defined as ≥1/2 complete encasement as a preoperative image finding, whereas simple microvascular or perineural invasion identified in the final pathological specimen was excluded.

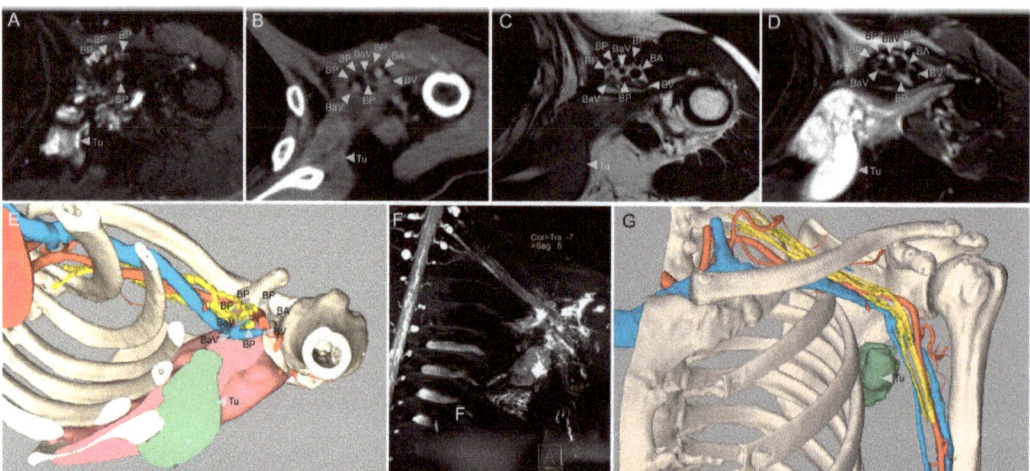

Figure 3. Classic images and their 3D reconstructions in a patient with liposarcoma. (**A**) MR hydrography image; (**B**) CT angiography image; (**C**) T1-weighted MRI; (**D**) T2-weighted MRI; (**E**) multimodality 3D reconstruction image with similar axial views as (**A–D**); (**F**) coronary view of MR hydrography image; (**G**) anterior view image of multimodality 3D reconstruction. Abbreviations: BA, brachial artery; BaV, basilic vein; BV, brachial vein; BP, brachial plexus; Tu, tumour.

The primary endpoints were the surgical margins and complications. The surgical margins were first documented by surgeons and later confirmed by an expert sarcoma pathologist using the Toronto Margin Context Classification (TMCC) [17–19]. The margins were classified into four categories: negative margins (R0 according to AJCC residual tumour classification); inadvertent positive margins (IPMs); planned close, but with an ultimately positive microscopic margin along a major bone or neurovascular structure; and positive margins after a second resection for patients treated initially elsewhere with inadequate margins. Surgical complications included injury to neurovascular structures and wound complications. Vascular injury was defined as an intraoperative inadvertent major vessel injury necessitating suture repair, and nerve injury as new postoperative limb function morbidity.

The secondary endpoints were operative time, blood loss, serum index of systemic inflammation, length of hospital stay, and limb function. Operative time and blood loss were dichotomised as less or more than the 75th percentile in both. The serum index of systemic inflammation encompassed C-reactive protein (CRP) and interleukin-6 (IL-6) levels recorded preoperatively and two days postoperatively to reflect the magnitude of surgical trauma [20,21]. Limb function was assessed using the Musculoskeletal Tumour Society (MSTS) and the Disabilities of the Arm, Shoulder, and Hand (DASH) scores both preoperatively and at six months postoperatively [22,23].

2.5. Statistical Analysis

Sample size calculation was not performed due to the limited availability of previously published data. Continuous variables were tested for normality using the Shapiro–Wilks test and presented as means (standard deviation) if normally distributed and were otherwise expressed as medians (interquartile range). Categorical variables were presented as proportions (percentage). Between-group comparisons were assessed using the independent-sample t-test for continuous variables and the Mann–Whitney U test and Fisher's exact test for categorical variables. R version 3.5.3 (R Foundation for Statistical Computing, Vienna, Austria) was used for the analyses; a two-sided $p < 0.05$ indicated statistical significance

2.6. Protocol Updates

This study was initially registered involving all bone and soft tissue tumours. Patients aiming for palliative surgery or amputation procedures were excluded to reduce heterogeneity in this report. The secondary indicator, tumour volume, was updated to the tumour size recorded at the maximum diameter during the first enrolment of the patient, since it was difficult to measure the volume in the non-3DMMI group. Performance status, another secondary indicator, was removed after the fifth enrolled case due to its low relevance.

3. Results

Between November 2019 and December 2020, 24 patients with axillary STS were identified, of which three were excluded (one had severe chronic pulmonary disease intolerant to anaesthesia and the other two underwent amputation after admission). Twenty-one patients (nine male, mean [standard deviation] age, 43.8 [16.0] years) were enrolled in this analysis, with nine in the non-3DMMI group and 12 in the 3DMMI group. The baseline characteristics indicating no statistical differences between groups are listed in Table 1.

Table 1. Baseline characteristics between groups who underwent limb salvage surgery with and without 3DMMI-based preoperative planning.

Characteristic	Participants, No. (%)		p Value
	Non-3DMMI (n = 9)	3DMMI (n = 12)	
Age, mean (SD), y	45.2 (18.8)	42.8 (14.3)	0.736 [d]
Male			>0.999 [e]
Male	4 (44)	5 (42)	
Female	5 (56)	7 (58)	
Histological type			0.885 [e]
Synovial sarcoma	2 (22)	3 (25)	
Liposarcoma	2 (22)	3 (25)	
Rhabdomyosarcoma	2 (22)	2 (17)	
Undifferentiated pleomorphic sarcoma	1 (11)	2 (17)	
Angiosarcoma	1 (11)	0	
Ewing	0	1 (8)	
Malignant fibrous histiocytoma	1 (11)	1 (8)	
FNCLCC grade			0.904 [f]
1	1 (11)	1 (8)	
2	3 (33)	4 (33)	
3	5 (56)	7 (58)	
Tumour Size [a], median (interquartile range), cm	8 (5.0)	8 (4.8)	0.902 [f]
Neurovascular Involvement			
Vessel	4 [b] (44)	4 [c] (33)	0.673 [e]
Nerve	5 [b] (56)	5 [c] (42)	0.670 [e]
Tumour Stage			0.864 [f]
IB	1 (11)	1 (8)	
IIIA	6 (67)	8 (67)	
IIIB	2 (22)	3 (25)	

[a] Tumour size was recorded at maximum diameter; [b] three patients had both vessel and neural involvement; [c] three patients had both vessel and neural involvement; [d] Student's T-test; [e] Fisher's exact test; [f] Wilcoxon rank sum test.

There were no statistically significant differences in the overall surgical margins ($p = 0.379$), IPM (1/12 vs. 3/9, $p = 0.272$), intraoperative complications ($p = 0.429$), and postoperative wound complications ($p = 0.788$). Moreover, there were no significant differences ≥75th percentile vs. <75th operative time percentile ($p = 0.331$) and blood loss ($p = 0.159$), or second postoperative day serum CRP ($p = 0.586$) and IL-6 levels ($p = 0.367$) between the groups. Further, MSTS and DASH showed no statistically significant differences ($p = 0.416$, and $p = 0.517$, respectively) at six months postoperatively. There were significant differences in operative time ($p = 0.048$), blood loss ($p = 0.038$), and length of stay ($p = 0.046$) (Table 2). One patient in each group underwent major vessel replacement for underlying gross tumour involvement, and no clavicle osteotomies were performed. The median time spent on model preparation was 3.5 h (range, 3.0–4.0 h) per patient.

Table 2. Comparative outcomes between groups who underwent limb salvage surgery with and without 3DMMI-based preoperative planning.

Outcome	Non-3DMMI (n = 9)	3DMMI (n = 12)	p Value
Surgical margin, No. (%)			0.379 [a]
Negative	3 (33)	5 (42)	
Planned close	3 (33)	6 (50)	
IPM	3 (33)	1 (8)	0.272 [b]
Surgical complications			
Intraoperative, vascular injury	3	1	0.429 [b]
Intraoperative, nerves injury	0	0	
Postoperative, wound complication	0	1	0.788 [b]
Operative time, mean (SD), min			
Mean (SD)	134.4 (35.75)	101.7 (34.60)	0.048 [c]
Median (IQR)	120 (60)	95 (37.5)	
≥75th percentile, participants, No. (%) [d]	4 (44)	2 (17)	0.331 [b]
Blood loss (mL)			
Mean (SD)	338.9 (89.4)	258.3 (76.4)	0.038 [c]
Median (IQR)	350 (150)	250 (100)	
≥75th percentile, participants, No. (%) [d]	5 (56)	2 (17)	0.159 [b]
Serum index of systemic inflammation			
CRP, preoperative, median (IQR), mg/L	3.77 (2.00)	3.99 (1.52)	0.602 [a]
IL-6, preoperative, median (IQR), pg/mL	2.56 (1.49)	2.86 (1.67)	0.754 [a]
CRP, at 2nd day, mean (SD), mg/L	40.11 (13.97)	37.63 (6.05)	0.586 [c]
IL-6, at 2nd day, mean (SD), pg/mL	36.56 (11.98)	32.89 (5.98)	0.367 [c]
Length of in-hospital stay, median (IQR)	8 (1.5)	7 (1)	0.046 [a]
Limb function			
MSTS, preoperative, median (IQR)	90 (13)	93 (9.3)	0.270 [a]
DASH, preoperative, median (IQR)	8 (18)	7.5 (10)	0.430 [a]
MSTS, at 6th month, median (IQR)	93 (8.5)	95 (7.0)	0.416 [a]
DASH, at 6th month, median (IQR)	8 (9)	5.5 (8.75)	0.517 [a]

[a] Wilcoxon rank sum test; [b] Fisher exact test; [c] Student's T-test; [d] 75th percentiles are defined as 150 min for operative time and 350 mL for blood loss. Abbreviations: IPM, inadvertent positive margins; CRP, C-reactive protein; IL-6, interleukin–6.

The median follow-up duration was 10 months (range, 6–18 months). One patient in the non-3DMMI group was lost to follow-up at six months postoperatively. No statistical differences were observed in MSTS (preoperative vs at six months) for the non-3DMMI ($p = 0.063$), 3DMMI group ($p = 0.063$), and DASH ($p = 0.156$, and $p = 0.055$).

4. Discussion

Axillary STS is challenging to resect because of its proximity to vital neurovascular bundles and occasional involvement. The literature related to axillary STS is limited since most studies have reported small cohorts of patients with STS in the axilla grouped with other locations [24–28]. Moreover, most of these studies emphasised patient demographics and treatment outcomes. However, this study explored ways to improve surgical outcomes from the perspective of preoperative planning based on multimodal images, which revealed these critical anatomical structures in 3D. The study found that 3DMMI can improve preoperative planning and surgical outcome for patients with axillary STS by reducing operative time, blood loss, and length of hospital stay and alleviating the risk of inadvertent residuals. Therefore, surgeons should consider 3D reconstruction from multimodal images when dealing with complicated STS, especially with neurovascular involvement.

A successful surgery depends mainly on the surgeon's skills and knowledge of anatomy. While the skills may remain constant, the anatomy varies owing to innate or tumour-related variations. Although sarcoma specialists may accomplish a limb salvage STS surgery well, even with large unexpected intraoperative anatomical variations, less experienced surgeons are more likely to injure the nerves and vessels or have prolonged operative time, especially in highly complicated cases. Therefore, preoperative images are used to detect these potential unexpected variations and tumour surroundings. In standard preoperative planning, surgeons need to recognise key anatomical structures from each image and roughly form an image of the tumour in the brain, and if necessary, communicate with radiologists in words, which is the usual method of so-called transdisciplinary collaboration. Despite being technically more capable of reading images than surgeons, especially young ones, radiologists cannot describe the image in complete detail, since words are always less intuitive and informative than a 3D representation. Hence, in a conventional setting when relying on the rough classic tumour image, surgeons may still face significant uncertainty, with unexpected details uncovered intraoperatively. However, most potential challenges can be resolved preoperatively rather than as an unexpected intraoperative encounter, based on improved preoperative planning using 3DMMI processed by a radiologist. This 3D image serves as the best tool for connecting surgeons and radiologists and facilitates better transdisciplinary teamwork. Surgeons may easily devise an improved surgical approach with a more detailed knowledge of patient-specific 3D anatomy, including the tumour and all adjacent critical structures, resulting in a minimised risk of major neurovascular injury and less time spent in dissection.

Apart from providing comprehensive knowledge of patient-specific anatomy, 3DMMI could also help with tailored individualised preoperative planning that can hardly be done with conventional separate images or which can be done in only a very rough manner. While surgeons have been trained to mentally integrate anatomical structures from different imaging modalities, a fused digital display of multimodal images is far more informative and diagnostically reliable [29]. Surgeons could design a detailed 3D surgical approach with this digital 3DMMI, including through which layer of anatomical structure the dissection/resection should be performed, in which plane the dissection should be performed with an involved major nerve or vessels, whether to perform an osteotomy to help the resection, and the exact position for the osteotomy. A recent study by Sambri et al. observed an increased local recurrence risk for STS close to major vessels immediately adjacent to or surrounded by the tumour, as compared with indirect vascular proximity to the tumour, indicating individualised limb salvage procedures [30]. To provide better local control and limit unnecessary trauma, 3DMMI can intuitively and easily help identify the surgical needs of patients, that is, whether to preserve or resect a major vessel and the appropriate site/length of resection, if necessary. The aforementioned preoperative planning can be difficult even for some experienced STS specialists, whereas, in most cases, especially among young and inexperienced surgeons, the surgical plan is designed after visualising the tumour surroundings intraoperatively. Therefore, with 3DMMI, the incidence of local recurrence associated with poor preoperative planning and operative time can be decreased, particularly for less experienced surgeons.

To evaluate outcomes related to surgical planning, TMCC was used to assess the resection margin, as it has a unique role in IPM residuals [18]. In this study, the percentage of IPMs in the 3DMMI group was a quarter of that in the non-3DMMI group (1/12 vs. 3/9); however, the difference was not statistically significant. We presumed that this was due to the small sample size. Nevertheless, this pilot study provides a rational basis for future multi-centre trials.

Achieving local control cannot not solely define a successful limb salvage STS operation; surgical metrics are also important. Despite similarities in intraoperative complications, inflammation index, and limb function between the two groups, operative time and blood loss were significantly improved in the 3DMMI group. Since it was impossible to limit bleeding in the axillary region by a tourniquet, faster surgery with a clear surgical field was necessary. By revealing critical anatomical structures and their relationships in 3D, 3DMMI facilitated preoperative decisions may help minimise surgical challenges related to uncertain anatomical parameters, especially in highly complicated cases, resulting in reduced operative time and intraoperative blood loss. Additionally, a shorter length of hospital stay was also observed, which may limit various potential in-hospital complications and additional costs, and may save healthcare resources [31]. Therefore, preoperative planning based on 3DMMI is promising for successful STS surgery in this setting.

In addition to the potential benefits previously mentioned for patients and hospitals, 3DMMI-based preoperative planning may also facilitate a reduced cognitive load on surgeons by simply decreasing the amount of information processing required for both experienced and young surgeons [32]. Cross-sectional images, such as CT and MRI, depict almost every element of the subject's anatomical information in grayscale, including structures irrelevant to surgical decision-making. Extraneous information may affect surgeons' cognition when interpreting imaging. Conversely, redundant structures that are less relevant to surgery are excluded from the 3DMMI representation. The vital structures and their spatial relationships are highlighted and visualised in 3D and colour. Thus, surgeons can focus on devising a personalised surgical plan with ease.

Even though 3DMMI features the advantages discussed above, the deviation between the medical images and the real anatomy of the human body should not be overlooked. Although 3D images may conform to the preoperative images, the different patient's positioning between preoperative imaging and surgery results in a 3D shift of all anatomical structures, especially in the lower limbs. The mean femoral artery shift is 3.28 mm for repeated supine positions and 14.72 mm for supine vs. right lateral decubitus position in the thigh, whereas the displacement of the tibial nerve is much less in the lower leg, ranging from 0.9 to 3.02 mm for all positions [7]. Although the sarcoma-involved neurovascular structures may stay in a relatively constant spatial location with the tumour, it is still recommended to capture preoperative images in the same position as the surgery to reduce the variability, especially when using 3DMMI images for surgical planning for STS from less rigid compartments.

Another issue that should be addressed is the time spent in 3D imaging processing. In this study, the median time was 3.5 h per patient even with semi-automatic algorithms including level-set, region-grow, and threshold control, which is much longer than writing a conventional medical image diagnostic report. However, it was conducted in the image post-processing Centre in our hospital instead of by a single radiologist from the conventional radiology department. We believe that the time spent was highly acceptable considering its benefits to patients, and potential value to personalised radiotherapy planning, rehabilitation procedures, and doctor–patient communication. Nevertheless, automatic algorithms are needed to reduce the time spent for 3D processing in the future.

Our study had some limitations. First, the sample size was small and uncalculated due to limited previously published data, and groups were heterogeneous with different histologies and grades. However, this was a prospective preliminary pilot study exploring the potential of a novel imaging technique for preoperative planning for a group of rare tumours encompassing over 100 histologic subtypes in unusual and challenging locations, which may lay the foundation for our future large-scale trials. Second, the follow-up period was relatively short. Nevertheless, the outcome measures were intraoperative findings and early clinical outcomes, which required a limited follow-up duration. However, follow-up on these patients will be continued and a standard survival analysis with special attention to local recurrence will be performed in the future. Third, the surgical margin was used to assess local control in this study, whereas the correlation between margin and local recurrence remains controversial, particularly in some specific STS histotypes with infiltrative growth patterns, such as myxofibrosarcoma and undifferentiated pleomorphic sarcoma [33–36]. Additionally, the "optimal" margin and its width have been debated in the literature [37]. However, the principal purpose of this preliminary study is to present a potentially useful 3D image-based tool. This may facilitate preoperative planning procedures and minimise unexpected surgical challenges related to neurovascular injury and IPM by giving comprehensive knowledge of patient-specific anatomy. This pilot study did not aim to directly establish correlations between 3DMMI and local recurrence. Nevertheless, our future large-scale trial will focus on local recurrence rather than on surgical margins only. Four, since the surgeries in this study were performed by 15-year-experience experts, the outcome measures and strength of 3DMMI might be underestimated when used by less experienced surgeons.

5. Conclusions

In summary, this study reported a real-world institutional experience of 3DMMI-based preoperative planning for patients with axillary STS, where different images synergistically contributed to more comprehensive guidance for surgical planning in three dimensions, especially for less experienced surgeons. These findings, while still preliminary, may affect the performance of preoperative planning for axillary STS. Furthermore, this planning may benefit patients, surgeons and hospitals in various ways. Improved outcomes for the patients were found, such as less intraoperative blood loss, shorter operative time, and a potentially lower risk of inadvertent residuals. The use of 3DMMI may also provide an intuitive and easy approach to improving surgical planning for surgeons, and hospitals would benefit from a shorter operative time and length of hospital stay. Overall, this pilot study yielded promising results that will support further studies in the future.

Author Contributions: Conceptualisation, X.F., Y.X., F.Y., W.Z. and H.D.; data curation, X.F., S.L., D.Y., Y.L., Y.Z., L.M., W.Z., C.T. and H.D.; funding acquisition, H.D., and Y.X.; methodology, X.F., Y.X. and F.Y.; resources, S.L., D.Y., Y.L., Y.Z., L.M., W.Z., C.T. and H.D.; supervision, W.Z. and H.D.; writing—original draft, X.F., Y.X. and F.Y.; writing—review and editing, X.F., Y.X., F.Y., S.L., D.Y., Y.L., Y.Z., L.M., W.Z., C.T. and H.D. All authors have read and agreed to the published version of the manuscript.

Funding: This work was funded by the West China Hospital Sichuan University Science Funds (NO. 141120752), and Health and Family Planning Commission research project of Sichuan Province (NO. 18PJ465). No benefits in any form have been or will be received from a commercial party directly or indirectly related to the subject of this manuscript.

Institutional Review Board Statement: The study was approved by the ethics committee of the Sichuan University West China Hospital (No. 2019-1062).

Informed Consent Statement: Written informed consent was obtained from all patients before this study. They gave permission for the materials to appear in print and online, and granted permission to third parties to reproduce these materials.

Data Availability Statement: The data presented in this study are available on Zenodo (https://doi.org/10.5281/zenodo.6471584). The corresponding authors will grant readers access to these data on reasonable request.

Acknowledgments: Special thanks to Jianqing Qiu from the Department of Epidemiology and Health Statistics, West China School of Public Health, Sichuan University, China, for the statistical assistance in this study.

Conflicts of Interest: The authors report no conflict of interest in this work.

References

1. Gamboa, A.C.; Gronchi, A.; Cardona, K. Soft-tissue sarcoma in adults: An update on the current state of histiotype-specific management in an era of personalized medicine. *CA Cancer J. Clin.* **2020**, *70*, 200–229. [CrossRef]
2. Siegel, R.L.; Miller, K.D.; Jemal, A. Cancer statistics, 2018. *CA Cancer J. Clin.* **2018**, *68*, 7–30. [CrossRef]
3. Blay, J.Y.; Honoré, C.; Stoeckle, E.; Meeus, P.; Jafari, M.; Gouin, F.; Anract, P.; Ferron, G.; Rochwerger, A.; Ropars, M.; et al. Surgery in reference centers improves survival of sarcoma patients: A nationwide study. *Ann. Oncol.* **2019**, *30*, 1143–1153. [CrossRef]

4. Hassan, H.; Elazar, A.; Takabe, K.; Datta, R.; Takahashi, H.; Seitelman, E. Scalp leiomyosarcoma: Diagnosis and treatment during a global pandemic with COVID-19. *World J. Oncol.* **2021**, *12*, 132–136. [CrossRef]
5. Ata, K.J.; Farsakh, H.N.; Rjoop, A.; Matalka, I.; Rousan, L.A. Alveolar soft part sarcoma of the extremity: Case report and literature review. *World J. Oncol.* **2014**, *5*, 47–51. [CrossRef]
6. Verga, L.; Brach Del Prever, E.M.; Linari, A.; Robiati, S.; De Marchi, A.; Martorano, D.; Boffano, M.; Piana, R.; Faletti, C. Accuracy and role of contrast-enhanced CT in diagnosis and surgical planning in 88 soft tissue tumours of extremities. *Eur. Radiol.* **2016**, *26*, 2100–2108. [CrossRef]
7. Kaiser, D.; Hoch, A.; Kriechling, P.; Graf, D.N.; Waibel, F.; Gerber, C.; Müller, D.A. The influence of different patient positions on the preoperative 3D planning for surgical resection of soft tissue sarcoma in the lower limb-a cadaver pilot study. *Surg. Oncol.* **2020**, *35*, 478–483. [CrossRef]
8. Li, L.; Zhang, K.; Wang, R.; Liu, Y.; Zhang, M.; Gao, W.; Ren, B.; Zhou, X.; Cheng, S.; Li, J. A study of three-dimensional reconstruction and printing models in two cases of soft tissue sarcoma of the thigh. *Int. J. Comput. Assist. Radiol. Surg.* **2021**, *16*, 1627–1636. [CrossRef]
9. Shemesh, S.S.; Garbrecht, E.L.; Rutenberg, T.F.; Conway, S.A.; Rosenberg, A.E.; Pretell-Mazzini, J. Unplanned excision of soft tissue sarcoma: Does it impact the accuracy of intra-operative pathologic assessment at time of re-excision? *Int. Orthop.* **2021**, *45*, 298–2991. [CrossRef]
10. Yu, Z.; Zhang, W.; Fang, X.; Tu, C.; Duan, H. Pelvic reconstruction with a novel three-dimensional-printed, multimodality imaging based endoprosthesis following enneking type I + IV resection. *Front. Oncol.* **2021**, *11*, 629582. [CrossRef]
11. Fang, X.; Yu, Z.; Xiong, Y.; Yuan, F.; Liu, H.; Wu, F.; Zhang, W.; Luo, Y.; Song, L.; Tu, C.; et al. Improved virtual surgical planning with 3D- multimodality image for malignant giant pelvic tumors. *Cancer Manag. Res.* **2018**, *10*, 6769–6777. [CrossRef]
12. Grajales, D.; Kadoury, S.; Shams, R.; Barkati, M.; Delouya, G.; Béliveau-Nadeau, D.; Nicolas, B.; Le, W.T.; Benhacene-Boudam, M.K.; Juneau, D.; et al. Performance of an integrated multimodality image guidance and dose-planning system supporting tumor-targeted HDR brachytherapy for prostate cancer. *Radiother. Oncol.* **2021**, *166*, 154–161. [CrossRef]
13. Nowell, M.; Rodionov, R.; Zombori, G.; Sparks, R.; Winston, G.; Kinghorn, J.; Diehl, B.; Wehner, T.; Miserocchi, A.; McEvoy, A.W.; et al. Utility of 3D multimodality imaging in the implantation of intracranial electrodes in epilepsy. *Epilepsia* **2015**, *56*, 403–413. [CrossRef]
14. Network NCC. *Soft Tissue Sarcoma. Version 2.2018. National Comprehensive Cancer Network.* 2018. Available online: https://www.nccn.org/guidelines/guidelines-detail?category=1&id=1464 (accessed on 6 March 2022).
15. Fedorov, A.; Beichel, R.; Kalpathy-Cramer, J.; Finet, J.; Fillion-Robin, J.C.; Pujol, S.; Bauer, C.; Jennings, D.; Fennessy, F.; Sonka, M.; et al. 3D Slicer as an image computing platform for the Quantitative Imaging Network. *Magn. Reson Imaging.* **2012**, *30*, 1323–1341. [CrossRef]
16. Trojani, M.; Contesso, G.; Coindre, J.M.; Rouesse, J.; Bui, N.B.; de Mascarel, A.; Goussot, J.F.; David, M.; Bonichon, F.; Lagarde, C. Soft-tissue sarcomas of adults; study of pathological prognostic variables and definition of a histopathological grading system. *Int. J. Cancer.* **1984**, *33*, 37–42. [CrossRef]
17. Gerrand, C.H.; Wunder, J.S.; Kandel, R.A.; O'Sullivan, B.; Catton, C.N.; Bell, R.S.; Griffin, A.M.; Davis, A.M. Classification of positive margins after resection of soft-tissue sarcoma of the limb predicts the risk of local recurrence. *J. Bone Joint. Surg. Br.* **2001**, *83*, 1149–1155. [CrossRef]
18. Gundle, K.R.; Kafchinski, L.; Gupta, S.; Griffin, A.M.; Dickson, B.C.; Chung, P.W.; Catton, C.N.; O'Sullivan, B.; Wunder, J.S.; Ferguson, P.C. Analysis of margin classification systems for assessing the risk of local recurrence after soft tissue sarcoma resection. *J. Clin Oncol.* **2018**, *36*, 704–709. [CrossRef]
19. O'Donnell, P.W.; Griffin, A.M.; Eward, W.C.; Sternheim, A.; Catton, C.N.; Chung, P.W.; O'Sullivan, B.; Ferguson, P.C.; Wunder, J.S. The effect of the setting of a positive surgical margin in soft tissue sarcoma. *Cancer* **2014**, *120*, 2866–2875. [CrossRef]
20. Zang, Y.F.; Li, F.Z.; Ji, Z.P.; Ding, Y.L. Application value of enhanced recovery after surgery for total laparoscopic uncut Roux-en-Y gastrojejunostomy after distal gastrectomy. *World J. Gastroenterol.* **2018**, *24*, 504–510. [CrossRef]
21. Watt, D.G.; Horgan, P.G.; McMillan, D.C. Routine clinical markers of the magnitude of the systemic inflammatory response after elective operation: A systematic review. *Surgery* **2015**, *157*, 362–380. [CrossRef]
22. Enneking, W.F.; Dunham, W.; Gebhardt, M.C.; Malawar, M.; Pritchard, D.J. A system for the functional evaluation of reconstructive procedures after surgical treatment of tumors of the musculoskeletal system. *Clin. Orthop. Relat. Res.* **1993**, *286*, 241–246. [CrossRef]
23. Hudak, P.L.; Amadio, P.C.; Bombardier, C. Development of an upper extremity outcome measure: The DASH (disabilities of the arm, shoulder and hand) [corrected]. The Upper Extremity Collaborative Group (UECG). *Am. J. Ind. Med.* **1996**, *29*, 602–608. [CrossRef]
24. Bell, R.S.; Ready, J.; Hudson, A.; O'Sullivan, B.; Mahoney, J.; Richards, R.; Davis, A.; Fornasier, V.L. Non-neurogenic soft tissue tumours of the axilla: Prospective review of 16 cases. *J. Surg. Oncol.* **1989**, *42*, 73–79. [CrossRef]
25. Verbeek, B.M.; Kaiser, C.L.; Larque, A.B.; Hornicek, F.J.; Raskin, K.A.; Schwab, J.H.; Chen, Y.L.; Lozano Calderón, S.A. Synovial sarcoma of the shoulder: A series of 14 cases. *J. Surg. Oncol.* **2018**, *117*, 788–796. [CrossRef]
26. Yang, R.S.; Lane, J.M.; Eilber, F.R.; Dorey, F.J.; al-Shaikh, R.; Schumacher, L.Y.; Rosen, G.; Forscher, C.A.; Eckardt, J.J. High grade soft tissue sarcoma of the flexor fossae. Size rather than compartmental status determine prognosis. *Cancer* **1995**, *76*, 1398–1405. [CrossRef]

27. Barr, L.C.; Robinson, M.H.; Fisher, C.; Fallowfield, M.E.; Westbury, G. Limb conservation for soft tissue sarcomas of the shoulder and pelvic girdles. *Br. J. Surg.* **1989**, *76*, 1198–1201. [CrossRef]
28. Karplus, G.; Krasin, M.J.; Rodriguez-Galindo, C.; McCarville, B.; Jenkins, J.; Rao, B.; Spyridis, G.; Spunt, S.L. Retrospective study of the surgical management and outcome of nonrhabdomyosarcoma soft tissue sarcomas of the groin and axilla in children. *J. Pediatr. Surg.* **2009**, *44*, 1972–1976. [CrossRef]
29. Piccinelli, M. Multimodality image fusion, moving forward. *J. Nucl. Cardiol.* **2020**, *27*, 973–975. [CrossRef]
30. Sambri, A.; Caldari, E.; Montanari, A.; Fiore, M.; Cevolani, L.; Ponti, F.; D'Agostino, V.; Bianchi, G.; Miceli, M.; Spinnato, P.; et al. Vascular proximity increases the risk of local recurrence in soft-tissue sarcomas of the thigh-a retrospective MRI study. *Cancers* **2021**, *13*, 6325. [CrossRef]
31. Iezzoni, L.I.; Daley, J.; Heeren, T.; Foley, S.M.; Fisher, E.S.; Duncan, C.; Hughes, J.S.; Coffman, G.A. Identifying complications of care using administrative data. *Med Care.* **1994**, *32*, 700–715. [CrossRef]
32. Shirk, J.D.; Thiel, D.D.; Wallen, E.M.; Linehan, J.M.; White, W.M.; Badani, K.K.; Porter, J.R. Effect of 3-dimensional virtual reality models for surgical planning of robotic-assisted partial nephrectomy on surgical outcomes: A randomized clinical trial. *JAMA Netw. Open.* **2019**, *2*, e1911598. [CrossRef]
33. Sambri, A.; Bianchi, G.; Righi, A.; Ferrari, C.; Donati, D. Surgical margins do not affect prognosis in high grade myxofibrosarcoma. *Eur. J. Surg. Oncol.* **2016**, *42*, 1042–1048. [CrossRef]
34. Sambri, A.; Caldari, E.; Fiore, M.; Zucchini, R.; Giannini, C.; Pirini, M.G.; Spinnato, P.; Cappelli, A.; Donati, D.M.; De Paolis, M. Margin assessment in soft tissue sarcomas: Review of the literature. *Cancers* **2021**, *13*, 1687. [CrossRef]
35. Bianchi, G.; Sambri, A.; Righi, A.; Dei Tos, A.P.; Picci, P.; Donati, D. Histology and grading are important prognostic factors in synovial sarcoma. *Eur. J. Surg. Oncol.* **2017**, *43*, 1733–1739. [CrossRef]
36. Sambri, A.; Bianchi, G.; Cevolani, L.; Donati, D.; Abudu, A. Can radical margins improve prognosis in primary and localized epithelioid sarcoma of the extremities? *J. Surg. Oncol.* **2018**, *117*, 1204–1210. [CrossRef]
37. Bilgeri, A.; Klein, A.; Lindner, L.H.; Nachbichler, S.; Knösel, T.; Birkenmaier, C.; Jansson, V.; Baur-Melnyk, A.; Dürr, H.R. The effect of resection margin on local recurrence and survival in high grade soft tissue sarcoma of the extremities: How far is far enough? *Cancers* **2020**, *12*, 2560. [CrossRef]

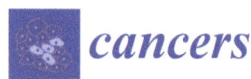

Article

Nomogram Predicting the Risk of Postoperative Major Wound Complication in Soft Tissue Sarcoma of the Trunk and Extremities after Preoperative Radiotherapy

Zhengxiao Ouyang [1,2], Sally Trent [3], Catherine McCarthy [2], Thomas Cosker [2], Duncan Whitwell [2], Harriet Branford-White [2] and Christopher Leonard Maxime Hardwicke Gibbons [2,*]

1. Department of Orthopedics, The Second Xiangya Hospital, Central South University, Changsha 410011, China
2. Nuffield Orthopaedic Centre, Oxford University Hospital Foundation Trust, Oxford OX3 7LD, UK
3. Department of Oncology, Churchill Hospital, Oxford University Hospital Foundation Trust, Oxford OX3 7LE, UK
* Correspondence: max.gibbons@ouh.nhs.uk; Tel.: +44-(0)7811186627

Simple Summary: Preoperative radiotherapy increases the risk of postoperative wound complication in the treatment of soft tissue sarcoma. This retrospective study evaluated risk factors and aimed to develop a nomogram for predicting major wound complication requiring secondary surgical intervention. We found that age, tumour size, and metastasis at presentation were independent risk factors of major wound complication. The nomogram constructed in the study effectively predicts and quantifies the risk of major wound complication.

Abstract: Preoperative radiotherapy increases the risk of postoperative wound complication in the treatment of soft tissue sarcoma (STS). This study aims to develop a nomogram for predicting major wound complication (MaWC) after surgery. Using the Oxford University Hospital (OUH) database, a total of 126 STS patients treated with preoperative radiotherapy and surgical resection between 2007 and 2021 were retrospectively reviewed. MaWC was defined as a wound complication that required secondary surgical intervention. Univariate and multivariate regression analyses on the association between MaWC and risk factors were performed. A nomogram was formulated and the areas under the Receiver Operating Characteristic Curves (AUC) were adopted to measure the predictive value of MaWC. A decision curve analysis (DCA) determined the model with the best discriminative ability. The incidence of MaWC was 19%. Age, tumour size, diabetes mellitus and metastasis at presentation were associated with MaWC in the univariate analysis. Age, tumour size, and metastasis at presentation were independent risk factors in the multivariate analysis. The sensitivity and specificity of the predictive model is 0.90 and 0.76, respectively. The AUC value was 0.86. The nomogram constructed in the study effectively predicts the risk of MaWC after preoperative radiotherapy and surgery for STS patients.

Keywords: soft tissue sarcoma; wound complication; preoperative radiotherapy; nomogram; limb preservation

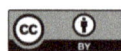

1. Introduction

Radiotherapy (RT) combined with surgery can reduce the risk of recurrent disease in high-grade soft tissue sarcoma (STS) and is the standard recommended treatment [1,2]. With the timing of RT, preoperative RT has several potential advantages over postoperative RT in reducing long-term function impairment (fibrosis, joint stiffness, fracture) with lower radiation dose and field, the ability to evaluate tumour response, and without treatment delay or cancellation [3,4]. While preserving the maximal function of the limb with preoperative RT, postoperative acute wound complications occur in 9–35% of cases, which is much lower in postoperative RT [5], and remain a major concern in the management of STS patients [6,7].

With the improvement of orthopaedic wound care techniques, the management of most postoperative wounds no longer requires surgical intervention, which has facilitated the use of preoperative RT [5,8]. Wound complications requiring repeat surgery attributed to preoperative RT is a significant concern for surgeons and one that significantly affects patients' quality of life. Thus, with an increasing demand for accurate and personalized risk assessment in major wound complication (MaWC), doctors require comprehensive and disease-specific knowledge. In this study, we aim to investigate the preoperative risk factors that relate to MaWC in patients with STS after preoperative RT, and to construct a nomogram to identify patients who are at a particularly high risk of MaWC and, ultimately, require reoperation and prolonged wound management.

2. Materials and Methods

A retrospective review of STS cases was carried out using the database of Oxford University Hospitals (OUH). After obtaining approval from our institutional review board and written informed consent from all patients, clinical, imaging and pathological data from 126 patients who underwent preoperative RT and resection of high-grade STS in the limb and trunk at Nuffield Orthopaedic Centre between 2007 and 2021 were collected. A total of 224 patients treated with postoperative RT, without surgery, or with retroperitoneal sarcoma were excluded. Positron emission tomography with fluorodeoxyglucose integrated with computed tomography (PET/CT) was used for disease staging preoperatively. All patients received preoperative RT with a total dose of 50 gray (Gy) in 25 daily fractions of 2 Gy each, five days a week. Surgery was performed between 3 and 6 weeks after the completion of preoperative RT. Following surgery, the patients were evaluated weekly until the wound was completely healed, then reviewed every 3 months for 2 years and every six months thereafter.

The data collected included patient gender, body mass index (BMI), smoking status, use of alcohol, mental status (depression and anxiety) and comorbidities (diabetes), as well as tumour site, size, volume, depth, histological subtype, maximum standardized uptake value (SUVmax) of PET/CT, metastasis at presentation and surgery type. Depression and anxiety were diagnosed by a GP (General Practitioner) before admission and recorded by nurses (the measurement of depression and anxiety self-assessment quiz is provided in the Supplementary File S1). Smoking and alcohol consumption data were collected by trained nurses and roughly classified as smoker or non-smoker and alcohol drinker or non-drinker if the patients had any historical smoking or drinking records. The tumour size was determined by the measurement of the maximal cross-sectional diameter obtained on axial magnetic resonance imaging (MRI). The tumour site was subdivided into upper extremity, proximal lower extremity, distal lower extremity and trunk. The tumour depth was evaluated as deep or superficial to fascia. The tumour volume was measured on planning three-dimensioned imaging before RT. Wound complication such as haematoma, seroma, erythema, infection, wound dehiscence and lymphoedema that ultimately required secondary surgery necessitating general anaesthesia, drainage of hematoma, wound debridement, drainage of seroma, secondary wound closure or orthoplastic composite flap repair were considered MaWC.

The characteristics of patients were displayed as counts (percentage) for categorical variables and mean (standard deviation) for continuous variables, and the p values were derived using the chi-square test and t-test, respectively. A univariate and multivariate logistic regression analysis was applied to find the significant risk variables for MaWC. Variables with p value < 0.05 in the univariate analysis were included in the multivariable analysis. The diagnostic odds ratio (OR) and 95% confidence interval (CI) of each independent factor were calculated. All variables were included for building the nomogram for predicting MaWC. A bootstrapping approach was used for internal validation on the original study sample. A receiver operating characteristic (ROC) curve was applied to evaluate model discrimination and tested using bootstrap resampling (500 times). A calibration curve was employed to assess the calibration of the nomogram [9]. All analyses were performed using Empower (R) (http://www.empowerstats.com (accessed on 28 May 2022), X&Y solutions, Inc., Boston, MA, USA) and R (http://www.R-project.org, accessed on 21 August 2022) [9]. Statistical tests with p value < 0.05 were considered significant.

3. Results

Patients were followed postoperatively for an average of 71.82 months (range, 10–186 months). Among the 126 patients, 24 cases had MaWC after preoperative RT and surgery, and the incidence of MaWC was 19% (24/126). The mean age was 62 years with 68.5 in the MaWC group and 57.9 in the non-MaWC group. The mean BMI was 28.7 with 27.4 in the MaWC group and 28.9 in the non-MaWC group. The most common tumour site was the proximal lower limb in both groups. Most tumours were located deep in the tissue (80.2%) with 80.4% in the non-MaWC group and 79.2% in the MaWC group. With respect to the mean tumour volume and SUVmax, it appears that they were much higher in the MaWC group than in the non-MaWC group (710.1 cm^3 vs. 434.6 cm^3, 19.6 vs. 13.9); however, they showed non-significance after the univariate analysis. The tumour size in the MaWC group was larger than in the non-MaWC group (13 vs. 9.5 cm). The most common histology subtype was unclassified pleomorphic sarcoma in both groups. There were 8.7% patients with metastasis at presentation, and this proportion was higher in the MaWC group compared with the non-MaWC group (20.8% vs. 5.9%). Most patients experienced primary closure (92.9%). It seems that more patients in the MaWC group experienced plastic surgery closure compared with the non-MaWC group (16.7% vs. 4.9%), but without significance after the univariate analysis. There were four patients who experienced R1 resection, but no significant difference could be seen in the comparison between the two groups (4.2% vs. 2.9%). Table 1 summarizes the clinical and pathological characteristics of the patients.

Table 1. Baseline characteristic of patients.

Category	Total, n	Non-MaWC n, %	MaWC, n, %	p-Value
Number of patients	126	102 (81.0%)	24 (19.0%)	
Gender				0.741
Female	51 (40.5%)	42 (41.2%)	9 (37.5%)	
Male	75 (59.5%)	60 (58.8%)	15 (62.5%)	
Mean age (year)	62.0	57.9 ± 17.1	68.5 ± 15.4	0.009
Mean BMI	28.7	28.9 ± 7.2	27.4 ± 5.9	0.361
Diabetes				0.048
Non-diabetes	110 (87.3%)	92 (90.2%)	18 (75.0%)	
Diabetes	16 (12.7%)	10 (9.8%)	6 (25.0%)	
Smoking				0.127
Non-smoking	80 (63.5%)	68 (66.7%)	12 (50.0%)	
Smoking	46 (36.5%)	34 (33.3%)	12 (50.0%)	
Alcohol				0.179
Non-alcohol	43 (34.1%)	32 (31.4%)	11 (45.8%)	
Alcohol	83 (65.9%)	70 (68.6%)	13 (54.2%)	
Depression or anxiety				0.467
Non-depression or anxiety	115 (91.3%)	94 (92.2%)	21 (87.5%)	
Depression or anxiety	11 (8.7%)	8 (7.8%)	3 (12.5%)	
Tumour site				0.181
Upper limb	11 (8.7%)	11 (10.8%)	0 (0.0%)	
Proximal lower limb	75 (59.5%)	60 (58.8%)	15 (62.5%)	
Distal lower limb	19 (15.1%)	13 (12.8%)	6 (25.0%)	
Trunk	21 (16.7%)	18 (17.6%)	3 (12.5%)	

Table 1. Cont.

Category	Total, n	Non-MaWC n, %	MaWC, n, %	p-Value
Tumour depth				0.892
Deep	101 (80.2%)	82 (80.4%)	19 (79.2%)	
Superficial	25 (19.8%)	20 (19.6%)	5 (20.8%)	
Mean tumour volume (mean ± SD, cm^3)	434.6	376.1 ± 173.7	710.1 ± 240.2	0.065
Mean tumour size (mean ± SD, cm)	10.2 ± 6.0	9.5 ± 5.3	13.0 ± 7.9	0.018
PETCT SUVmax (Mean ± SD)	15.0 ± 13.8	13.9 ± 9.7	19.6 ± 16.7	0.090
Histology type				0.686
Myxoid liposarcoma	23 (18.3%)	19 (18.6%)	4 (16.7%)	
Other liposarcoma	8 (6.4%)	5 (4.9%)	3 (12.5%)	
Myxoidfibrosarcoma	19 (15.1%)	16 (15.7%)	3 (12.5%)	
Synovial sarcoma	11 (8.7%)	10 (9.8%)	1 (4.2%)	
Undifferentiated pleomorphic sarcoma	13 (10.3%)	11 (10.8%)	2 (8.3%)	
Leiomyosarcoma	12 (9.5%)	11 (10.8%)	1 (4.2%)	
Unclassified pleomorphic sarcoma	25 (19.8%)	20 (19.6%)	5 (20.8%)	
Unclassified spindle-cell sarcoma	6 (4.8%)	4 (3.9%)	2 (8.3%)	
Others	9 (7.1%)	6 (5.9%)	3 (12.5%)	
Metastasis at presentation				0.028
Non-metastasis	115 (91.3%)	96 (94.1%)	19 (79.2%)	
Metastasis	11 (8.7%)	6 (5.9%)	5 (20.8%)	
Type of surgery				0.066
Primary closure	117 (92.9%)	97 (95.1%)	20 (83.3%)	
Plastic surgery closure	9 (7.1%)	5 (4.9%)	4 (16.7%)	
Surgery margin				0.758
R0	122 (96.8%)	99 (97.1%)	23 (95.8%)	
R1	4 (3.2%)	3 (2.9%)	1 (4.2%)	

Others including rhabdomyosarcoma, malignant peripheral nerve sheath tumour, angiosarcoma.

After univariate and multivariate study, we found that age (OR: 1.04, 95%CI: 1.01–1.08, p = 0.009); diabetes (OR: 3.07, 95%CI: 1.01–9.71, p = 0.048); metastasis at presentation (OR: 4.21, 95%CI:1.17–15.22, p = 0.028); and tumour size (OR: 1.09, 95% CI: 1.01–1.17, p = 0.018) are risk factors in the univariate analysis. Age (OR: 1.08, 95%CI: 1.02–1.13, p = 0.004); metastasis at presentation (OR: 9.12, 95%CI: 1.21–68.67, p = 0.032); and tumour size (OR: 1.12, 95%CI: 1.01–1.24, p = 0.032) are independent risk factors of MaWC in the multivariate study. The variables for the univariate and multivariate study are summarized in Table 2. All the variates that could be evaluated preoperatively (age, gender, tumour site, SUVmax, metastasis at presentation, BMI, diabetes, smoking, alcohol, type of surgery, tumour size and tumour depth) were included in the predictive model and were incorporated into the nomogram. Due to the limited number of cases, when we set the tumour site according to four locations as we previously analysed, the nomogram could not be modelled. Thus, the tumour site was set as the lower limb vs. other location in nomogram 1, and proximal lower limb vs. other location in nomogram 2. As PETCT is not uniformly used worldwide and factors such as smoking, use of alcohol, anxiety and depression are not quantitatively defined, we built a simplified nomogram 3 without PETCT and these parameters.

Table 2. Univariate and multivariate analysis of significant predictors of wound complications.

Risk Factor	Univariate Analysis			Multivariable Analysis		
	OR	95%CI	p-Value	OR	95%CI	p-Value
Age	1.04	1.01–1.08	0.009	1.08	1.02–1.13	0.004
Diabetes	3.07	1.01–9.71	0.048	2.46	0.57–10.42	0.226
Metastasis at presentation	4.21	1.17–15.22	0.028	9.12	1.21–68.67	0.032
Tumour size (cm)	1.09	1.01–1.17	0.018	1.12	1.01–1.24	0.032

The ROC curve for the predictive nomograms 1 and 2 are presented in Figure 1. The area under the ROC curve (AUC) and the corresponding 95% CI were estimated by bootstrap resampling (times = 500). It was 0.855 (95% CI: 0.770–0.917) with a sensitivity and specificity of 0.905 and 0.750 in nomogram 1 and 0.831 (95% CI: 0.742–0.898) with a sensitivity and specificity of 0.762 and 0.794 in nomogram 2, respectively. To further evaluate the discriminative ability and net benefits of the two models, a decision curve analysis (DCA) was performed. The DCA results of the two nomograms are shown in Figure 2. In general, nomogram 1 showed the highest net benefit. Therefore, nomogram 1 exhibited the best accuracy for risk prediction and the highest net benefit. Based on model 1 (Figure 3), the predictive model formula was as follows:

$$\text{Logit (MaWC)} = -10.32344 - 0.75211 \times \text{gender} + 0.07223 \times \text{age} + 2.01095 \times \text{site} + 0.04656 \times \text{SUVmax} + 2.60662 \times \text{metastasis at presentation} - 0.00630 \times \text{BMI} + 0.88274 \times \text{smoking} + 0.40016 \times \text{diabetes} + 1.86011 \times \text{depression or anxiety} - 0.16794 \times \text{alcohol} + 1.37350 \times \text{type of surgery} + 0.08594 \times \text{tumour size} - 0.29359 \times \text{tumour depth} \quad (1)$$

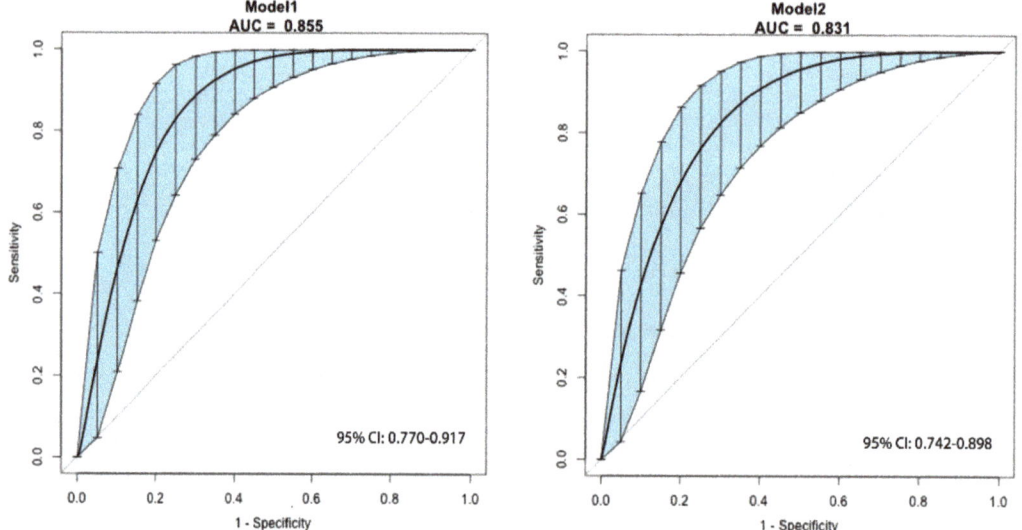

Figure 1. The ROC curve for the predictive model 1 and 2 using bootstrap resampling (times = 500). Shading shows the bootstrap estimated 95% CI with the AUC. ROC, receiver operating characteristic; AUC, area under the curve; CI, confidence interval.

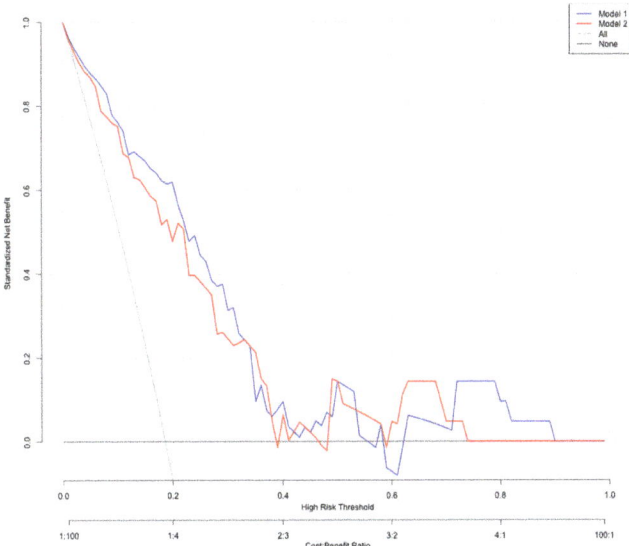

Figure 2. Decision curve analysis results of the nomograms. Net benefit curves of two predictive models. "None" line means net benefit when no participant is considered as having the outcome (major wound complication); "All" line means net benefit when all participants are considered as having the outcome. The preferred model is the model with the highest net benefit at any given threshold.

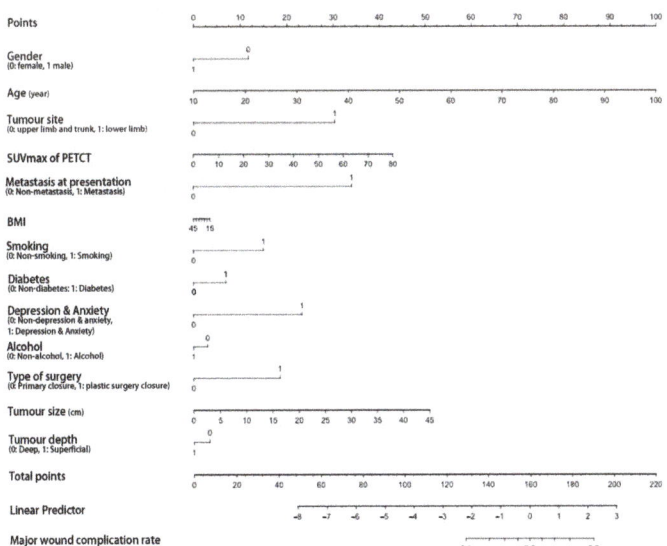

Figure 3. Nomogram 1 for prediction of postoperative major wound complication after preoperative radiotherapy and surgery. The point of each predictor could be assessed at the first line (Points) and the total points then could be calculated by summing up the points of each predictor and identified on the penultimate line. At last, the rate of MaWC could be assessed by the corresponding total points at the last line. BMI, body mass index.

The ROC curve for the predictive nomograms 3 are presented in Figure 4 and the area under the ROC curve (AUC) and the corresponding 95% CI were 0.822 (95% CI: 0.732–0.893) with a sensitivity and specificity of 0.917 and 0.637, respectively. Based on model 3 (Figure 5), the predictive model formula was as follows:

$$\text{Logit (MaWC)} = -7.23569 - 0.19839 \times \text{gender} + 0.04977 \times \text{age} + 1.91307 \times \text{site} + 2.27947 \times \text{metastasis at presentation} - 0.01091 \times \text{BMI} + 0.40016 \times \text{diabetes} + 1.92471 \times \text{type of surgery} + 0.07427 \times \text{tumour size} - 0.35312 \times \text{tumour depth} \quad (2)$$

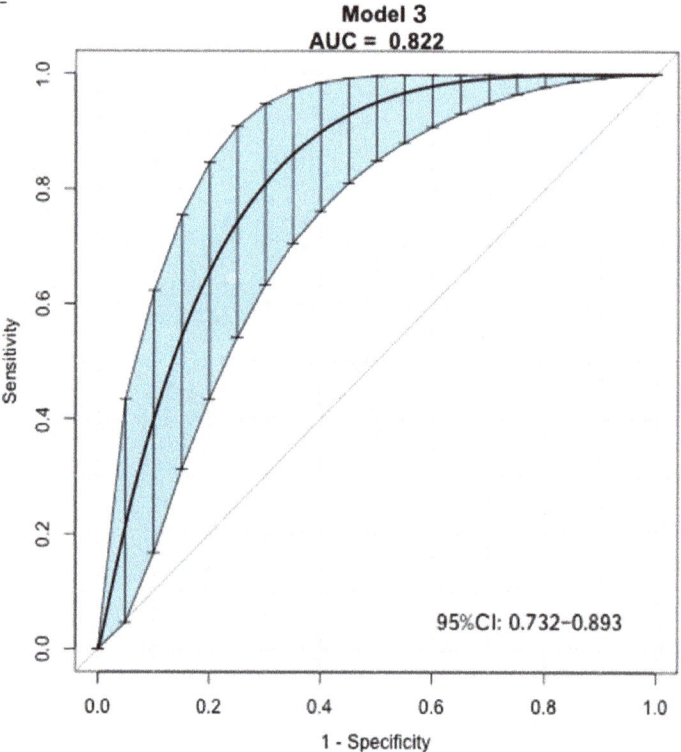

Figure 4. The ROC curve for the nomogram 3 using bootstrap resampling (times = 500). Shading shows the bootstrap estimated 95% CI with the AUC. ROC, receiver operating characteristic; AUC, area under the curve; CI, confidence interval.

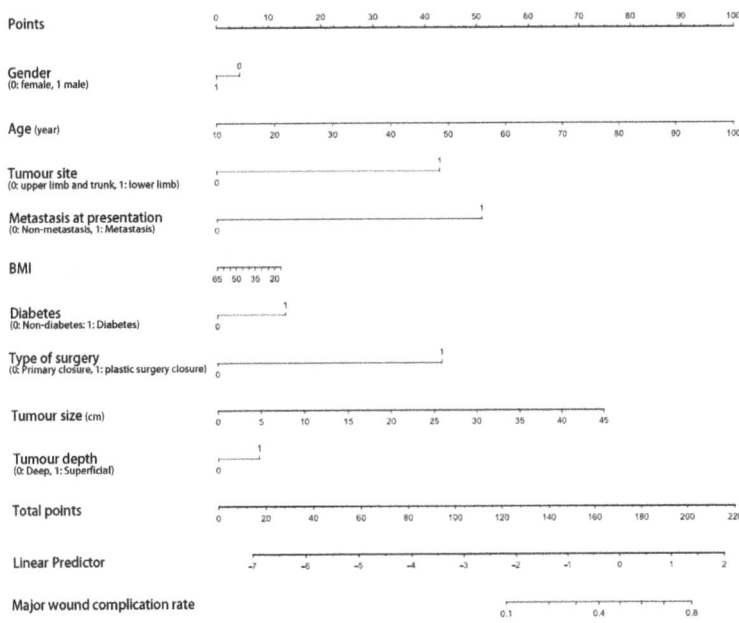

Figure 5. Nomogram 3 (without smoking, use of alcohol, anxiety and depression, SUVmax of PET-CT) for prediction of postoperative major wound complication after preoperative radiotherapy and surgery.

4. Discussion

Previous studies showed that RT combined with surgery could significantly reduce the rate of local recurrence in high-grade STS [4,5], meaning that the completion of the local treatment of STS is of utmost importance. In postoperative RT studies, it is reported that 15% of patients did not complete the combination treatment as planned due to MaWC [3]. A 12-week delay rate in receiving postoperative RT is 26% reported by Casabianca et al. [10] and 15% reported by Miller et al. [11]. In respect of oncological prognosis, preoperative RT would be preferable for the completion of local treatment without interruption from wound complication. However, the high risk of postoperative wound complication in preoperative RT compared with postoperative RT remains a substantial challenge [7,12,13]. With respect to the quality of life, function and oncologic outcomes, it is believed that MaWC needing a secondary procedure should be assessed separately. As with the development of integrated wound care, most wound complications have little effect on patients' daily life. In this study, the rate of MaWC is 19%, which is consistent with the rate of 18% reported by Hui et al. [14], and is slightly higher than reported by Rosenberg et al. [15] and O'Sullivan et al. [5]. In these studies, the rate of secondary surgery considered as "a true clinically significant major complication" is 16%. The difference might be due to the different study group, as we only included patients with a high-grade tumour located in the trunk and limb, and they only included limb STS of both high and low grade. Studies also reported the rate of 11% of the secondary operation, in which only patients with a tumour located in the upper limb and who received a lower RT volume were included. Thus, the rate of 19% might be more accurate, according to the guideline which recommended RT application in high-grade sarcoma [1,2].

Given the complex and multifactorial nature of wound complications, recent studies examined whether specific clinical predictors could better identify patients at the greatest risk. Rosenberg et al. reported female gender, radiation outside their institution and low grade as independent risk factors for a secondary operation [15]. In this study, age, diabetes, tumour size and metastasis at presentation are risk factors for MaWC in the univariate analysis. In the multivariate regression analysis, age, metastasis at presentation and tumour size are independent risk factors. It is widely accepted that larger tumours were associated with a higher rate of complications, but there was wide variation in how tumour size was defined, which resulted in a high degree of heterogeneity [6,16]. Thus, tumour volume that was calculated by an oncologist before RT could consider more information than tumour size was also analysed in this study. However, we did not find it a risk factor for MaWC and it was not included in the nomogram, as we tested and found that the nomogram including the tumour volume had a lower AUC compared with the current one. This might because of the limitation of case numbers and the wide range of tumour volume.

To avoid MaWC, studies also suggested the important effect of immediate flap reconstruction on the postoperative wound [16–18], while others found the difference with or without plastic surgery to be non-significant [15,19,20]. Consistent with the latter, we did not find that the type of surgery was a significant risk factor for MaWC. However, for patients with a high risk of MaWC, Moor et al. reported that a substitution of irradiated soft tissue for healthy and well-vascularized soft tissue would be reasonable, especially with a tumour located in the adductor compartment of the thigh [16].

Adam et al. reported that patients with tumours located in the lower extremity with vascular involvement should be considered for immediate vascularized tissue transfer [8], which confirms the important effect of tumour site on MaWC. We did not find that tumour site was a significant risk factor for MaWC. This might be largely due to the stratification method, in which we divided tumour site into four groups according to guidelines, and made some adjustments to the recent literature that considers the proximal lower limb to be the most important risk factor [3,8,16]. As it is difficult to construct a nomogram with such stratification, a two categories method was applied in this study. Both lower limb vs. other location and proximal lower limb vs. other location were applied in the nomogram, and a better AUC was observed in nomogram 1 with the classification of tumour location by lower limb vs. other location.

Metastasis at presentation is an independent risk factor for MaWC. Though it is recommended in guideline [1] that with metastatic disease, surgery and chemotherapy are first-line management, selected patients were treated with preoperative RT and surgery in this study. It is sometimes difficult to confirm whether the suspected lung or other site lesion is metastatic with staging and PETCT. Thus, for patients in which suspected metastatic disease cannot be excluded, caution should be made on MaWC.

With these results, we developed a prediction model to evaluate the MaWC risk in STS patients treated with preoperative RT and resection. Gender, age, smoking, alcohol, BMI, diabetes, depression and anxiety, tumour site, size and depth, SUVmax, metastasis at presentation and type of surgery, which were considered significant risk predictors in previous studies, were included in the model [6]. The AUC of the model is 0.855, indicating a good predictive value for MaWC. To our knowledge, this is the first study describing a nomogram for the prediction of MaWC based on preoperative factors.

This study had limitations. Some data (smoking and the use of alcohol, anxiety and depression) were not clearly and quantitatively defined, and PET-CT is not routinely used in the diagnostic work-up for all STS; thus, we developed a nomogram 3 without these parameters with lower AUC (0.822) for wider application. The data presented may be underpowered to detect a significant association of the variables with MaWC due to the potential for selection bias, particularly with respect to tumour type and for the indication of radiation. As noted previously, patients who underwent preoperative RT were those who were thought to be at a high risk for local recurrence. This was a single-centre multivariate prediction model development study, which may affect the accuracy and generalizability of the results. However, we used bootstrap resampling (time = 500) to estimate the AUC and the corresponding 95% CI to improve the accuracy of the model's predictive value. In future studies, this established model should be applied in a multicentre study to validate its generalizability. The methodology in this study may be practical in clinical research and can be applied in different populations.

5. Conclusions

In conclusion, this study focuses on the impact of multiple personal variables and the synergistic interaction between variables that can increase the rate of postoperative MaWC. Age, tumour size and metastasis at presentation are independent risk factors. The nomogram showing a good predictive value for MaWC is an intuitive tool that provides clinicians with a graphical calculation of each predictor to assess the risk of MaWC. Clinicians can use this model easily and rapidly to clinically evaluate the risk of MaWC and administer an individualized strategy for STS patients.

Supplementary Materials: The following supporting information can be downloaded at: https://www.mdpi.com/article/10.3390/cancers14174096/s1. File S1: Patient Health Questionnaire (PHQ-9).

Author Contributions: Conceptualization, Z.O. and C.L.M.H.G.; methodology, Z.O.; software, Z.O.; validation, S.T., C.M. and C.L.M.H.G.; formal analysis, Z.O.; investigation, Z.O.; resources, S.T.; data curation, Z.O.; writing—original draft preparation, Z.O.; writing—review and editing, S.T., C.M., T.C., D.W. and H.B.-W.; supervision, C.L.M.H.G.; project administration, C.L.M.H.G.; funding acquisition, Z.O. All authors have read and agreed to the published version of the manuscript.

Funding: This research was funded in part by the Visiting Scholar Project from the China Scholar Council, grant number 202006375045, and the Natural Science Foundation of Hunan Province of Outstanding Young Scholars, grant number 2021JJ20086.

Institutional Review Board Statement: The study was conducted in accordance with the Declaration of Helsinki and was internally reviewed by senior management and found to comply with all regulatory requirements. As no regulatory issues were identified, a full ethical review was not required and exempted.

Informed Consent Statement: Informed consent was obtained from all subjects involved in the study. Written informed consent has been obtained from the patients to publish this paper.

Data Availability Statement: The data presented in this study are available on request from the corresponding author. The data are not publicly available due to privacy restrictions.

Acknowledgments: The authors would like to thank Nicholas Athanasou and Barbara Marks for their help with the manuscript.

Conflicts of Interest: The authors declare no conflict of interest. The funders had no role in the design of the study; in the collection, analyses, or interpretation of data; in the writing of the manuscript; or in the decision to publish the results.

References

1. Gronchi, A.; Miah, A.; Dei Tos, A.; Abecassis, N.; Bajpai, J.; Bauer, S.; Biagini, R.; Bielack, S.; Blay, J.; Bolle, S. Soft tissue and visceral sarcomas: ESMO–EURACAN–GENTURIS Clinical Practice Guidelines for diagnosis, treatment and follow-up☆. *Ann. Oncol.* **2021**, *32*, 1348–1365. [CrossRef] [PubMed]
2. von Mehren, M.; Kane, J.M.; Bui, M.M.; Choy, E.; Connelly, M.; Dry, S.; Ganjoo, K.N.; George, S.; Gonzalez, R.J.; Heslin, M.J. NCCN guidelines insights: Soft tissue sarcoma, version 1.2021: Featured updates to the NCCN guidelines. *J. Natl. Compr. Cancer Netw.* **2020**, *18*, 1604–1612. [CrossRef] [PubMed]
3. Rene, N.J.; Castiglioni, A.; Coccaro, N.; Scheitlin, B.; Papa, L. Soft Tissue Sarcomas: Is Pre-operative Radiotherapy Associated With More Acute Wound Complications? *Cureus* **2021**, *13*, e15654. [CrossRef] [PubMed]
4. Kungwengwe, G.; Clancy, R.; Vass, J.; Slade, R.; Sandhar, S.; Dobbs, T.D.; Bragg, T.W.H. Preoperative versus Post-operative Radiotherapy for Extremity Soft tissue Sarcoma: A Systematic Review and Meta-analysis of Long-term Survival. *J. Plast. Reconstr. Aesthet. Surg.* **2021**, *74*, 2443–2457. [CrossRef] [PubMed]
5. O'Sullivan, B.; Davis, A.M.; Turcotte, R.; Bell, R.; Catton, C.; Chabot, P.; Wunder, J.; Kandel, R.; Goddard, K.; Sadura, A.; et al. Preoperative versus postoperative radiotherapy in soft-tissue sarcoma of the limbs: A randomised trial. *Lancet* **2002**, *359*, 2235–2241. [CrossRef] [PubMed]

6. Slump, J.; Bastiaannet, E.; Halka, A.; Hoekstra, H.J.; Ferguson, P.C.; Wunder, J.S.; Hofer, S.O.P.; O'Neill, A.C. Risk factors for postoperative wound complications after extremity soft tissue sarcoma resection: A systematic review and meta-analyses. *J. Plast. Reconstr. Aesthet. Surg.* **2019**, *72*, 1449–1464. [CrossRef] [PubMed]
7. Callaghan, C.M.; Hasibuzzaman, M.M.; Rodman, S.N.; Goetz, J.E.; Mapuskar, K.A.; Petronek, M.S.; Steinbach, E.J.; Miller, B.J.; Pulliam, C.F.; Coleman, M.C.; et al. Neoadjuvant Radiotherapy-Related Wound Morbidity in Soft Tissue Sarcoma: Perspectives for Radioprotective Agents. *Cancers* **2020**, *12*, 2258. [CrossRef] [PubMed]
8. Schwartz, A.; Rebecca, A.; Smith, A.; Casey, W.; Ashman, J., Gunderson, L., Curtis, K., Chang, Y.H.; Beauchamp, C. Risk factors for significant wound complications following wide resection of extremity soft tissue sarcomas. *Clin. Orthop. Relat. Res.* **2013**, *471*, 3612–3617. [CrossRef] [PubMed]
9. Liu, J.; Liang, C.; Wang, X.; Sun, M.; Kang, L. A computed tomography-based nomogram to predict pneumothorax caused by preoperative localization of ground glass nodules using hook wire. *Br. J. Radiol.* **2021**, *94*, 20200633. [CrossRef] [PubMed]
10. Casabianca, L.; Kreps, S.; Helfre, S.; Housset, M.; Anract, P.; Biau, D.J. Optimal post-operative radiation after soft-tissue sarcoma resection is achieved in less than two thirds of cases. *Int. Orthop.* **2017**, *41*, 2401–2405. [CrossRef] [PubMed]
11. Miller, E.D.; Mo, X.; Andonian, N.T.; Haglund, K.E.; Martin, D.D.; Liebner, D.A.; Chen, J.L.; Iwenofu, O.H.; Chakravarti, A.; Scharschmidt, T.J.; et al. Patterns of major wound complications following multidisciplinary therapy for lower extremity soft tissue sarcoma. *J. Surg. Oncol.* **2016**, *114*, 385–391. [CrossRef] [PubMed]
12. Clark, M.A.; Fisher, C.; Judson, I.; Thomas, J.M. Soft-tissue sarcomas in adults. *N. Engl. J. Med.* **2005**, *353*, 701–711. [CrossRef] [PubMed]
13. Elswick, S.M.; Curiel, D.A.; Wu, P.; Akhavan, A.; Molinar, V.E.; Mohan, A.T.; Sim, F.H.; Martinez-Jorge, J.; Saint-Cyr, M. Complications after thigh sarcoma resection. *J. Surg. Oncol.* **2020**, *121*, 945–951. [CrossRef] [PubMed]
14. Hui, A.C.; Ngan, S.Y.; Wong, K.; Powell, G.; Choong, P.F. Preoperative radiotherapy for soft tissue sarcoma: The Peter MacCallum Cancer Centre experience. *Eur. J. Surg. Oncol.* **2006**, *32*, 1159–1164. [CrossRef] [PubMed]
15. Rosenberg, L.A.; Esther, R.J.; Erfanian, K.; Green, R.; Kim, H.J.; Sweeting, R.; Tepper, J.E. Wound complications in preoperatively irradiated soft-tissue sarcomas of the extremities. *Int J. Radiat. Oncol. Biol. Phys.* **2013**, *85*, 432–437. [CrossRef] [PubMed]
16. Moore, J.; Isler, M.; Barry, J.; Mottard, S. Major wound complication risk factors following soft tissue sarcoma resection. *Eur. J. Surg. Oncol.* **2014**, *40*, 1671–1676. [CrossRef] [PubMed]
17. Slump, J.; Hofer, S.O.P.; Ferguson, P.C.; Wunder, J.S.; Griffin, A.M.; Hoekstra, H.J.; Bastiaannet, E.; O'Neill, A.C. Flap reconstruction does not increase complication rates following surgical resection of extremity soft tissue sarcoma. *Eur. J. Surg. Oncol.* **2018**, *44*, 251–259. [CrossRef] [PubMed]
18. Chao, A.H.; Chang, D.W.; Shuaib, S.W.; Hanasono, M.M. The effect of neoadjuvant versus adjuvant irradiation on microvascular free flap reconstruction in sarcoma patients. *Plast. Reconstr. Surg.* **2012**, *129*, 675–682. [CrossRef]
19. Cannon, C.P.; Ballo, M.T.; Zagars, G.K.; Mirza, A.N.; Lin, P.P.; Lewis, V.O.; Yasko, A.W.; Benjamin, R.S.; Pisters, P.W. Complications of combined modality treatment of primary lower extremity soft-tissue sarcomas. *Cancer* **2006**, *107*, 2455–2461. [CrossRef] [PubMed]
20. Temple, C.L.; Ross, D.C.; Magi, E.; DiFrancesco, L.M.; Kurien, E.; Temple, W.J. Preoperative chemoradiation and flap reconstruction provide high local control and low wound complication rates for patients undergoing limb salvage surgery for upper extremity tumors. *J. Surg. Oncol.* **2007**, *95*, 135–141. [CrossRef] [PubMed]

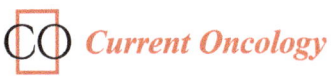

Article

Gastrointestinal Stromal Tumors: 10-Year Experience in Cancer Center—The Ottawa Hospital (TOH)

Abdulhameed Alfagih [1,2,*], Abdulaziz AlJassim [1], Bader Alshamsan [1,3], Nasser Alqahtani [1,4] and Timothy Asmis [1]

1. Division of Medical Oncology, Department of Medicine, The Ottawa Hospital, The University of Ottawa, Ottawa, ON K1H 8L6, Canada
2. Medical Oncology Department, Comprehensive Cancer Center, King Fahad Medical City, Riyadh 11525, Saudi Arabia
3. Department of Medicine, College of Medicine, Qassim University, Qassim 51452, Saudi Arabia
4. King Abdulaziz Hospital, Ministry of National Guard Health Affairs, Al Ahsa 36427, Saudi Arabia
* Correspondence: aalfaqih@kfmc.med.sa

Abstract: (1) Background: The management of gastrointestinal stromal tumors (GIST) has significantly evolved over the last two decades, with the introduction of tyrosine kinase inhibitors (TKI). We aim to report 10 years of experience of GIST management at a regional cancer center in Canada. (2) Methods: We retrospectively analyzed the records of 248 consecutive patients diagnosed with GIST between 2011 and 2021. We describe the clinical and pathological data, management, and outcome, including survival. (3) Results: The most common GIST sites were the stomach 63% (156), followed by the small bowel 29% (73). At diagnosis, 83% (206) of patients had localized disease (stage I–III). According to the modified National Institutes of Health consensus criteria (NIH) for GIST, around 45% (90) had intermediate or high-risk disease. Most patients, 86% (213), underwent curative surgical resection. Forty-nine patients received adjuvant imatinib, while forty-three patients had advanced disease and received at least one line of TKI. With a median follow-up of 47 months, the 5-year recurrence-free survival (RFS) rates for very low and low risk were 100% and 94%, respectively, while those for intermediate and high risk were 84% and 51%, respectively. The 5-year overall survival (OS) rates for very low and low risk were 100% and 94%, while intermediate, high risk, and advanced were 91%, 88%, and 65%, respectively. Using the Kaplan–Meier method, there were statistically significant differences in RFS and OS between NIH risk groups, $p < 0.0005$. In univariate analysis, ECOG, site, mitosis, secondary malignancy, and size were predictors for OS. High mitosis and large size (>5 cm) were associated with worse RFS. (4) Conclusions: Curative surgical resection remains the gold standard management of GIST. Our results are comparable to the reported literature. Further research is needed to explore histology's role in risk stratification and initiating adjuvant TKI.

Keywords: gastrointestinal stromal tumors; GIST; C-Kit; imatinib mesylate; survival

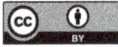

1. Introduction

Gastrointestinal stromal tumors (GIST) are rare non-epithelial tumors derived from mesenchymal tissues. They originate from interstitial Cajal cells or the stem cell precursors of these cells, located around the myenteric plexus throughout the gastrointestinal tract [1,2]. GIST account for 1–3% of all GI tumors. In 1983, two pathologists, Mazur and Clark, introduced the term GIST. Subsequently, further research led to a considerable understanding of the pathogenesis and biology of this type of tumor [3]. Identifying c-KIT mutation was a breakthrough that allowed for better characterization and identification of GIST, based on molecular studies. Further studies of the c-KIT pathway identified many important mutations with clinical and therapeutic significance, including exons 11, 9, 13, and 17 and platelet-derived growth factor receptor alpha gene (PDGFRA) [4,5].

Surgical resection is the standard treatment for localized GIST, while debulking surgery may be considered for symptomatic advanced bulky tumors. For small asymptomatic GIST, watchful waiting may be a reasonable option. The introduction of imatinib, a selective inhibitor of the KIT protein tyrosine kinase, in the management of GIST, revolutionized the treatment approaches [6,7]. Adjuvant imatinib has substantially improved recurrence-free survival in many phase III trials, particularly in the intermediate and high-risk groups [8].

In advanced GIST, many TKIs are shown to improve PFS and OS. In KIT-positive GISTs, imatinib is considered the standard first-line treatment [9]. Resistance due to secondary KIT mutations is expected despite the remarkable responses achieved with imatinib [10]. Sunitinib is an appropriate second-line option for patients who progressed on imatinib or had intolerance or resistance to imatinib [11]. Regorafenib improved PFS, when used after imatinib, and sunitinib failure, based on the phase III GRID trial result [12]. Ripretinib, as a fourth-line therapy, showed improvement in PFS over a placebo in the INVICTUS trial. Many evolving options have improved PFS, based on phase II trials, such as Sorafenib, nilotinib, avapritinib, and dasatinib [13–17].

The management of GIST has had a significant evolution over the last two decades. The data from real world practice from Canada on GIST are limited. Our study aims to report a 10-year experience in the management of GISTs in a regional cancer Centre in Canada- The Ottawa Hospital (TOH).

2. Materials and Methods

This is an observational retrospective cohort study. We identified GIST cases by searching hospital databases using ICD 10 codes. We examined records of all GIST cases referred to/or diagnosed in TOH between 1 January 2011 and 31 December 2021. Only patients with biopsy-proven and immunohistochemistry-confirmed diagnoses of GIST were included in the study. Details of the tumor site, risk assessments, and clinical, pathological, management, and outcomes data were recorded.

Risk assessment was estimated according to modified NIH and Miettinen risk criteria. Data were collected from the electronic medical records (Epic) on the access database. Results were analyzed using MS Excel and SPSS 25.0 software. Descriptive statistics are used to summarize data and synthesize and report patients' demographic and clinico-pathological data. Qualitative variables were analyzed by χ^2 test and Fisher's exact test. Survival data (RFS, PFS, OS) were analyzed using Kaplan–Meier methods and compared by log-rank test. OS was calculated from the date of tissue diagnosis to the date of death or last follow-up. Recurrence-free survival (RFS) was calculated from the date of surgical intervention to the date of recurrence or death or last follow-up. PFS for imatinib was calculated from the date of starting imatinib to the date of confirmed progressive disease (including escalated dose) or death or last follow-up. Potential prognostic factors were analyzed using the Cox proportional hazard model for multivariate analysis. Two-tailed p-values were reported and were considered to be statistically significant when $p < 0.05$.

3. Results

3.1. Patient Characteristics

The patient's' characteristics are shown in Table 1. In total, 248 patients were identified with a median age of 64 (range 28–90); males and females were a 1:1 ratio. An average of 23 cases were diagnosed per year (range 16–32).

Table 1. Baseline patients' characteristics.

		Total n = 248 (Percentage %)	
Age	Median	64 (Range 28–90)	
Gender	Male	124	50%
	Female	124	50%

Table 1. *Cont.*

		Total *n* = 248 (Percentage %)	
Comorbidities	HTN	103	41.5%
	DM	49	19.8%
	DLP	75	30.2%
	GERD	25	10%
	IHD	28	11.3%
	Neurofibromatosis	4	1.6%
	Other	104	42%
Clinical presentation	Incidental	87 *	35%
	Abdominal pain	84	34%
	GI bleeding	59	24%
	Anemia	48	19%
	Bowel obstruction	7	2.8%
	Perforation	3	1.2%
	Other	56	23%
Duration of symptom **	<14 days	41	16.5%
	>14 day	32	12.9%
	>2 months	38	15.3%
	>6 months	32	12.9%
	NA	24	9.7%
ECOG	0	100	40.3%
	1	77	31%
	2	7	2.8%
	3	4	1.6%
	NA	22	8.9%
Mode of initial diagnosis	CT	123	49.5%
	Endoscopy	63	25%
	Surgical exploration	14	5.6%
	EUS	13	5.2%
	MRI	10	4%
	Other	11	4%
Curative surgical resection		213	85.9%

* Eighty-one patients were lacking symptoms, while six patients presented with non-specific abdominal pain (e.g., flank pain). ** not including incidental diagnosis. HTN: hypertension, DM: diabetes mellitus, DLP: dyslipidemia, GERD: gastroesophageal reflux disease, IHD: ischemic heart disease, ECOG: Eastern Cooperative Oncology Group performance status, CT: computed tomography, EUS: endoscopic ultrasound, MRI: magnetic resonance imaging.

3.2. Sites

Sites and pathology data are shown in Table 2. The most common GIST sites were the stomach (156 patients, 63%), followed by the small bowel (73 patients, 29%). Other sites, including the esophagus, appendix, colon and rectum, and mesentery, collectively comprise 8% (19). The duodenum and jejunum represent around 52% of small bowel GIST (*n* = 19, 26% for each), while the ileum represents 17% (13).

Table 2. GIST sites and the pathology data.

		Total n = 248 (Percentage %)	
Site	Esophagus	1	0.4%
	Stomach	156	62.9%
	Small bowel	73	29.4%
	Duodenum	19	7.7%
	Jejunum	19	7.7%
	Ileum	13	5.2%
	Unspecified	22	8.9%
	Appendix	1	0.4%
	Colon	2	0.8%
	Rectum	5	2%
	Diffuse/overlapping	8	3.2%
	Mesentery	2	0.8%
Miettinenrisk class	None	23	11%
	None–rare **	5	2%
	Very low	44	22%
	Low	68	33%
	Moderate	39	19%
	High	24	12%
Modified NIH risk class	Very low	29	14%
	Not defined **	5	2%
	Low	78	38%
	Intermediate	48	24%
	High	42	21%
Histology	Spindle cell	159	64.1%
	Epithelioid	18	7.3%
	Mixed	39	15.7%
	NA *	32	12.9%
Size	<2 cm	37	14.9%
	2–5	91	36.7%
	5–10	70	28.2%
	>10	31	12.5%
	NA	19	7.7%
Mitosis	≤5 hpf	177	71.4%
	>5 hpf	45	18.1%
	NA	26	10.5%
Grade	1	159	64.1%
	2	36	14.5%
	3	5	2%
	Unknown	48	19.4%

Table 2. Cont.

		Total n = 248 (Percentage %)	
	No study	237	95.6%
	Study	11	4.4%
	KIT Exon 11	3	1.2%
Mutation	PDGFR Exon 18	4	1.6%
	PDGFR c.2525A	1	0.4%
	SDHB	2	0.8%
	Other	1	0.4%
	I	131	52.8%
	II	50	20.2%
TNM stage	III	25	10.1%
	IV	32	12.9%
	NA	10	4%

* NA: no available data. ** This category not defined clearly in Miettinen or NIH criteria (size $\leq$ 2 cm, and mitotic rate > 5 per 50 HPFs).

3.3. Clinical Presentation

The most common presentation was an incidental finding during workup for another clinical problem, followed by abdominal pain, representing 35% (87) and 34% (84), respectively. GI bleeding and anemia were the main presenting symptoms, representing 24% (59) and 19% (48), respectively. Only 4% (10) of patients presented with bowel obstruction or perforation. Among those presenting with symptoms, 13% (32) had symptoms for more than six months. Around 17% (41) had acute symptoms (less than 14 days). In addition, 71% (177) of patients had an excellent performance status, ECOG 0 to 1. Three cases had familial GIST. A CT scan made the provisional diagnosis in around half of the cases. Moreover, 30% (76) were diagnosed by either endoscopy or EUS. Nearly 53% (131) had TNM stage I disease at presentation, while 13% (32) had stage IV disease. Using a chi-squared test, there was a statistically significant association between gender* TNM stage ($\chi^2(4)$ = 10.4, p = 0.034) and gender* NIH risk class ($\chi^2(6)$ = 13.5, p = 0.036). Males had more advanced and higher-risk disease compared to females.

3.4. Pathology Data

The majority, 64% (159), had spindle cell histology, followed by mixed and epithelioid histology, 16% (39) and 7% (18), respectively. Very small tumors (less than 2 cm) were found in 15% (37). At the same time, larger tumors of more than 10 cm were seen in 13% (31). The majority has a low mitosis rate—less than five mitoses per HPF, 71% (177).

3.5. Risk Assessment

According to NIH criteria for nonmetastatic GIST, 24% (48) and 21% (42) had intermediate or high-risk diseases. While using the Miettinen criteria, 19% (39) and 12% (24) had moderate or high-risk diseases.

3.6. Molecular Data

Mutation testing is not routinely done. Only 11 patients had mutational analysis. Among them, four have PDGFR mutation, and three have KIT exon 11 mutation.

3.7. Management Data and TKI Use

The OS based on management approach is shown in Figure 1. In total, 86% (n = 213) underwent curative surgical resection, including eight patients with advanced/metastatic disease. Forty-nine patients received adjuvant imatinib. Among the NIH intermediate and high-risk groups (90 patients), only 40 patients (44%) received adjuvant imatinib, and only 15/40 (38%) completed three years of adjuvant imatinib. Seventeen patients (7%) had recurrence after curative treatment, including adjuvant TKI. Thirteen patients were treated with neoadjuvant imatinib. Forty-three patients (17%) received at least one line of palliative TKI. Seven patients received three lines of TKI. TKI use is shown in Table 3.

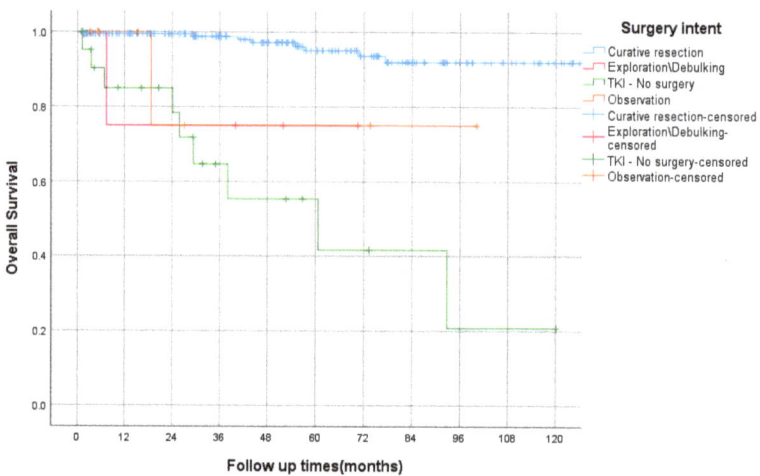

Figure 1. Overall survival based on management approach using Kaplan–Meier curve.

Table 3. Utilization of TKI in the study population.

		Total n = 248 (Percentage %)	
Adjuvant Imatinib		49 *	19.8
Neoadjuvant Imatinib		13	5.2%
Palliative TKI	Imatinib	41	16.5%
	Sunitinib	13	5.2%
	Regorafenib	7	2.8%
	Ripertinib	3	1.2%
	TKI alone (no surgery)	22	8.9%

* Forty patients had intermediate or high-risk disease, while three patients had low risk. Four patients had resected metastatic disease and two patients had unknown risk.

3.8. Survival

The median follow-up was 47 months (range 1–137). The OS, by TNM stage, is shown in Figure 2. In the entire study cohort, death was documented in 18 cases (8%). The 5-years recurrence-free survival (RFS) rates for very low and low risk were 100% and 94%, respectively, while those for intermediate and high risks were 84% and 51%, respectively, as shown in Figure 3. Among the intermediate/high-risk group, patients who did not receive adjuvant imatinib had longer RFS than those who received adjuvant IM with 5-year RFS rates of 89% and 54%, respectively, p = 0.059, HR = 0.34 (95% CI, 0.11–1.04). The median PFS of first-line imatinib was 40 months (95% CI, 12 to 69 months). The 2- and 5-year PFS rates were 51% and 39%, respectively. The 5-year overall survival (OS) rate was 100%, that of very low and low risk was 94%, while those of intermediate, high risk, and advanced were 91%, 88%, and 65%, respectively. Using the Kaplan–Meier method, there were statistically significant differences in RFS and OS between NIH risk groups, both p < 0.0005.

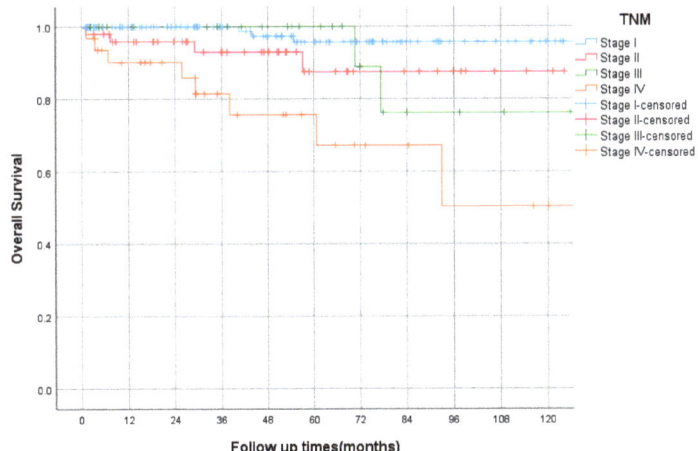

Figure 2. Overall survival by TNM stage using Kaplan–Meier curve.

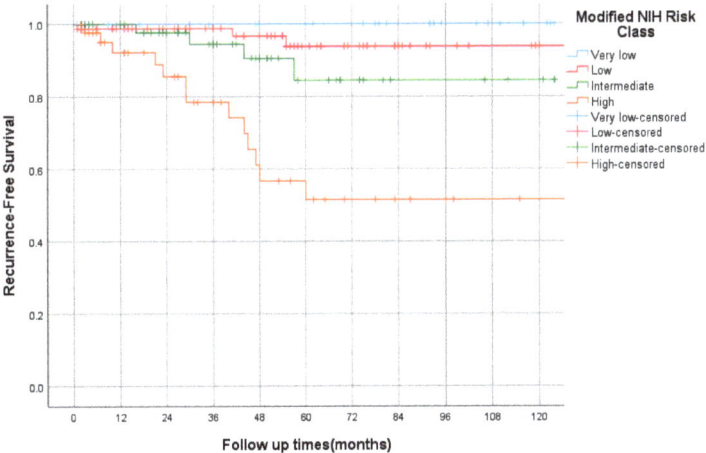

Figure 3. Recurrence-free survival by NIH risk class using Kaplan–Meier curve.

In univariate analysis, ECOG at diagnosis, site, mitosis, secondary malignancy, and size were significant predictors for OS. By multivariate analysis, poor performance status (ECOG 3) was a predictor for shorter OS ($p < 0.005$). The other factors analyzed (patient gender, site, histology, size, mitosis, and presence of secondary malignancy) were insignificant. In univariate and multivariate analysis, high mitosis and large size (>5 cm) were associated with worse RFS, for both $p < 0.002$ and $p < 0.016$, respectively.

4. Discussion

Although many clinical trials evaluate the various treatment options for GIST, available documentation of the outcomes in the real-world data from Canada is limited. The present study explores the outcomes and clinicopathological features of 248 GIST cases treated at the Ottawa Hospital over the past 10 years. In our study, the most common GIST locations were the stomach (63%) and small bowel (29%). Nearly 35% of patients were asymptomatic at the time of diagnosis, and their tumors were found incidentally. This finding is comparable to other reports and could be explained by the small size of the tumors, less than 5 cm, and the indolent course of these tumors [18]. Although males and females were equally distributed, males have a more aggressive and higher-risk disease. In contrast, an Asian study reported higher recurrence or metastasis in females than males [19]. Around 13% presented with de novo metastasis, similar to a study from British Columbia [20].

Unlike solid organ tumors, the behavior of GIST is variable, though it is always malignant if it measures more than 2 cm. Therefore, risk assessment tools were developed to predict malignant potential [21]. Modified NIH and Miettinen criteria are commonly used assessment tools. In this study, nearly 68% and 54% had no or low-risk disease, respectively, using Miettinen and NIH criteria. This is comparable with the described risk classes in other studies [22,23]. There are limited data about the optimal risk assessment tool; however, we observed overlapping between low and moderate risk using Miettinen criteria, while NIH appeared more accurate in predicting the outcome. Epithelioid histology looked to have a more favorable prognosis than spindle cell or mixed histology. However, there is no statistically significant association between type of histology and risk of recurrence ($p = 0.41$).

Surgical resection remains the only curative intervention for localized GIST tumors. Patients with bulky or limited metastases could benefit from surgical management. In this study, around 86% had curative surgical resection with a 5-year survival rate of 94%. This is significantly better than the outcome of surgery in the pre-imatinib era (5-year OS of ~54%) and comparable to reported data in the imatinib era [23,24].

Adjuvant imatinib has substantially improved recurrence-free survival in many phase III trials, particularly in intermediate and high-risk groups. The Scandinavian Sarcoma Group (SSG XVIII/AIO) trial is a phase III trial that compared 36 vs. 12 months of adjuvant imatinib and showed significant improvement in the 5-year RFS and OS rates in patients who received 36 months of adjuvant imatinib compared to 12 months. The 5-year RFS rates were 71.1% vs. 52.3%, respectively; $p < 0.001$; the 5-year OS rates were 91.9% vs. 85.3%, respectively; $p = 0.036$. A recent update showed that the 10-year RFS rates were 52.5% vs. 41.8%, respectively. Further exploratory analysis showed that patients with KIT exon 11 deletion mutations benefit most from the longer duration of adjuvant imatinib [7,8,25,26].

In our study, the 5-year RFS rate for intermediate and high risk were 84% and 51%, respectively, comparable to the clinical trials. However, 56% (50/90) did not receive adjuvant imatinib. Interestingly, by comparing subgroups, we found that patients who received adjuvant IM had a trend toward shorter RFS; however, HR was not significant. Although there is no clear explanation, possible reasons could be the relatively small sample size; shorter adjuvant duration, as only 15/40 (38%) completed three years of adjuvant imatinib; and more inclusion of intermediate risk (35%, 14) in the adjuvant group. At the same time, the no-adjuvant group has a predominantly intermediate risk (68%, 34), a lack of mutational testing, and more deaths than the adjuvant group. Moreover, there was no statistically significant difference in OS between those who did or did not receive adjuvant imatinib, with a p-value of 0.151. This is also similar to the COSOG Z9001 study, a phase III trial that evaluated imatinib 400 mg vs. a placebo for one year, as adjuvant treatment, which did not show OS benefit. Moreover, this emphasizes the importance of 3 years of adjuvant imatinib. Less than three years of adjuvant imatinib were evaluated in the EORTC-62024 study: the 5-year imatinib failure-free survival (IFFS) rate did not reach significance, at 87% vs. 84% (HR, 0.79; 98.5% CI, 0.50–1.25; $p = 0.21$).

Unresectable or metastatic KIT-positive GISTs are common, and imatinib is considered the standard first-line treatment. The Intergroup S0033 study evaluated two doses of imatinib (400 mg daily) vs. a high dose (800 mg) and found that the median OS rates were 55 and 51 months, respectively, after a median follow-up of 4.5 years. The high-dose arm had more grade 3, 4, and 5 toxicities [9]. In this study, the median PFS of first-line imatinib was 40 months (95%CI, 12 to 69 months). The 2- and 5-year PFS rates were 51% and 39%, respectively. These are slightly better than the data reported in the Intergroup S0033 study. Blanke CD et al. reported a 5-year survival rate of 55%, in patients with advanced GIST who were treated with imatinib, regardless of a 400 or 600 mg/d starting dose [27]. In contrast, this study showed that the 5-year overall survival (OS) rate was 65% for the same group of patients; this could be explained by the availability of other TKI options after imatinib failure.

Treatment options for GIST are expanding with evolving sequencing technology. There is growing evidence of the cost-effectiveness of precision-medicine-assisted imatinib treatment, compared with empirical treatment. T. Patterson et al. conducted a population-based study in British Columbia. They found that mutational analysis (MA) was ordered in 41% of patients and MA use increased after 2015, especially in the metastatic setting. In our hospital, MA is not routinely performed; however, despite limited use of MA, OS remains comparable to the reported literature [20,28].

Our study has limitations, including the retrospective design and lack of MA data. It could not collect the complete toxicity data of TKI. Other limitations include the relatively limited sample size, especially for patients who received TKI.

5. Conclusions

Curative surgical resection remains the gold standard management of GIST. Our results are comparable to the reported literature. Further research is needed to explore histology's role in risk stratification and initiating adjuvant TKI.

Author Contributions: A.A. (Abdulhameed Alfagih): conceptual development of the study, literature search, statistical analysis, analysis and interpretation of results, drafting the manuscript, and final approval of the manuscript; A.A. (Abdulaziz AlJassim), B.A. and N.A.: data collection, review of the manuscript, and final approval of the manuscript; T.A.: conceptual development of the study, critical review of the manuscript, and final approval of the manuscript. All authors have read and agreed to the published version of the manuscript.

Funding: This research received no external funding.

Institutional Review Board Statement: The Ottawa Hospital Research Institute (OHRI) approved the study—20210769-01H.

Informed Consent Statement: Patient consent was waived due to the retrospective design of the study.

Data Availability Statement: The data that support the findings of this study are available from the corresponding author upon reasonable request.

Conflicts of Interest: The authors have no relevant financial or non-financial interests to disclose.

References

1. Sircar, K.; Hewlett, B.R.; Huizinga, J.D.; Chorneyko, K.; Berezin, I.; Riddell, R.H. Interstitial Cells of Cajal as Precursors of Gastrointestinal Stromal Tumors. *Am. J. Surg. Pathol.* **1999**, *23*, 377–389. [CrossRef]
2. Corless, C.L.; Barnett, C.M.; Heinrich, M. Gastrointestinal stromal tumours: Origin and molecular oncology. *Nat. Cancer* **2011**, *11*, 865–878. [CrossRef]
3. Mazur, M.T.; Clark, H.B. Gastric stromal tumors Reappraisal of histogenesis. *Am. J. Surg. Pathol.* **1983**, *7*, 507–519. [CrossRef] [PubMed]
4. Hirota, S.; Isozaki, K.; Moriyama, Y.; Hashimoto, K.; Nishida, T.; Ishiguro, S.; Kawano, K.; Hanada, M.; Kurata, A.; Takeda, M.; et al. Gain-of-Function Mutations of c-kit in Human Gastrointestinal Stromal Tumors. *Science* **1998**, *279*, 577–580. [CrossRef]
5. Miettinen, M.; Lasota, J. Gastrointestinal Stromal Tumors: Review on Morphology, Molecular Pathology, Prognosis, and Differential Diagnosis. *Arch. Pathol. Lab. Med.* **2006**, *130*, 1466–1478. [CrossRef] [PubMed]
6. Reichardt, P.; Blay, J.-Y.; Boukovinas, I.; Brodowicz, T.; Broto, J.M.; Casali, P.G.; Decatris, M.; Eriksson, M.; Gelderblom, H.; Kosmidis, P.; et al. Adjuvant therapy in primary GIST: State-of-the-art. *Ann. Oncol.* **2012**, *23*, 2776–2781. [CrossRef] [PubMed]
7. Joensuu, H.; Eriksson, M.; Hall, K.S.; Reichardt, A.; Hermes, B.; Schütte, J.; Cameron, S.; Hohenberger, P.; Jost, P.J.; Al-Batran, S.-E.; et al. Survival Outcomes Associated with 3 Years vs 1 Year of Adjuvant Imatinib for Patients with High-Risk Gastrointestinal Stromal Tumors. *JAMA Oncol.* **2020**, *6*, 1241–1246. [CrossRef]
8. Joensuu, H.; Wardelmann, E.; Sihto, H.; Eriksson, M.; Hall, K.S.; Reichardt, A.; Hartmann, J.T.; Pink, D.; Cameron, S.; Hohenberger, P.; et al. Effect of KIT and PDGFRA Mutations on Survival in Patients with Gastrointestinal Stromal Tumors Treated with Adjuvant Imatinib: An Exploratory Analysis of a Randomized Clinical Trial. *JAMA Oncol.* **2017**, *3*, 602–609. [CrossRef] [PubMed]

9. Blanke, C.D.; Rankin, C.; Demetri, G.D.; Ryan, C.W.; von Mehren, M.; Benjamin, R.S.; Raymond, A.K.; Bramwell, V.H.; Baker, L.H.; Maki, R.G.; et al. Phase III Randomized, Intergroup Trial Assessing Imatinib Mesylate at Two Dose Levels in Patients with Unresectable or Metastatic Gastrointestinal Stromal Tumors Expressing the Kit Receptor Tyrosine Kinase: S0033. *J. Clin. Oncol.* **2008**, *26*, 626–632. [CrossRef]
10. Goettsch, W.G.; Bos, S.; Breekveldt-Postma, N.; Casparie, M.; Herings, R.M.; Hogendoorn, P. Incidence of gastrointestinal stromal tumours is underestimated: Results of a nation-wide study. *Eur. J. Cancer* **2005**, *41*, 2868–2872. [CrossRef] [PubMed]
11. Demetri, G.D.; van Oosterom, A.T.; Garrett, C.R.; Blackstein, M.E.; Shah, M.H.; Verweij, J.; McArthur, G.; Judson, I.R.; Heinrich, M.C.; Morgan, J.A.; et al. Efficacy and safety of sunitinib in patients with advanced gastrointestinal stromal tumour after failure of imatinib: A randomised controlled trial. *Lancet* **2006**, *368*, 1329–1338. [CrossRef]
12. Demetri, G.D.; Reichardt, P.; Kang, Y.-K.; Blay, J.-Y.; Rutkowski, P.; Gelderblom, H.; Hohenberger, P.; Leahy, M.; Von Mehren, M.; Joensuu, H.; et al. Efficacy and safety of regorafenib for advanced gastrointestinal stromal tumours after failure of imatinib and sunitinib (GRID): An international, multicentre, randomised, placebo-controlled, phase 3 trial. *Lancet* **2013**, *381*, 295–302. [CrossRef]
13. Von Mehren, M.; Serrano, C.; Bauer, S.; Gelderblom, H.; George, S.; Heinrich, M.; Schöffski, P.; Zalcberg, J.; Chi, P.; Jones, R.L.; et al. INVICTUS: A phase III, interventional, double-blind, placebo-controlled study to assess the safety and efficacy of ripretinib as fourth-line therapy in advanced GIST who have received treatment with prior anticancer therapies (NCT03353753). *Eur. Soc. Med. Oncol.* **2019**, *30*, v925–v926. [CrossRef]
14. Montemurro, M.; Schöffski, P.; Reichardt, P.; Gelderblom, H.; Schütte, J.; Hartmann, J.; von Moos, R.; Seddon, B.; Joensuu, H.; Wendtner, C.; et al. Nilotinib in the treatment of advanced gastrointestinal stromal tumours resistant to both imatinib and sunitinib. *Eur. J. Cancer* **2009**, *45*, 2293–2297. [CrossRef]
15. Montemurro, M.; Gelderblom, H.; Bitz, U.; Schütte, J.; Blay, J.; Joensuu, H.; Trent, J.; Bauer, S.; Rutkowski, P.; Duffaud, F.; et al. Sorafenib as third- or fourth-line treatment of advanced gastrointestinal stromal tumour and pretreatment including both imatinib and sunitinib, and nilotinib: A retrospective analysis. *Eur. J. Cancer* **2013**, *49*, 1027–1031. [CrossRef]
16. Atiq, M.A.; Davis, J.L.; Hornick, J.L.; Dickson, B.C.; Fletcher, C.D.M.; Fletcher, J.A.; Folpe, A.L.; Mariño-Enríquez, A. Mesenchymal tumors of the gastrointestinal tract with NTRK rearrangements: A clinicopathological, immunophenotypic, and molecular study of eight cases, emphasizing their distinction from gastrointestinal stromal tumor (GIST). *Mod. Pathol.* **2020**, *34*, 95–103. [CrossRef]
17. Kelly, C.M.; Sainz, L.G.; Chi, P. The management of metastatic GIST: Current standard and investigational therapeutics. *J. Hematol. Oncol.* **2021**, *14*, 2. [CrossRef]
18. Mucciarini, C.; Rossi, G.; Bertolini, F.; Valli, R.; Cirilli, C.; Rashid, I.; Marcheselli, L.; Luppi, G.; Federico, M. Incidence and clinicopathologic features of gastrointestinal stromal tumors. A population-based study. *BMC Cancer* **2007**, *7*, 230. [CrossRef]
19. Li, Y.-H.; Shi, Y.-H.; Song, X.-Y.; Wang, H.; Li, M.-Z.; Yang, X.-F.; Wang, T.-Q.; Zhao, Q.-J.; Xu, W.-J.; Dong, P.-D.; et al. Multicenter analysis of gastrointestinal stromal tumors in inner Mongolia of China: A study of 804 cases. *Asian J. Surg.* **2021**, *45*, 718–724. [CrossRef]
20. Patterson, T.; Chai, J.; Li, H.; de Bruyns, A.; Cleversey, C.; Lee, C.-H.; Yip, S.; Simmons, C.; Hart, J.; Pollock, P.; et al. Utilization of Mutational Analysis (MA) in Gastrointestinal Stromal Tumor (GIST) Management in British Columbia (BC) Between January 2008 to December 2017: A Retrospective Population-Based Study. *J. Gastrointest. Cancer* **2021**, *53*, 709–717. [CrossRef]
21. Joensuu, H. Risk stratification of patients diagnosed with gastrointestinal stromal tumor. *Hum. Pathol.* **2008**, *39*, 1411–1419. [CrossRef] [PubMed]
22. Verschoor, A.J.; The PALGA group; Bovée, J.V.M.G.; Overbeek, L.I.H.; Hogendoorn, P.C.W.; Gelderblom, H. The incidence, mutational status, risk classification and referral pattern of gastro-intestinal stromal tumours in the Netherlands: A nationwide pathology registry (PALGA) study. *Virchows Arch.* **2018**, *472*, 221–229. [CrossRef] [PubMed]
23. Wang, M.; Xu, J.; Zhang, Y.; Tu, L.; Qiu, W.-Q.; Wang, C.-J.; Shen, Y.-Y.; Liu, Q.; Cao, H. Gastrointestinal stromal tumor: 15-years' experience in a single center. *BMC Surg.* **2014**, *14*, 93. [CrossRef]
24. DeMatteo, R.P.; Lewis, J.J.; Leung, D.H.Y.; Mudan, S.S.; Woodruff, J.M.; Brennan, M. Two Hundred Gastrointestinal Stromal Tumors. *Ann. Surg.* **2000**, *231*, 51–58. [CrossRef] [PubMed]
25. Joensuu, H.; Eriksson, M.; Hall, K.S.; Hartmann, J.T.; Pink, D.; Schütte, J.; Ramadori, G.; Hohenberger, P.; Duyster, J.; Al-Batran, S.-E.; et al. One vs Three Years of Adjuvant Imatinib for Operable Gastrointestinal Stromal Tumor. *JAMA* **2012**, *307*, 1265–1272. [CrossRef]
26. Joensuu, H.; Eriksson, M.; Hall, K.S.; Reichardt, A.; Hartmann, J.T.; Pink, D.; Ramadori, G.; Hohenberger, P.; Al-Batran, S.-E.; Schlemmer, M.; et al. Adjuvant Imatinib for High-Risk GI Stromal Tumor: Analysis of a Randomized Trial. *J. Clin. Oncol.* **2015**, *34*, 244–250. [CrossRef]
27. Blanke, C.D.; Demetri, G.D.; von Mehren, M.; Heinrich, M.C.; Eisenberg, B.; Fletcher, J.A.; Corless, C.L.; Fletcher, C.D.; Roberts, P.J.; Heinz, D.; et al. Long-Term Results from a Randomized Phase II Trial of Standard-Versus Higher-Dose Imatinib Mesylate for Patients with Unresectable or Metastatic Gastrointestinal Stromal Tumors Expressing KIT. *J. Clin. Oncol.* **2008**, *26*, 620–625. [CrossRef]
28. Feng, M.; Yang, Y.; Liao, W.; Li, Q. Cost-Effectiveness Analysis of Tyrosine Kinase Inhibitors in Gastrointestinal Stromal Tumor: A Systematic Review. *Front. Public Health* **2022**, *9*, 2244. [CrossRef]

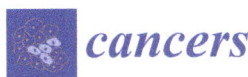

Article

Trabectedin for Patients with Advanced Soft Tissue Sarcoma: A Non-Interventional, Prospective, Multicenter, Phase IV Trial

Viktor Grünwald [1,*], Daniel Pink [2,3], Gerlinde Egerer [4], Enrico Schalk [5], Marinela Augustin [6], Christoph K. W. Deinzer [7], Viola Kob [8], Dietmar Reichert [9], Maxim Kebenko [10], Stephan Brandl [11], Dennis Hahn [12], Lars H. Lindner [13], Mathias Hoiczyk [14], Uta Ringsdorf [15], Lars C. Hanker [16], Dirk Hempel [17], Beatriz De Rivas [18], Tobias Wismann [19] and Philipp Ivanyi [20]

1. Innere Klinik (Tumorforschung) und Klinik für Urologie, Universitätsklinikum Essen, 45147 Essen, Germany
2. Helios Klinikum Bad-Saarow, Klinik für Onkologie und Palliativmedizin, Sarkomzentrum Berlin-Brandenburg, 15526 Bad Saarow, Germany
3. Innere Medizin C, Universitätsmedizin Greifswald, 17489 Greifswald, Germany
4. Klinik für Hämatologie, Onkologie, Rheumatologie, Universitätsklinikum Heidelberg, 69120 Heidelberg, Germany
5. Medical Center, Otto-von-Guericke University Magdeburg, 39106 Magdeburg, Germany
6. Klinikum Nürnberg Nord, Schwerpunkt Onkologie/Hämatologie, Klinik für Innere Medizin 5, Paracelsus Medizinische Privatuniversität, 90419 Nürnberg, Germany
7. Hämatologie und Internistische Onkologie, Medizinische Klinik und Poliklinik II, Universitätsklinikum Würzburg, 97078 Würzburg, Germany
8. Schwerpunktpraxis Hämatologie/Onkologie Volksdorf, MVZ für Immunologie Lokstedt GmbH, 20251 Hamburg, Germany
9. Gemeinschaftspraxis für Hämatologie und Onkologie, Kuhlenstraße 53d, 26655 Westerstede, Germany
10. Klinik für Hämatologie und Onkologie, Universitätsklinikum Schleswig-Holstein, 23538 Lübeck, Germany
11. Überörtliche Gemeinschaftspraxis Bergedorf, 21029 Hamburg, Germany
12. Klinik für Hämatologie, Onkologie und Palliativmedizin, Klinikum Stuttgart, 70174 Stuttgart, Germany
13. Medizinische Klinik und Poliklinik III, LMU Klinikum-Campus Großhadern, 81377 München, Germany
14. Medizinischen Klinik II, Marien-Hospital Wesel gGmbH, 46483 Wesel, Germany
15. Lahn-Dill-Kliniken GmbH, Gynäkologischen Tumorzentrums Lahn-Dill, 35578 Wetzlar, Germany
16. Klinik für Frauenheilkunde und Geburtshilfe (Gynäkologie), Universitätsklinikum Schleswig-Holstein, 23538 Lübeck, Germany
17. Onkologisches Zentrum, 86609 Donauwörth, Germany
18. Medical Affairs, PharmaMar, S.A., Colmenar Viejo, 28770 Madrid, Spain
19. Praxis für Onkologie und Urologie, 26389 Wilhelmshaven, Germany
20. Hämostaseologie, Onkologie und Stammzelltransplantation, Klinik für Hämatologie, Claudia von Schilling Zentrum Comprehensive Cancer Center, Medizinische Hochschule Hannover, 30625 Hannover, Germany
* Correspondence: viktor.gruenwald@uk-essen.de; Tel.: +49-201-723-2637

Citation: Grünwald, V.; Pink, D.; Egerer, G.; Schalk, E.; Augustin, M.; Deinzer, C.K.W.; Kob, V.; Reichert, D.; Kebenko, M.; Brandl, S.; et al. Trabectedin for Patients with Advanced Soft Tissue Sarcoma: A Non-Interventional, Prospective, Multicenter, Phase IV Trial. *Cancers* 2022, *14*, 5234. https://doi.org/10.3390/cancers14215234

Academic Editors: Shinji Miwa, Po-Kuei Wu and Hiroyuki Tsuchiya

Received: 12 September 2022
Accepted: 23 October 2022
Published: 25 October 2022

Publisher's Note: MDPI stays neutral with regard to jurisdictional claims in published maps and institutional affiliations.

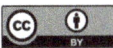

Copyright: © 2022 by the authors. Licensee MDPI, Basel, Switzerland. This article is an open access article distributed under the terms and conditions of the Creative Commons Attribution (CC BY) license (https:// creativecommons.org/licenses/by/ 4.0/).

Simple Summary: Active therapeutic options in advanced soft tissue sarcoma (STS), able to induce durable objective responses, are limited beyond first-line chemotherapy. Although results obtained in clinical trials suggest there is a high probability for patients with STS to benefit from treatment with trabectedin (Yondelis®), there is still a paucity of robust real-life data in more diverse patient populations. The prospective, non-interventional phase IV YON-SAR trial (NCT02367924) was designed to evaluate treatment effects of trabectedin in patients with advanced STS in real-life clinical practice across Germany. The efficacy results of this trial, conducted in 128 patients from 19 sites across Germany, further support trabectedin as a standard of care for a second- or further-line treatment of patients with advanced STS in routine clinical practice (median progression-free survival: 5.2 months; median overall survival: 15.2 months). The safety profile of trabectedin was manageable and in line with those observed in previous studies.

Abstract: This non-interventional, prospective phase IV trial evaluated trabectedin in patients with soft tissue sarcoma (STS) in real-life clinical practice across Germany. The primary endpoints were progression-free survival (PFS) rates at 3 and 6 months, as defined by investigators. Overall, 128 patients from 19 German sites were evaluated for efficacy and 130 for safety. Median age was

58.5 years (range: 23–84) and leiomyosarcoma was the most frequent histotype (n = 45; 35.2%). Trabectedin was mostly used as second/third-line treatment (n = 91; 71.1%). Median PFS was 5.2 months (95% CI: 3.3–6.7), with 60.7% and 44.5% of patients free from progression at 3 and 6 months, respectively. Median overall survival was 15.2 months (95% CI: 9.6–21.4). One patient achieved a complete and 14 patients a partial response, conferring an objective response rate of 11.7%. Decreases in white blood cells (27.0% of patients), platelets (16.2%) and neutrophils (13.1%) and increased alanine aminotransferase (10.8%) were the most common trabectedin-related grade 3/4 adverse drug reactions. Two deaths due to pneumonia and sepsis were considered trabectedin-related. Trabectedin confers clinically meaningful activity in patients with multiple STS histotypes, comparable to that previously observed in clinical trials and other non-interventional studies, and with a manageable safety profile.

Keywords: trabectedin; STS; sarcoma; non-interventional; prospective

1. Introduction

Soft tissue sarcomas (STS) are a heterogeneous group of rare malignancies with mesenchymal origin that comprise approximately 1% of adult and 7% of pediatric malignancies [1–3]. Once metastatic or unresectable, prognosis for advanced STS is poor, and patients are not considered curable. For patients with advanced STS, systemic chemotherapy has been a cornerstone of treatment, although local therapies such as surgery and radiation therapy may achieve prolonged survival in selected patients [4].

Trabectedin (Yondelis®) is an alkylating agent with a multifaceted mechanism of action, which, apart from being a DNA-binding agent, also has selective anti-inflammatory, immunomodulatory and anti-angiogenic properties [5–7]. In 2007, trabectedin was the first marine-derived antineoplastic drug approved in the European Union for treatment of patients with advanced STS after failure of anthracyclines and ifosfamide, or who are unsuited to receive these agents [8]. Since 2015, following the analysis of a pivotal, active-controlled, randomized phase III trial in patients with advanced liposarcoma or leiomyosarcoma (commonly abbreviated as L-sarcomas) after failure of prior anthracycline-containing chemotherapy, trabectedin was also approved by the U.S. Food and Drug Administration [9]. Trabectedin was reported to be active in non-L-sarcomas as well since it has demonstrated efficacy in patients with a variety of sarcoma histotypes [10–13]. In a clinical trial setting, the efficacy of trabectedin compared to best supportive care is also supported by the results of trials conducted in patients with histologically different sarcoma subtypes [14,15]. In addition, trabectedin has a manageable safety profile and is without cumulative toxicities, including those in patients treated for prolonged periods [16].

Although results obtained in clinical trials suggest there is a high probability for patients with STS to benefit from treatment with trabectedin, at the time this study was launched, there was a paucity of robust real-life data on a more diverse patient population than that recruited in clinical trials. Indeed, such observational studies can provide useful insights into the real-life efficacy, safety and management of patients who may be underrepresented in clinical trials due to more restrictive eligibility criteria. Recently, one European and two national observational studies on the real-life use of trabectedin in patients with advanced STS reported clinically meaningful long-term benefits in patients with multiple STS histotypes, largely comparable to those previously reported in selected populations from clinical trials, and with a manageable safety profile [17–19].

Currently, data on the real-life use of trabectedin for STS in Germany are limited [20]. The constant change in patient selection and novel therapies applied in advanced STS mandate re-evaluation of real-life management in this evolving treatment landscape. Therefore, the prospective, non-interventional YON-SAR trial (http://www.ClinicalTrials.gov Identifier: NCT02367924) was designed with the aim of evaluating treatment effects of trabectedin in patients with advanced STS across a contemporary treatment landscape in Germany.

2. Materials and Methods

This non-interventional, prospective, multicenter phase IV study evaluated trabectedin in routine clinical practice in patients with advanced STS in Germany [21]. Treatment decisions, dosing, monitoring as well as diagnostic or therapeutic procedures were at the discretion of the investigator, were performed according to routine care and were not mandated by the observational plan.

Eligible participants included adults ($\geq$18 years old) with histologically diagnosed advanced STS and who signed an informed consent document. All eligible patients had either progressive disease following therapy with anthracyclines and ifosfamide or were unsuited to receive these agents, and were suitable to undergo treatment with trabectedin according to the Summary of Product Characteristics (SmPC). Patients with contraindications for treatment with trabectedin according to SmPC were excluded.

Trabectedin was administered in agreement with the marketing authorization, standard local clinical practice, and the treating clinician's discretion. The recommended dose of trabectedin for the treatment of STS is 1.5 mg/m^2 body surface area, given intravenously over 24 h every 3 weeks. There were no predefined limits of administered trabectedin cycles, and treatment could continue until disease progression, intolerance or consent withdrawal.

The observational period for each patient enrolled in this study consisted of the treatment period and the follow-up period. The treatment period began from the date of the first administration of trabectedin until progressive disease, death or treatment termination (whichever occurred first). After the end of treatment, patients were followed up for at least 12 months. After trabectedin treatment discontinuation, patients could have been treated with subsequent anticancer therapies or supportive care as per the treating clinician's clinical judgment.

All study procedures were conducted in accordance with the ethical standards as laid down in the 1964 Declaration of Helsinki and its later amendments, guidelines for Good Clinical Practice and local regulations on clinical trials, and were approved by the independent ethics committee.

The primary endpoint of this study was to assess the number of patients free from progression at 3 and 6 months after treatment (i.e., progression-free survival [PFS] rate at 3 and 6 months) as measured by institutional routine clinical standards. Secondary efficacy endpoints included unconfirmed disease control rate (DCR), defined as the percentage of patients with a complete response (CR) or partial response (PR) and/or stable disease (SD), PFS, overall survival (OS) and OS rates at 3 and 6 months after treatment. Secondary endpoints also included an assessment of the treatment with trabectedin and employed doses, treatment duration, causes for treatment discontinuation, and safety profile. The PFS was defined as the time interval from the first administration of trabectedin to the date of disease progression or death, regardless of cause (whichever occurred first), whereas OS was defined as the time between the start of trabectedin and patient death from any cause. Patients not experiencing an event or death or considered lost to follow-up were censored with the date of last contact or with the beginning of the following therapy (whichever occurred first). Response evaluations (i.e., CR, PR and SD) were measured according to local institutional standards, being preferred according to Response Evaluation Criteria in Solid Tumors (RECIST) 1.1 [22] or Choi criteria [23]. Adverse events (AE) were reported according to CTCAE 4.03 and their relationship to trabectedin. Treatment-related AEs were followed until resolution or start of new therapy. Documentation of AEs and serious AEs (SAE) occurred until 30 days after the last dose.

All collected parameters were analyzed in a descriptive manner. Categorical variables were expressed as absolute and relative frequencies, and continuous variables were described by number of observations, median, and range (minimum to maximum). Frequency tables ware prepared for categorical variables and checked for dependencies by Fisher's exact test. The exact binomial estimator and its 95% confidence interval (CI) were used in the analysis of categorical outcome parameters (e.g., tumor control rate). Time-to-event endpoints (i.e., PFS and OS) and their fixed-time estimations were estimated according to the Kaplan–Meier method and were compared using the log-rank test, while Cox regression models were performed for covariate analyses. All p-values were descriptive in nature and the significance level selected was 0.05. All statistical analyses were performed by means of SAS version 9.4 software (SAS Institute Inc., Cary, NC, USA). The efficacy analyses were based on the modified intention-to-treat (mITT) population, defined as all patients who received at least one dose of trabectedin, signed informed consent, and did not violate any inclusion or exclusion criterion. The analysis of safety was performed on the Safety Analysis Set (SAS) that included all enrolled patients who received at least one dose of trabectedin and provided consent to participate in the study.

3. Results

3.1. Patient Disposition and Characteristics

Between 16 July 2015 and 22 January 2019, a total of 130 patients from 19 medical centers in Germany were enrolled and received at least one dose of trabectedin (SAS). Two patients were excluded due to lack of STS diagnosis, and therefore, 128 patients were included in the mITT (Figure 1).

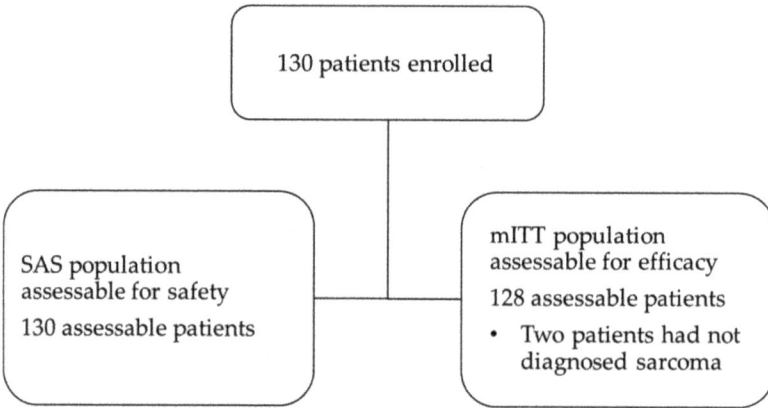

Figure 1. Description of included patients.

The mITT included 65 females (50.8%) and 63 males (49.2%) with a median age of 58.5 years (range: 23–84) (Table 1). An Eastern Cooperative Oncology Group (ECOG) performance status score of 0–1 was recorded in 100 (78.2%) patients. The most prevalent histological type of sarcoma was leiomyosarcoma (n = 45, 35.2%), followed by liposarcoma (n = 23, 18.0%) and pleomorphic undifferentiated sarcoma (n = 20, 15.6%), mostly being localized in lower extremity (n = 23, 18.0%), abdomen (retroperitoneal) (n = 20, 15.6%), upper extremity (n = 17, 13.3%) or uterus (n = 15, 11.7%). The most common tumor grade was grade 3 both in patients assessed according to FNCLCC (n = 34, 45.3%) and UICC (n = 23, 42.6%) system grading, and most had stage IV sarcoma as per AJCC staging system (Table 1). The majority of patients had metastatic disease (n = 79, 61.7%), mostly being localized in the lung (n = 59, 74.7%), liver (n = 25, 31.7%), or bones (n = 22, 27.9%).

Previous therapies included surgery in 111 (86.7%) patients, while 64 (50%) patients were treated with radiotherapy. The majority of patients received systemic therapy (n = 101; 78.9%), mostly with doxorubicin (n = 87, 86.1%) and/or ifosfamide (n = 63, 62.4%). Twenty-seven (21.1%) patients were chemotherapy-naïve (Table 2). Most patients received one or two lines of prior systemic therapy (n = 91; 71.1%). Overall, 113 patients (88.3%) reported relevant concomitant disease, mainly being arterial hypertension ($n = 54$, 47.8%), other cardiac diseases ($n = 29$, 25.7%) or thyropathy ($n = 25$, 22.1%).

Table 1. Patient and disease characteristics at baseline.

Patients	Modified Intent-to-Treat Set (mITT) [1] $n = 128$	
Age at study entry (years)	Median (range)	58.5 (23–84)
	≤60 years	70 (54.7%)
	>60 years	58 (45.3%)
	≤70 years	99 (77.3%)
	>70 years	29 (22.7%)
Gender	Female	65 (50.8%)
	Male	63 (49.2%)
Histology	Leiomyosarcoma	45 (35.2%)
	Liposarcoma	23 (18.0%)
	Pleomorphic undifferentiated sarcoma	20 (15.6%)
	Synovial sarcoma	8 (6.3%)
	Fibrosarcoma	8 (6.3%)
	Angiosarcoma	1 (0.8%)
	Other	23 (18.0%)
Site of primary tumor	Lower extremity	23 (18.0%)
	Abdomen (retroperitoneal)	20 (15.6%)
	Upper extremity	17 (13.3%)
	Uterus	15 (11.7%)
	Abdomen (intraperitoneal)	11 (8.6%)
	Other	42 (32.8%)
Eastern Cooperative Oncology Group (ECOG) performance status	0	34 (26.6%)
	1	66 (51.6%)
	2	10 (7.8%)
	3	1 (0.8%)
	4	1 (0.8%)
	Missing	16 (12.5%)
Tumor grade according to the French Federation of Cancer Centers Sarcoma Group grading systems (FNCLCC) [2]	Grade 1	13 (17.3%)
	Grade 2	21 (28.0%)
	Grade 3	34 (45.3%)
	Grade X [3]	6 (8.0%)
	Missing	1 (1.3%)
According to the Union for International Cancer Control (UICC) [2]	Grade 1	5 (9.3%)
	Grade 2	9 (16.7%)
	Grade 3	23 (42.6%)
	Grade 4	3 (5.6%)
	Grade X [3]	13 (24.1%)
	Missing	1 (1.9%)

Table 1. Cont.

Patients		Modified Intent-to-Treat Set (mITT) [1] n = 128
Tumor stage according to the American Joint Committee on Cancer (AJCC)	Ia	3 (2.3)
	Ib	7 (5.5)
	IIa	4 (3.1)
	IIb	5 (3.9)
	III	15 (11.7)
	IV	26 (20.3)
	Unknown	68 (53.1)
Time from first diagnosis to first treatment (months); n = 125	Median (range)	0.4 (0.0–149.7)
Time from diagnosis to last treatment before trabectedin (months); n = 125	Median (range)	15.9 (0.0–250.2)
Time from last progression to trabectedin treatment (months); n = 95	Median (range)	0.9 (0.0–2.5)

[1] Modified intent-to-treat set (mITT) included all patients who received at least one dose of trabectedin, signed informed consent and did not violate any inclusion or exclusion criterion. [2] One patient had no documented grading according to both FNCLCC and UICC and was counted in both grading categories as missing. [3] Tumor grade could not be assessed.

Table 2. Prior treatments.

Patients		Modified Intent-to-Treat Set (mITT); n = 128
Prior treatments	Prior surgery	111 (86.7%)
	Prior radiotherapy	64 (50.0%)
	Prior chemotherapy/ targeted treatments	101 (78.9%)
No. of lines of prior chemotherapy/targeted treatments, n = 128	0 lines	27 (21.1%)
	1 line	66 (51.6%)
	2 lines	25 (19.5%)
	≥3 lines (3 to 6 lines)	10 (7.8%)
Types of prior chemotherapy/targeted treatments, n = 101 (≥4% of patients)	Doxorubicin	87 (86.1%)
	Ifosfamide	63 (62.4%)
	Dacarbazine (DTIC)	18 (17.8%)
	Trophosphamide	16 (15.8%)
	Gemcitabine	13 (12.9%)
	Docetaxel	12 (11.9%)
	Epirubicin	12 (11.9%)
	Olaratumab	10 (9.9%)
	Pazopanib	8 (7.9%)
Best response to last prior chemotherapy/targeted treatments, n = 101	Complete response (CR)	2 (2.0%)
	Partial response (PR)	22 (21.8%)
	Stable disease (SD)	39 (38.6%)
	Progressive disease (PD)	22 (21.8%)
	Non evaluated (NE)	16 (15.8%)

Subsequent antineoplastic therapies were given to 78 (60.8%) patients, which consisted of gemcitabine (n = 34, 43.6%), pazopanib (n = 31, 39.7%), dacarbazine (n = 24, 30.8%) or other treatments (n = 33, 42.3%).

3.2. Extent of Exposure

Although all patients were suitable to undergo treatment with trabectedin according to SmPC, therapy deviated from the approved label in 67 patients (52.3%), commonly due to a reduced starting dose lower than 1.5 mg/m^2 (n = 53, 41.4%), use of aprepitant as premedication at first cycle (n = 14, 10.9%), and lack of baseline biochemistry or hematology in 10 (7.8%) and 5 patients (3.9%), respectively.

Patients received a median of four trabectedin cycles, with 52 (40.6%) patients receiving ≥6 cycles and up to a maximum of 44 cycles (Table 3). Of note, four patients received >24 cycles of treatment (approximately 18 months), one of whom reached 44 cycles of treatment with trabectedin (Table S1). Patients received a median cumulative total dose of 10.7 mg/m^2 (range: 1.8–110.9) over a median infusion duration of 24 h (range: 3.0–24.2). Premedication consisted of corticosteroids in 96.7% and antiemetics in 75.0% or more patients in each trabectedin cycle. The use of aprepitant was registered in 4.4% to 20.0% of patients during the study.

Table 3. Trabectedin exposure.

Treatment Delivery	Modified Intent-to-Treat Set (mITT); n = 128	
Number of cycles received per patient	Median (range)	4 (1–44)
	<6 cycles	76 (59.4%)
	≥6 cycles	52 (40.6%)
Dose reductions (per patient)	0 cycle	62 (48.4%)
	1 cycle	17 (13.3%)
	2 cycles	21 (16.4%)
	>2 cycles	18 (14.1%)
	Unknown [1]	10 (7.8%)
Cycle delays (per patient)	0 cycle	49 (38.3%)
	1 cycle	22 (17.2%)
	2 cycles	8 (6.3%)
	>2 cycles	44 (34.4%)
	Unknown [1]	5 (3.9%)

Data shown are numbers and percentages of patients or median and range values with available data. [1] Patients who started the treatment with trabectedin before the signed informed consents and with unknown starting dose.

Dose reductions occurred in 61 patients (47.7%), and dose delays in 76 patients (59.4%). Among 125 (97.7%) patients who discontinued trabectedin, the most frequent reason for treatment discontinuation was progression (n = 77, 60.2%), followed by death or other reason (n = 12, 9.4% each), patient's wish (n = 10, 7.8%) and trabectedin-related adverse drug reactions (ADRs) (n = 9, 7.0%).

3.3. Primary Efficacy Endpoint

The analysis of the primary endpoint revealed that 60.7% (95% CI: 51.5–68.8) and 44.5% (95% CI: 35.5–53.1) of patients were free from progression at 3 and 6 months after treatment, respectively (Figure 2).

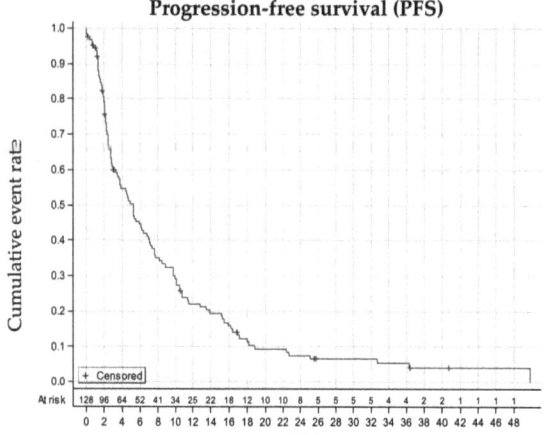
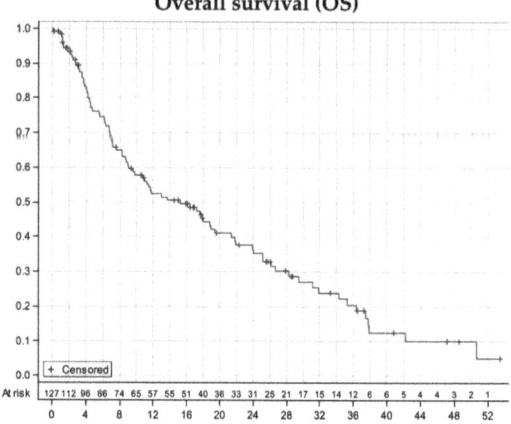

Parameter	mITT, $n = 128$
Censored [a]	15 (11.7%)
Patients with events	113 (88.3%)
Progressive disease (PD)	92 (81.4%)
Death, any cause	21 (18.6%)
Median PFS (months), (95% CI)	5.2 (3.3–6.7)
PFS at 3 months: (95% CI)	60.7% (51.5–68.8)
PFS at 6 months: (95% CI)	44.5% (35.5–53.1)
PFS at 12 months: (95% CI)	22.1% (15.1–30.0)

[a] Patients who had not died and did not have an assessment of progressive disease were censored.

Parameter	mITT, $n = 127$ *
Censored [a]	40
Death events	87 (68.5%)
Median OS (months), (95% CI)	15.2 (9.6–21.4)
OS at 3 months: (95% CI)	89.3% (82.2–93.6)
OS at 6 months: (95% CI)	74.5% (65.6–81.5)
OS at 12 months: (95% CI)	52.4% (42.9–61.1)

* One patient died with unknown date of death. [a] Patients who had not died were censored.

CI, confidence interval; mITT, modified intention-to-treat population; OS, overall survival; PFS, progression-free survival.

Figure 2. Kaplan–Meier plot of progression-free survival and overall survival.

3.4. Secondary Efficacy Endpoint

In the mITT after a median follow-up of 28.7 months (range 0.07–53.5), a total of 113 progression or death events (88.3% of patients) were recorded, whereas 15 (11.7%) patients who were alive or not assessed for disease progression at the time of this analysis were censored. Median PFS was 5.2 months (95% CI: 3.3–6.7) (Figure 2).

Median PFS was similar between patients with reduced dosing during the study (i.e., patients who received at least one trabectedin dose <1.5 mg/m^2 throughout the study) and in those with reduced starting dose (7.1 months, 95% CI: 4.8–9.8 vs. 5.4 months, 95% CI: 3.7–9.8), as well as in patients fully treated according to the SmPC and those who had treatment deviations from the SmPC recommendations (4.6 months, 95% CI: 2.7–7.1 vs. 5.2 months, 95% CI: 3.3–7.3). Similarly, there were no statistically significant differences in median PFS ($p = 0.41$) among patients who received trabectedin as first- (6.4 months, 95% CI: 2.7–10.8), second (5.3 months, 95% CI: 2.8–7.7), third (4.0 months, 95% CI: 2.0–6.2) and ≥fourth- (3.4 months, 95% CI: 0.7–9.8) line of treatment. After 87 death events (68.5% of patients), treatment with trabectedin resulted in a median OS of 15.2 months (95% CI: 9.6–21.4), with 89.3%, 74.5%, and 52.4% of patients alive 3, 6 and 12 months after treatment (Figure 2), respectively. No statistical difference was detected for OS in patients with reduced dosing during the study (18.9 months, 95% CI: 11.6–25.1) and in those with reduced starting dose (13.7 months, 95% CI: 8.3–26.6) and according to trabectedin treatment line (first-line: 24.0 months, 95% CI: 8.9-not reached; second-line: 15.2 months, 95% CI: 6.9–21.8; third-line: 11.0 months, 95% CI: 6.1–19.4; and ≥fourth-line: 17.5 months, 95% CI: 3.5-not reached; $p = 0.1558$).

Regarding the overall trabectedin activity, one patient (0.8%) had a CR, and 14 (10.9%) patients achieved a PR, reaching the ORR of 11.7%. Additionally, 43 (33.6%) patients had SD as a best result for a DCR of 45.3% (Table 4). Conversely, comparable DCR was observed between patients treated with trabectedin in different treatment lines, and a logistic regression analysis also revealed that presence or absence of tumor metastases at baseline was not statistically associated with DCR outcomes (odds ratio: 0.53, 95% CI: 0.23–1.24, p = 0.1421). The ORR and DCR were similar among patients <70 and ≥70 years old (ORR: 12.1% in <70 years and 10.3% in ≥70 years; DCR: 45.4% in <70 years and 41.4% in ≥70 years; post-hoc analysis). Regarding histology, CR was observed in one patient with liposarcoma, and PR was recorded in six patients with liposarcoma, in four patients with other histologies, and in two patients with leiomyosarcoma and synovial sarcoma, while stable disease was observed in patients with several histologies (Table S2).

Table 4. Best response rate according to investigator assessment by number of treatment cycles.

Best Response to Trabectedin per Patient (Unconfirmed)	Modified Intent-to-Treat Set (mITT); n = 128		
	<6 Cycles n = 76	≥6 Cycles n = 52	Total n = 128
Complete response (CR)	-	1 (1.9%)	1 (0.8%)
Partial response (PR)	1 (1.3%)	13 (25.0%)	14 (10.9%)
Stable disease (SD)	10 (13.2%)	33 (63.5%)	43 (33.6%)
Progressive disease (PD)	35 (46.1%)	3 (5.8%)	38 (29.7%)
Not evaluable	4 (5.3%)	2 (3.9%)	6 (4.7%)
Not done	26 (34.2%)	-	26 (20.3%)
Objective response rate (ORR; CR + PR)	1 (1.3%)	14 (26.9%)	15 (11.7%)
Disease control rate (DCR; ORR + SD)	11 (14.5%)	47 (89.4%)	58 (45.3%)
Fisher's exact test (p-value) [1]	<0.0001		-

[1] Unevaluated patients and those with missing best responses were excluded from the comparison.

Additionally, throughout the study, ECOG performance status improved by 1 in 10 (7.8%) patients, deteriorated by 1 in 38 (29.7%), and remained unchanged in 64 (50.0%) patients.

3.5. Safety

A total of 86 (66.2%) patients had at least one grade ≥3 AE. Most common (≥10% of patients) grade-3/4 AEs were decreased white blood cell count (n = 35, 26.9% of patients), decreased platelet count (n = 22, 16.9%), decreased neutrophil count (n = 17, 13.1%), increased alanine aminotransferase and anemia (n = 14, 10.8% each), and increased gamma-glutamyl transferase (n = 13, 10%). Nine (6.9%) patients experienced 10 grade-5 AEs, namely sepsis (n = 4, 3.1%), pneumonia, a combination of pneumonia and other infections and infestations, acute coronary syndrome, death not otherwise specified, and benign, malignant and unspecified neoplasm in one patient each (n = 1, 0.8% each). Forty-two (32.3%) patients had at least one SAE.

A total of 105 (80.8%) patients had at least one trabectedin-related ADR of any grade, 71 (54.6%) of whom experienced grade ≥3 ADRs (Table 5). Forty-four patients (33.8%) have grade ≥3 ADRs leading to dose modifications. Treatment-emergent serious ADRs (SADR) were uncommon, as a total of 19 (14.6%) patients presented with at least one SADR. No new or unexpected safety concerns were identified for trabectedin.

Table 5. Treatment-related adverse drug reactions (ADRs) in at least ≥3% of patients and all grade-5 ADRs as reported by the investigators (all treated patients).

Treatment-Related ADR as per NCI-CTC, Worst Grade per Patient (≥3% of Patients)	Safety Analysis Set [1,2] n = 130											
	Grade 1 n = 79		Grade 2 n = 73		Grade 3 n = 67		Grade 4 n = 23		Grade 5 n = 2		Total n = 105	
	n	%	n	%	n	%	n	%	n	%	n	%
ALT increased	9	6.9	11	8.5	14	10.8	-	-	-	-	34	26.2
AP increased	5	3.9	3	2.3	1	0.8	-	-	-	-	9	6.9
Anemia	10	7.7	16	12.3	12	9.2	-	-	-	-	38	29.2
Anorexia	15	11.5	5	3.9	3	2.3	-	-	-	-	23	17.7
Arthralgia	2	1.5	2	1.5			-	-	-	-	4	3.1
AST increased	9	6.9	9	6.9	5	3.9	-	-	-	-	23	17.7
Leukopenia	2	1.5	3	2.3	1	0.8	-	-	-	-	6	4.6
Constipation	16	12.3	2	1.5			-	-	-	-	18	13.9
Diarrhea	4	3.1	4	3.1	2	1.5	-	-	-	-	10	7.69
Dry skin	4	3.1	-	-	-	-	-	-	-	-	4	3.1
Dysgeusia	5	3.85	2	1.5	-	-	-	-	-	-	7	5.4
Dyspnea	3	2.3	2	1.5	-	-	1	0.8	-	-	6	4.6
Edema limbs	3	2.3	-	-	1	0.8	-	-	-	-	4	3.1
Fatigue	24	18.5	19	14.6	3	2.3	-	-	-	-	46	35.4
Febrile neutropenia	-	-	-	-	4	3.1	1	0.8	-	-	5	3.9
Fever	7	5.4	1	0.8					-	-	8	6.2
Night sweating	4	3.1	-	-	-	c	-	-	-	-	4	3.1
GGT increased	7	5.4	3	2.3	11	8.5	1	0.8	-	-	22	16.9
Headache	5	3.9	1	0.8	-	-	-	-	-	-	6	4.6
Hypoalbuminemia	3	2.3	1	0.8	-	-	-	-	-	-	4	3.1
Pneumonia [3]	-	-	-	-	2	1.5			1	0.8	3	2.3
Mucositis oral	2	1.5	1	0.8	3	2.3	-	-	-	-	6	4.6
Myalgia	3	2.3	1	0.8	1	0.8	-	-	-	-	5	3.9
Nausea	33	25.4	16	12.3	5	3.9	-	-	-	-	54	41.5
Neutrophil count decreased	2	1.5	5	3.9	10	7.7	7	5.4	-	-	24	18.5
Peripheral sensory neuropathy	3	2.3	1	0.8	1	0.8			-	-	5	3.9
Platelet count decreased	14	10.8	5	3.9	13	10.0	8	6.2	-	-	40	30.8
Sepsis [3]	-	-	-	-	-	-	2	1.5	1	0.8	3	2.3
Vomiting	16	12.3	7	5.4	3	2.3			-	-	26	20.0
White blood cell decreased	7	5.4	12	9.2	27	20.8	8	6.2	-	-	54	41.4

[1] Safety Analysis Set included all patients who signed informed consent and received at least one dose of trabectedin. [2] The percentages relate to the number of patients in the Safety Analysis Set. [3] Grade-5 adverse drug reactions. ADR, adverse drug reactions; ALT, alanine aminotransferase; AP, alkaline phosphatase; AST, aspartate aminotransferase; GGT, Gamma-glutamyltransferase; NCI-CTC, National Cancer Institute Common Toxicity Criteria.

4. Discussion

YON-SAR was the first prospective, multicenter, non-interventional, phase IV study that evaluated trabectedin's outcomes in routine clinical practice in patients with advanced STS in Germany. While randomized controlled clinical trials are the cornerstone standard of medical evidence, their generalizability to daily clinical practice in a diverse and unselected patient populations always should be verified in non-interventional studies [24]. Of note, considering that in our study we included data from 130 patients from 19 sites across Germany, our data can surely provide a good representation of German real-life clinical practice.

The results of this study corroborate that trabectedin is an active treatment that offers clinical benefits to patients with multiple STS histotypes. In our study, trabectedin administration resulted in a median PFS of 5.2 months with 3- and 6-month PFS rates (primary endpoint) of 60.7% and 44.5%, respectively, which largely exceeded the 3- and 6-month PFS rate thresholds (i.e., 39% and 14%, respectively) established by the EORTC for active agents for the treatment of unselected STS [25] and are either close to or even exceed the new benchmarks proposed only for advanced/metastatic liposarcoma (63% and 44%) and synovial sarcoma (60% and 41%) [26]. However, the nature of our study may limit the interpretation of these observations. Recognizing that direct comparisons cannot be established, the efficacy outcomes of the present study are comparable with the reported median PFS previously reported in phase II (range: 3.3–7.2 months) [8,14,27] and phase III (range: 3.1–4.2 months) trials [9,15]. Furthermore, the results are in line with other observational studies investigating trabectedin in STS (Table 6). In TrObs and RetrospectYon studies, a tendency toward better PFS in patients treated in an early treatment line was demonstrated [18,19]. Although YON-SAR did not observe significant differences in median PFS with respect to treatment lines, PFS estimates indicate that higher PFS may be achieved in earlier lines. Unfortunately, the small sample size of these subgroups is a major limitation and precludes drawing definite conclusions. Conversely, retrospective data from 101 German patients with advanced STS revealed a similar finding [20]. A median PFS of 2.1 months was reported in that study. However, the majority of patients received trabectedin as third or later line (73%). In the fraction of patients who received trabectedin as first or second line, the median PFS was 5.7 months.

Table 6. Relevance of the YON-SAR results within the context of trabectedin treatment for recurrent advanced STS.

Median (95% CI)	Advanced Sarcoma	PFS (Months)	PFS-3/6 (%)	OS (Months)	ORR (%)	SD (%)	DCR (%)
	Retrospective, Non-Interventional Studies						
French RetrospectYon database Le Cesne et al., 2015 [19]	STS; $n = 804$	4.4 (3.9–4.9)	59.0/40.0	12.2 (11.0–13.3)	16.5	50.1	66.7
	L-sarcoma; $n = 481$	5.7 (4.9–6.5)	64–69.0/NA	15.0 (13.2–16.8)	18.6	54.0	72.6
TrObs study Palmerini et al., 2021 [18]	STS; $n = 512$	5.1 (4.1–6.7)	NA/46.0	21.6 (19.3–25.0)	13.7 (11.2–17.2)	33.0	46.7 (43.2–51.9)
	L-sarcoma; $n = 348$	8.3 (6–10.1)	NA/55.0	25.9 (22.4–33.4)	16.6	37.4	53.4
	non-L-sarcoma; $n = 164$	2.4 (1.8–3.4)	NA/26.0	11.3 (8.1–16.3)	9.0	23.8	32.3
German retrospective study Hoiczyk M et al., 2013 [20]	STS; $n = 101$	2.1	NA	NA	NA	NA	NA
	L-sarcoma; $n = 46$	3.1	51/38	NA	NA	NA	55
	non-L-sarcoma; $n = 55$	1.6	36/16	NA	NA	NA	34
	Prospective, Non-Interventional Studies						
Y-IMAGE study Buonadonna et al., 2017 [17]	STS; $n = 218$	5.9 (4.9–7.8)	70.0/49.0	21.3 (18.8–24.3)	26.6 (20.9–33)	39.0	65.6 (58.9–71.9)
YON-SAR study Grünwald et al., 2022	STS; $n = 128$	5.2 (3.3–6.7)	60.7/44.5	15.2 (9.6–21.4)	11.7	33.6	45.3

Results of time-to-event endpoints show median and 95% confidence intervals with available data. CI; confidence intervals; DCR, disease control rate; h, hour; L-sarcoma, liposarcoma or leiomyosarcoma; NA, not available; NR, not reached; ORR, objective response rate; OS, overall survival; PFS, progression-free survival; PFS-3/-6, PFS rate at 3/6 months; SD, stable disease; STS, soft tissue sarcoma.

YON-SAR reported a median OS of 15.2 months (95% CI: 9.6–21.4). Median OS in this observational study tended to be slightly longer than previously reported in phase II and III trials (12.4–13.9 months) [8,9,15,28] and observational study RetrospectYon (12.2 months) [19]. However, other observational studies reported comparatively longer median OS of 21.3 months and 21.6 months [17,18] (Table 6). This variance in survival is likely explained by differences in patient populations. Several studies of trabectedin indicated that median OS is longer in L-sarcoma patients than in those with other histologies [29]. Conversely, the fraction of liposarcoma patients varied among studies (YON-SAR: 18.0%; Y-IMAGE: 23.4% [17]; TrObs: 30.3% [18]) and, thus, may contribute to differences in outcomes.

In our study, treatment duration was an important factor for long-term outcomes. Patients who received ≥6 trabectedin cycles obtained higher response rates than those who received <6 cycles (Table 3). This observation has been previously reported, and protracted trabectedin treatment beyond 6 cycles is supported both in retrospective [19,30] and prospective series, such as in phase II T-DIS study [26,31]. Clearly, a selection bias applies in this subgroup of patients, and contributing factors other than treatment duration cannot be excluded. However, our data indicate that patients who achieve disease control and tolerate trabectedin treatment can be safely treated beyond 6 cycles, until progression.

Furthermore, in our study nearly 60% of patients reported either improved or unchanged ECOG performance status during the study period. These data could indicate a low disease-related worsening during the treatment with trabectedin, and when the symptoms worsened, this was largely caused by the natural course of disease, since 60% of patients discontinued the treatment due to disease progression.

Although all enrolled patients were suitable to undergo treatment with trabectedin, we observed that therapy deviated from the approved label according to SmPC in 67 patients (52.3%). It is important to note that deviation from SmPC did not affect the efficacy of trabectedin in term of PFS. As per investigator decision, trabectedin was given to 53 (41.4%) patients at a lower dose than that recommended (i.e., 1.5 mg/m^2). Moreover, in the present study, median PFS and OS were similar between patients treated with reduced starting trabectedin dose and those with reduced dosing during the study; however, comparison of different trabectedin dosages was not the objective of this study. Although our data did not indicate major differences in outcomes among patients with reduced trabectedin doses, the putative effectivity of full-dose trabectedin remains unknown in these patients. This regimen yielded more tumor shrinkage and superior time to progression compared to a weekly regimen. Although we believe it is imperative to use the recommended starting dose of trabectedin and consider treatment modifications only during therapy as specified in the SmPC, our data indicated that in selected cases, and always based on clinical judgment to optimize patient outcomes, reduced doses may be used.

Although aprepitant is not recommended as premedication for trabectedin, 10.9% of patients received aprepitant prior to the first cycle of trabectedin, and 4.4% to 20.0% of patients during therapy. Aprepitant was recognized to potentially increase trabectedin exposure and exert thereby an additional risk of toxicity if given concomitantly [32]. In such cases, close monitoring is required and appropriate dose adjustments should be applied in the event of toxicities.

The safety profile of trabectedin was in line with prior experience and reports, characterized by myelosuppression and hepatic toxicities [16]. In our study, trabectedin demonstrated a favorable safety profile over long-term treatment, as >40% of patients received ≥6 cycles of trabectedin and up to a maximum of 44 cycles of treatment. This is consistent with previous reports where comparable numbers of patients were treated with ≥6 cycles (e.g., RetrospectYon: 34.4%; TrObs: 36.5%; Y-IMAGE: 56.9% of patients) [17–19].

According to the non-interventional nature of this study, the exact time points and method of response assessment were not previously fixed but were determined according to the clinician's discretion and with no central radiological review and response confirmation; thus, our data must be interpreted with caution. Moreover, missing or unavailable data can additionally hamper the interpretation of the results. Nevertheless, in spite of these limitations, our real-life study complements well the findings from the clinical trials with trabectedin, as it provides information on unselected patient characteristics treated in routine treatment practices.

5. Conclusions

In conclusion, the findings of this non-interventional and prospective phase IV study in Germany consistently support that trabectedin is an active treatment in a routine clinical setting. The overall data observed in our study are in line with those observed in clinical and non-interventional studies and further support the use of trabectedin for patients with multiple sarcoma histotypes.

Supplementary Materials: The following supporting information can be downloaded at: https://www.mdpi.com/article/10.3390/cancers14215234/s1, Table S1. Characteristics of patients treated with prolonged trabectedin treatment (>24 cycles); Table S2. Best responses by patient and disease characteristics at baseline (post hoc analysis).

Author Contributions: Conceptualization, V.G., D.P. and B.D.R.; methodology, V.G., D.P. and B.D.R.; formal analysis and data curation, V.G., D.P. and B.D.R.; investigation, V.G., D.P., G.E., E.S., M.A., C.K.W.D., V.K., D.R., M.K., S.B., D.H. (Dennis Hahn), L.H.L., M.H., U.R., L.C.H., D.H. (Dirk Hempel), B.D.R., T.W. and P.I.; writing—original draft preparation, V.G., D.P. and B.D.R.; writing—review and editing, V.G., D.P, G.E., E.S., M.A., C.K.W.D., V.K., D.R., M.K., S.B., D.H. (Dennis Hahn), L.H.L., M.H., U.R., L.H.L., D.H. (Dirk Hempel), B.D.R., T.W. and P.I.; supervision, V.G. All authors have read and agreed to the published version of the manuscript.

Funding: This research was funded by PharmaMar, S.A., Madrid, Spain.

Institutional Review Board Statement: All study procedures were carried out in accordance with the Declaration of Helsinki and its later amendments and local regulations on clinical trials, and were approved by the institutional review boards of each participating center (Landesärztekammer Baden-Württemberg, Ethik-Kommission, F-2013-044).

Informed Consent Statement: Informed consent was obtained from all subjects involved in the study.

Data Availability Statement: The data underlying this article will be shared on reasonable request to the corresponding author.

Acknowledgments: This study was sponsored by PharmaMar, S.A., Madrid, Spain. The authors acknowledge Adnan Tanović for providing writing and editorial assistance for the manuscript (funded by PharmaMar, S.A.).

Conflicts of Interest: V.G. declares ownership interests in MSD, Bristol-Myers Squibb, AstraZeneca, Seagen, and Genmab, declares having received payment honoraria from Bristol-Myers Squibb, Pfizer, Novartis, Ipsen, Eisai, MSD, Merck Serono, Roche, AstraZeneca, EUSA Pharma, Janssen-Cilag, Apogepha, Nanobiotix, ClinSol, and Ono Pharmaceutical, fees from advisory boards from Bristol-Myers Squibb, Pfizer, Novartis, MSD, Ipsen, Janssen-Cilag, Onkowissen, CORE2ED, Eisai, and Debiopharm, and fees from speaker's bureau from Novartis, Amgen, MSD, Bristol-Myers Squibb, Seattle Genetics, Ipsen, Bristol-Myers Squibb, Pfizer, and Astra Zeneca. D.P. declares fees from speaker's bureau from Blueprint and PharmaMar and declares having received consulting fees and payment honoraria from Boehringer Ingelheim, PharmaMar, Roche, Advisory, Novartis, PharmaMar, Roche, Bristol-Myers Squibb, EUSA-Pharma, and Lilly. C.D., D.H. (Dennis Hahn), M.K. and V.K. declare fees from speaker's bureau from PharmaMar. L.H. declares having received payment honoraria from Amgen, Astra Zeneca, Clovis, Eisai, GSK, MSD, Pharma Mar, and Roche. Beatriz De Rivas is an employee and stockholder of PharmaMar. The other authors indicated no financial relationships.

References

1. Lahat, G.; Lazar, A.; Lev, D. Sarcoma Epidemiology and Etiology: Potential Environmental and Genetic Factors. *Surg. Clin. N. Am.* **2008**, *88*, 451–481. [CrossRef] [PubMed]

2. Burningham, Z.; Hashibe, M.; Spector, L.; Schiffman, J.D. The Epidemiology of Sarcoma. *Clin. Sarcoma Res.* **2012**, *2*, 14. [CrossRef] [PubMed]
3. Montella, L.; Altucci, L.; Sarno, F.; Buonerba, C.; De Simone, S.; Facchini, B.; Franzese, E.; De Vita, F.; Tafuto, S.; Berretta, M.; et al. Toward a Personalized Therapy in Soft-Tissue Sarcomas: State of the Art and Future Directions. *Cancers* **2021**, *13*, 2359. [CrossRef] [PubMed]
4. Casali, P.G.; Abecassis, N.; Aro, H.T.; Bauer, S.; Biagini, R.; Bielack, S.; Bonvalot, S.; Boukovinas, I.; Bovee, J.V.M.G.; Brodowicz, T.; et al. Soft tissue and visceral sarcomas: ESMO-EURACAN Clinical Practice Guidelines for diagnosis, treat-ment and follow-up. *Ann. Oncol.* **2018**, *29* (Suppl. S4), iv268–iv269. [CrossRef]
5. Larsen, A.K.; Galmarini, C.M.; D'Incalci, M. Unique features of trabectedin mechanism of action. *Cancer Chemother. Pharmacol.* **2015**, *77*, 663–671. [CrossRef] [PubMed]
6. D'Incalci, M. Trabectedin mechanism of action: What's new? *Future Oncol.* **2013**, *9* (Suppl. S12), 5–10. [CrossRef]
7. D'Incalci, M.; Galmarini, C.M. A Review of Trabectedin (ET-743): A Unique Mechanism of Action. *Mol. Cancer Ther.* **2010**, *9*, 2157–2163. [CrossRef]
8. Demetri, G.D.; Chawla, S.P.; von Mehren, M.; Ritch, P.; Baker, L.H.; Blay, J.Y.; Hande, K.R.; Keohan, M.L.; Samuels, B.L.; Schuetze, S.; et al. Efficacy and safety of trabectedin in patients with advanced or metastatic liposarcoma or leiomyo-sarcoma after failure of prior anthracyclines and ifosfamide: Results of a randomized phase II study of two different schedules. *J. Clin. Oncol.* **2009**, *27*, 4188–4196. [CrossRef]
9. Demetri, G.D.; von Mehren, M.; Jones, R.L.; Hensley, M.L.; Schuetze, S.M.; Staddon, A.; Milhem, M.; Elias, A.; Ganjoo, K.; Tawbi, H.; et al. Efficacy and Safety of Trabectedin or Dacarbazine for Metastatic Liposarcoma or Leiomyosarcoma After Failure of Conventional Chemotherapy: Results of a Phase III Randomized Multicenter Clinical Trial. *J. Clin. Oncol.* **2016**, *34*, 786–793. [CrossRef]
10. Casali, P.G.; Blay, J.-Y. Soft tissue and visceral sarcomas: ESMO Clinical Practice Guidelines for diagnosis, treatment and follow-up. *Ann. Oncol.* **2014**, *25* (Suppl. S3), iii102–iii112.
11. De Sanctis, R.; Marrari, A.; Marchetti, S.; Mussi, C.; Balzarini, L.; Lutman, F.R.; Daolio, P.; Bastoni, S.; Bertuzzi, A.F.; Quagliuolo, V.; et al. Efficacy of trabectedin in advanced soft tissue sarcoma: Beyond lipo- and leiomyosarcoma. *Drug Des. Dev. Ther.* **2015**, *9*, 5785–5791. [CrossRef] [PubMed]
12. Reichardt, P.; Grünwald, V.; Kasper, B.; Schuler, M.; Gelderblom, H. Efficacy of trabectedin in patients with some rare advanced soft tissue sarcoma subtypes other than liposarcoma and leiomyosarcoma. *J. Med. Drug Rev.* **2015**, *5*, 33–42.
13. Serdà, P.C.; Terés, R.; Sebio, A.; Bagué, S.; Orellana, R.; Moreno, M.E.; Riba, M.; López-Pousa, A. Single-Center Experience with Trabectedin for the Treatment of Non-L-sarcomas. *Adv. Ther.* **2022**, *39*, 1596–1610. [CrossRef] [PubMed]
14. Kawai, A.; Araki, N.; Sugiura, H.; Ueda, T.; Yonemoto, T.; Takahashi, M.; Morioka, H.; Hiraga, H.; Hiruma, T.; Kunisada, T.; et al. Trabectedin monotherapy after standard chemotherapy versus best supportive care in patients with advanced, translocation-related sarcoma: A randomised, open-label, phase 2 study. *Lancet Oncol.* **2015**, *16*, 406–416. [CrossRef]
15. Le Cesne, A.; Blay, J.-Y.; Cupissol, D.; Italiano, A.; Delcambre, C.; Penel, N.; Isambert, N.; Chevreau, C.; Bompas, E.; Bertucci, F.; et al. A randomized phase III trial comparing trabectedin to best supportive care in patients with pre-treated soft tissue sarcoma: T-SAR, a French Sarcoma Group trial. *Ann. Oncol.* **2021**, *32*, 1034–1044. [CrossRef]
16. Le Cesne, A.; Yovine, A.; Blay, J.-Y.; Delaloge, S.; Maki, R.G.; Misset, J.-L.; Frontelo, P.; Nieto, A.; Jiao, J.J.; Demetri, G.D. A retrospective pooled analysis of trabectedin safety in 1132 patients with solid tumors treated in phase II clinical trials. *Investig. New Drugs* **2012**, *30*, 1193–1202. [CrossRef]
17. Buonadonna, A.; Benson, C.; Casanova, J.; Kasper, B.; López Pousa, A.; Mazzeo, F.; Thomas, B.; Nicolas, P. A noninterventional, multicenter, prospective phase IV study of trabectedin in patients with ad-vanced soft tissue sarcoma. *Anticancer Drugs* **2017**, *28*, 1157–1165. [CrossRef]
18. Palmerini, E.; Sanfilippo, R.; Grignani, G.; Buonadonna, A.; Romanini, A.; Badalamenti, G.; Ferraresi, V.; Vincenzi, B.; Comandone, A.; Pizzolorusso, A.; et al. Trabectedin for Patients with Advanced Soft Tissue Sarcoma: A Non-Interventional, Retrospective, Multicenter Study of the Italian Sarcoma Group. *Cancers* **2021**, *13*, 1053. [CrossRef]
19. Le Cesne, A.; Ray-Coquard, I.; Duffaud, F.; Chevreau, C.; Penel, N.; Nguyen, B.B.; Piperno-Neumann, S.; Delcambre, C.; Rios, M.; Chaigneau, L.; et al. Trabectedin in patients with advanced soft tissue sarcoma: A retrospective national analysis of the French Sarcoma Group. *Eur. J. Cancer* **2015**, *51*, 742–750. [CrossRef]
20. Hoiczyk, M.; Grabellus, F.; Podleska, L.; Ahrens, M.; Schwindenhammer, B.; Taeger, G.; Pöttgen, C.; Schuler, M.; Bauer, S. Trabectedin in metastatic soft tissue sarcomas: Role of pretreatment and age. *Int. J. Oncol.* **2013**, *43*, 23–28. [CrossRef]
21. Grünwald, V.; Pink, D.; Egerer, G.; Schalk, E.; Augustin, M.; Deinzer, C.; Kob, V.; Reichert, D.; Kebenko, M.; Brandl, S.; et al. 1496P Trabectedin for patients with advanced soft tissue sarcoma: A non-interventional, prospective, multicenter study. *Ann. Oncol.* **2022**, *33* (Suppl. S7), S1231. [CrossRef]
22. Eisenhauer, E.A.; Therasse, P.; Bogaerts, J.; Schwartz, L.H.; Sargent, D.; Ford, R.; Dancey, J.; Arbuck, S.; Gwyther, S.; Mooney, M.; et al. New response evaluation criteria in solid tumours: Revised RECIST guideline (version 1.1). *Eur. J. Cancer* **2009**, *45*, 228–247. [CrossRef] [PubMed]
23. Choi, H.; Charnsangavej, C.; Faria, S.C.; Macapinlac, H.A.; Burgess, M.A.; Patel, S.R.; Chen, L.L.; Podoloff, D.A.; Benjamin, R.S. Correlation of computed tomography and positron emission tomography in patients with metastatic gas-trointestinal stromal

tumor treated at a single institution with imatinib mesylate: Proposal of new computed tomography response criteria. *J. Clin. Oncol.* **2007**, *25*, 1753–1759. [CrossRef] [PubMed]
24. Mishra, D.; Vora, J. Non interventional drug studies in oncology: Why we need them? *Perspect. Clin. Res.* **2010**, *1*, 128–133. [CrossRef]
25. Van Glabbeke, M.; Van Oosterom, A.T.; Oosterhuis, J.W.; Mouridsen, H.; Crowther, D.; Somers, R.; Verweij, J.; Santoro, A.; Buesa, J.; Tursz, T. Prognostic factors for the outcome of chemotherapy in advanced soft tissue sarcoma: An analysis of 2,185 patients treated with anthracycline-containing first-line regimens-a European Organization for Research and Treatment of Cancer Soft Tissue and Bone Sarcoma Group Study. *J. Clin. Oncol.* **1999**, *17*, 150–157.
26. Kantidakis, G.; Litière, S.; Neven, A.; Vinches, M.; Judson, I.; Blay, J.Y.; Wardelmann, E.; Stacchiotti, S.; D'Ambrosio, L.; Marréaud, S.; et al. New benchmarks to design clinical trials with advanced or metastatic liposarcoma or synovial sar-coma patients: An EORTC-Soft Tissue and Bone Sarcoma Group (STBSG) meta-analysis based on a literature review for soft-tissue sarcomas. *Eur. J. Cancer* **2022**, *174*, 261–276. [CrossRef]
27. Le Cesne, A.; Blay, J.Y.; Domont, J.; Tresch-Bruneel, E.; Chevreau, C.; Bertucci, F.; Delcambre, C.; Saada-Bouzid, E.; Piperno-Neumann, S.; Bay, J.-O.; et al. Interruption versus continuation of trabectedin in patients with soft-tissue sarcoma (T-DIS): A ran-domised phase 2 trial. *Lancet Oncol.* **2015**, *16*, 312–319. [CrossRef]
28. Patel, S.; von Mehren, M.; Reed, D.R.; Kaiser, P.; Charlson, J.; Ryan, C.W.; Rushing, D.; Livingston, M.; Singh, A.; Seth, R.; et al. Overall survival and histology-specific subgroup analyses from a phase 3, randomized controlled study of trabectedin or dacarbazine in patients with advanced liposarcoma or leiomyosarcoma. *Cancer* **2019**, *125*, 2610–2620. [CrossRef]
29. Le Cesne, A. Making the Best of Available Options for Optimal Sarcoma Treatment. *Oncology* **2018**, *95* (Suppl. S1), 11–20. [CrossRef]
30. Blay, J.-Y.; Italiano, A.; Ray-Coquard, I.; Le Cesne, A.; Duffaud, F.; Rios, M.; Collard, O.; Bertucci, F.; Bompas, E.; Isambert, N.; et al. Long-term outcome and effect of maintenance therapy in patients with advanced sarcoma treated with trabectedin: An analysis of 181 patients of the French ATU compassionate use program. *BMC Cancer* **2013**, *13*, 64. [CrossRef]
31. Kotecki, N.; Le Cesne, A.; Tresch-Bruneel, E.; Mir, O.; Chevreau, C.; Bertucci, F.; Delcambre, C.; Saada-Bouzid, E.; Piperno-Neumann, S.; Bay, J.-O.; et al. Update of the T-DIS randomized phase II trial: Trabectedin rechallenge verus continuation in patients (pts) with advanced soft tissue sarcoma (ASTS). *Ann. Oncol.* **2016**, *27* (Suppl. S6), vi486. [CrossRef]
32. Yondelis Summary of Product Characteristics. Available online: https://www.ema.europa.eu/en/medicines/human/EPAR/yondelis#product-information-section (accessed on 1 October 2022).

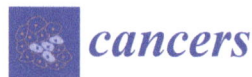

Article

Small Gastric Stromal Tumors: An Underestimated Risk

Jintao Guo [1,†], Qichao Ge [1,2,†], Fan Yang [1], Sheng Wang [1], Nan Ge [1], Xiang Liu [1], Jing Shi [1], Pietro Fusaroli [3], Yang Liu [1,2,*] and Siyu Sun [1,*]

[1] Department of Gastroenterology, Shengjing Hospital of China Medical University, Shenyang 110004, China
[2] Innovative Research Center for Integrated Cancer Omics, Shengjing Hospital of China Medical University, Shenyang 110004, China
[3] Gastroenterology Unit, Hospital of Imola, University of Bologna, 40126 Imola, Italy
* Correspondence: liuy21@sj-hospital.org (Y.L.); sunsy@sj-hospital.org (S.S.); Tel.: +86-24-88483780 (Y.L.); +86-189-4025-1329 (S.S.); Fax: +86-24-88483780 (Y.L.); +86-24-23892617 (S.S.)
† These authors contributed equally in this work.

Simple Summary: In this study, the high oncogenic mutation frequency (96%) of small GISTs is identified by whole-exome sequencing and targeted sanger sequencing in the entire cohort ($n = 76$) of a Chinese population. The BRAF-V600E hotspot mutation was present in ~15% small GISTs. Positive surgical or endoscopic resection should be considered for small GISTs because of their universal oncogenic mutation and undefined prognosis.

Abstract: Background and Objectives: Small gastrointestinal stromal tumors (GISTs) are defined as tumors less than 2 cm in diameter, which are often found incidentally during gastroscopy. There is controversy regarding the management of small GISTs, and a certain percentage of small GISTs become malignant during follow-up. Previous studies which used Sanger targeted sequencing have shown that the mutation rate of small GISTs is significantly lower than that of large tumors. The aim of this study was to investigate the overall mutational profile of small GISTs, including those of wild-type tumors, using whole-exome sequencing (WES) and Sanger sequencing. Methods: Thirty-six paired small GIST specimens, which were resected by endoscopy, were analyzed by WES. Somatic mutations identified by WES were confirmed by Sanger sequencing. Sanger sequencing was performed in an additional 38 small gastric stromal tumor samples for examining hotspot mutations in KIT, PDGFRA, and BRAF. Results: Somatic C-KIT/PDGFRA mutations accounted for 81% of the mutations, including three novel mutation sites in *C-KIT* at exon 11, across the entire small gastric stromal tumor cohort ($n = 74$). In addition, 15% of small GISTs harbored previously undescribed BRAF-V600E hotspot mutations. No significant correlation was observed among the genotype, pathological features, and clinical classification. Conclusions: Our data revealed a high overall mutation rate (~96%) in small GISTs, indicating that genetic alterations are common events in early GIST generation. We also identified a high frequency of oncogenic BRAF-V600E mutations (15%) in small GISTs, which has not been previously reported.

Keywords: gastrointestinal stromal tumor; next-generation sequencing; small GIST; endoscopic resection

Citation: Guo, J.; Ge, Q.; Yang, F.; Wang, S.; Ge, N.; Liu, X.; Shi, J.; Fusaroli, P.; Liu, Y.; Sun, S. Small Gastric Stromal Tumors: An Underestimated Risk. *Cancers* **2022**, *14*, 6008. https://doi.org/10.3390/cancers14236008

Academic Editor: Shinji Miwa

Received: 30 September 2022
Accepted: 5 December 2022
Published: 6 December 2022

Publisher's Note: MDPI stays neutral with regard to jurisdictional claims in published maps and institutional affiliations.

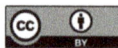

Copyright: © 2022 by the authors. Licensee MDPI, Basel, Switzerland. This article is an open access article distributed under the terms and conditions of the Creative Commons Attribution (CC BY) license (https://creativecommons.org/licenses/by/4.0/).

1. Introduction

Gastrointestinal stromal tumors (GISTs) are the most common mesenchymal tumors of the gastrointestinal tract and have phenotypic similarities with interstitial cells of Cajal (ICCs) [1,2]. GISTs are commonly present in the stomach (60%) and small intestine (25%) [1]. GISTs with a diameter <2 cm are defined as small GISTs, which can be subdivided into mini- (1–2 cm) and micro-GISTs (<1 cm). The annual age-adjusted incidence averaged 6.8 per 1,000,000, and GISTs are more common in males, non-Hispanics, Blacks, and Asians/Pacific Islanders [3]. Most GISTs are usually asymptomatic and incidentally discovered during endoscopy or surgery. The diagnosis and classification of small GISTs are currently based on pathological features and imaging methods, such as computed tomography and endoscopic ultrasound (EUS). The management (endoscopic resection or follow-up) of small GISTs is controversial, and there are no consensus-based guidelines [1,4–6]. Current clinical guidelines recommend surgical or endoscopic resection for small GISTs with high-risk EUS presentations. For other small GISTs, EUS surveillance every 6–12 months is recommended [6,7]. The current prognostic factors and risk indices for GISTs are commonly based on the modified NIH (M-NIH) classification [8], which focuses on the tumor size (2, 5, or 10 cm), mitotic index, primary tumor sites, and tumor rupture. Low-risk or benign tumors are defined as those <2 cm with a mitotic index of <5 mitoses per 50 high-power fields [9]. Most small GISTs are generally considered low risk, but the potential malignancy of small GISTs should not be ignored. A population-based epidemiological and mortality investigation illustrated that the 5-year mortality for small GISTs is 12%, and that some of these tumors might progress and become life-threatening [10].

Large cohort studies have shown that small GISTs have a high incidence in the stomach, with some of these tumors not being benign, as they are associated with worse gastrointestinal symptoms during regular surveillance [11–13]. Owing to the continuously increasing rate of small GIST detection and the earlier time of onset, their surveillance and management have been deemed controversial, with a lack of evidence-based approaches [14]. Moreover, an explanation of the epidemiology, risk factors, and etiology of these small tumors is lacking [15]. Previous studies have shown that the overall frequency of KIT/PDGFRA mutations (<76%) is significantly lower in small GISTs than that in large GISTs (85–95%) [13,16,17]. However, the Sanger sequencing used in previous studies was typically based on limited primers, likely leading to an underestimation of the mutation frequency of driver genes. Therefore, more advanced sequencing methods are required to profile the mutation status of small GISTs and understand their molecular basis. In this study, we aimed to investigate potential driver genes in small GISTs using whole-exome sequencing (WES) and targeted Sanger sequencing, which will contribute to an increase in the understanding of small GISTs.

2. Patients and Methods

2.1. Clinical Samples

We primary collected 40 paired small GIST samples from the gastric muscularis propria layer obtained from the lesion sample library (January 2022–June 2022) of the Shengjing Hospital of China Medical University (Shenyang, China). Paired blood samples were used as negative controls to differentiate somatic mutations using WES. The selection criteria included the tumor size (<2 cm), definite pathological diagnosis (according to the Chinese Society of Clinical Oncology (CSCO) criteria), and endoscopic resection methods (endoscopic submucosal dissection (ESD) or endoscopic full-thickness resection (EFTR)). Four patients with an actual tumor volume >2 cm or those who did not meet the pathological diagnostic criteria were excluded. For validating the sequencing results of WES, we collected another 60 formalin fixed, paraffin embedded (FFPE) small GIST tissue samples (June 2021–December 2021) from the Department of Pathology of Shengjing Hospital for targeted Sanger sequencing (Figure 1).

2.2. Ethics Statement

The study and tumor tissues for sequencing and clinical information collected were reviewed and approved by the Ethics Review Committee of Shengjing Hospital of China Medical University (No: 2022PS049K).

2.3. Whole-Exome Sequencing

Genomic DNA was extracted and sequenced according to standard protocols for next-generation sequencing (Novogene Co., Ltd., Beijing, China). Briefly, paired-end DNA was obtained according to the manufacturer's instructions (Agilent Technologies). The adapter-modified gDNA fragments were enriched by polymerase chain reaction (PCR).

Whole-exome capture was conducted using the Agilent SureSelect Human All Exon V5 Kit. A total of 60 MB of DNA sequences from 33,4378 exons of 20,965 samples was captured. After DNA quality evaluation, the samples were sequenced on an Illumina HiSeq PE150 for paired-end 150 bp reads. The average sequencing depth was 224×. The coverage of the target region was 99.6%, and 96.5% of the target bases were covered to a depth of at least 20×.

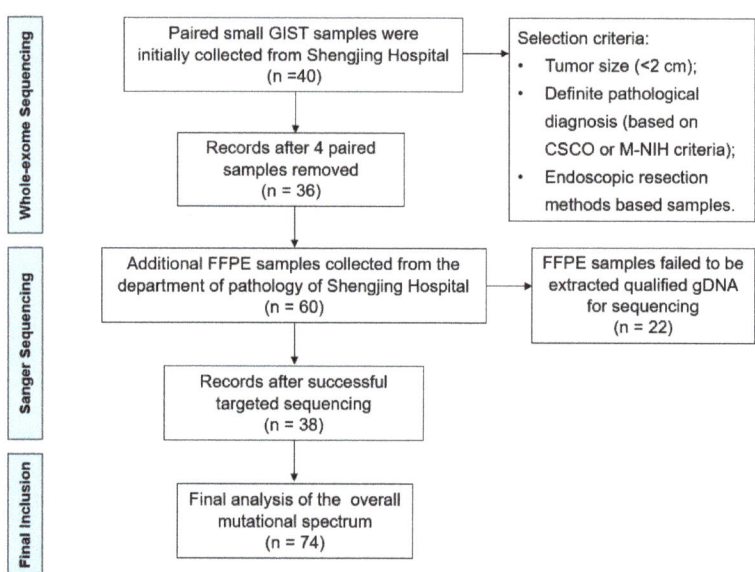

Figure 1. Flow chart of the selection procedure.

2.4. Validation of Variants by Sanger Sequencing

Sanger sequencing was used to verify the suspected somatic variants identified by WES and further determine the mutation rate in the supplementary FFPE samples. Briefly, primers were designed using Primer Premier 5, and gDNA was extracted from FFPE tissues and blood samples (Takara, 9782). The Invitrogen™ Platinum™ Green Hot Start PCR 2X Master Mix (Invitrogen, Carlsbad, CA, USA) was used for PCR amplification, and the PCR products were sent for automatic DNA sequencing (Takara). PCR thermocycling conditions were as follows: activation at 94 °C for 2 min, followed by 35 cycles of denaturation at 94 °C for 30 s, annealing at 55 °C for 30 s, elongation at 72 °C for 1 min, and final elongation at 72 °C for 5 min. The nucleotide sequences of primers used for Sanger sequencing are shown in Table 1.

Table 1. Nucleotide sequences of primers used for Sanger sequencing.

Primers	Sequence
KIT-Exon9-F	CCTTTAGATGCTCTGCTTC
KIT-Exon9-R	GGTAGACAGAGCCTAAACATC
KIT-Exon11-F	GTGCTCTAATGACTGAGACAAT
KIT-Exon11-R	AGGAAGCCACTGGAGTTC
KIT-Exon13-F	TGCATGCGCTTGACATCAGTTTG
KIT-Exon13-R	AGGCAGCTTGGACACGGCTT
KIT-Exon14-F	GTCTGATCCACTGAAGCTG
KIT-Exon14-R	ACCCCATGAACTGCCTGTC
KIT-Exon17-F	TGGTTTTCTTTTCTCCTCCAACC
KIT-Exon17-R	GCAGGACTGTCAAGCAGAG

Table 1. *Cont.*

Primers	Sequence
PDGFRA-Exon12-F	TCCAGTCACTGTGCTGCTTC
PDGFRA-Exon 12-R	GCAAGGGAAAAGGGAGTCTT
PDGFRA-Exon14-F	GGTAGCTCAGCTGGACTGAT
PDGFRA-Exon14-R	GGATGGAGAGTGGAGGATTT
PDGFRA-Exon18-F	TCAGCTACAGATGGCTTGATC
PDGFRA-Exon18-R	TGAAGGAGGATGAGCCTGACC
BRAF Exon15-F	CTTCATAATGCTTGCTCTG
BRAF-Exon15-R	GTAACTCAGCAGCATCTCAG

2.5. In Silico Analysis

Somatic mutations were evaluated for their predicted pathogenic effects using in silico tools, including SIFT (http://sift.jcvi.org/, accessed on 1 January 2022) and PolyPhen (http://genetics.bwh.harvard.edu/pph/, accessed on 1 January 2022).

3. Results

3.1. Clinical Features

A total of 36 paired small GISTs samples were collected for WES (labeled P1–P36), and 38 FFPE samples were successfully extracted as qualified gDNA for targeted Sanger sequencing (labeled P36–P74) (Figure 1). The clinical features and mutation information for the 74 patients are presented in Supplementary Table S1. The age of the patients ranged from 30 to 75 years, with a median age of 56 years (Table 2). Primary tumor distributions showed that the fundus of the stomach (51.3%) and gastric body (39.2%) were the most frequent sites of small GISTs. Micro- and mini-GISTs accounted for 37.8% and 62.2% of the samples, respectively, most of which were classified as very low or low risk based on the modified NIH criteria. These small GISTs were diagnosed by endoscopy, EUS, and pathological presentations involving hematoxylin and eosin staining and positive immunohistochemical features, such as CD117(+) and CD34(+). All enrolled patients were predominantly treated with ESD and partly with EFTR.

Table 2. Clinicopathological characteristics of 74 patients with small gastrointestinal stromal tumors.

Clinical Pathological Characteristics	Number (%)
Sex	
Male	27 (36.5)
Female	47 (63.5)
Age	
Median, years	56
Range, years	30–75
30–50 years	22 (29.7)
51–60 years	24 (32.4)
61–75 years	28 (37.9)
Primary site	
Fundus	38 (51.3)
Junction of the fundus and body	5 (6.8)
Body	29 (39.2)
Antrum	2 (2.7)
Tumor size	
<1 cm (micro-GIST)	28 (37.8)
1–2 cm (mini-GIST)	46 (62.2)
Classification of risk	
Very low	58 (78.4)
Low	12 (16.2)
Intermediate	3 (4.1)
High	1 (1.3)

3.2. Molecular Analysis

Small GISTs with KIT/PDGFRA Mutations

WES was performed to explore the genetic variation in small GISTs. Among the 36 patients, 30 (83%) KIT mutations and 1 (3%) PDGFRA mutation were identified (Figure 2A). The most common mutation area of *KIT* was exon 11 (72%), which encodes the intracellular juxtamembrane domain, whereas other mutated sites of *KIT* were related to exon 9 (8%) and exon 17 (3%). *PDGFRA* mutations accounted for only 3% (1/36) of the mutations, occurring in exon 18. Other probable driver genes selected through a comparison with a public database (Cancer Gene Census513) are shown in Figure 2A. Among the 36 small GIST samples, the most common form of missense substitutions was C > T/G > A. The distribution of KIT mutations is shown in the molecular structure diagram (Figure 2B). The only somatic mutation in the *PDGFRA* gene was a single nucleotide change in exon 18, c.2523A > T p.D842V, which is mainly involved in the activation loop. Direct Sanger sequencing was subsequently performed on 38 additional small GIST samples. Among these samples, 68.4% (26/38) contained missense mutations in KIT and 7.9% (3/38) contained missense mutations in PDGFRA. Most *KIT* mutations were detected in exons 11 and 9, similar to the results of the WES. Two cases harbored single-nucleotide changes in *PDGFRA* at exon 18, including c.2543A > C p.N848T and c.C2544A p.N848K. Another case harboring a *PDGFRA* mutation was determined to be c.1698_1712del p. S566E571delinsR at exon 12. No mutations were detected at exon 14 of the *PDGFRA* gene. In this study, the total KIT/PDGFRA mutation rate was 81% (Figure 3).

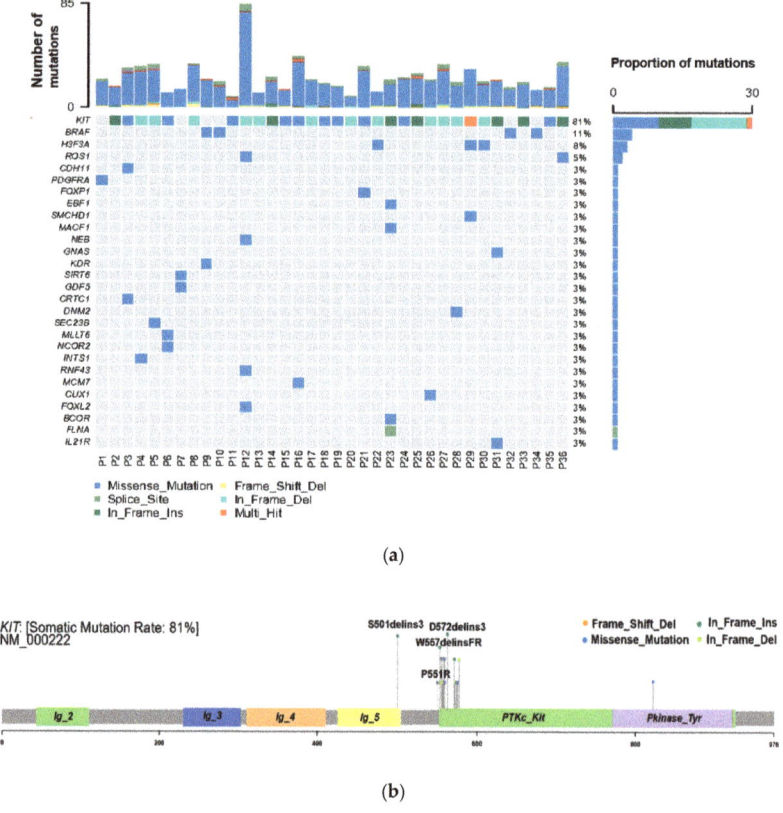

Figure 2. High frequency of oncogenic mutations in 36 small gastrointestinal stromal tumor (GIST) samples identified by whole-exome sequencing (WES). (**a**) Selected driver genes, by comparing somatic

mutations and known driver genes in the database; (**b**) mutation distribution in the KIT molecular structure diagram, with novel mutations marked.

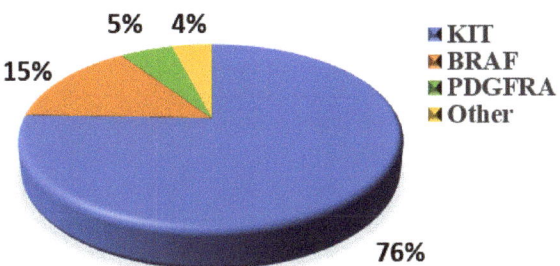

Figure 3. Percentage of classic oncogenic mutations in all 74 samples.

The novel KIT mutations identified in the small GISTs included c.1716_1717insCCAACA p.(Asp572delins3), c.1502_1503insTGCCTA p.(Ser501delins3), and c.1669_1670insTTC p.(W557 delinsFR), all of which were verified by Sanger sequencing (Figure 3). One patient harboring double KIT somatic single-nucleotide variants, including C1652G p. (Pro551Arg) and c.T1679C p. (Val560Ala), was identified (Figure 4a). Furthermore, these two mutations have been considered tumor-promoting factors (COSM7342419 and COSM36302), whereas P551R, usually associated with colon carcinoma, has never been reported to be associated with GIST development.

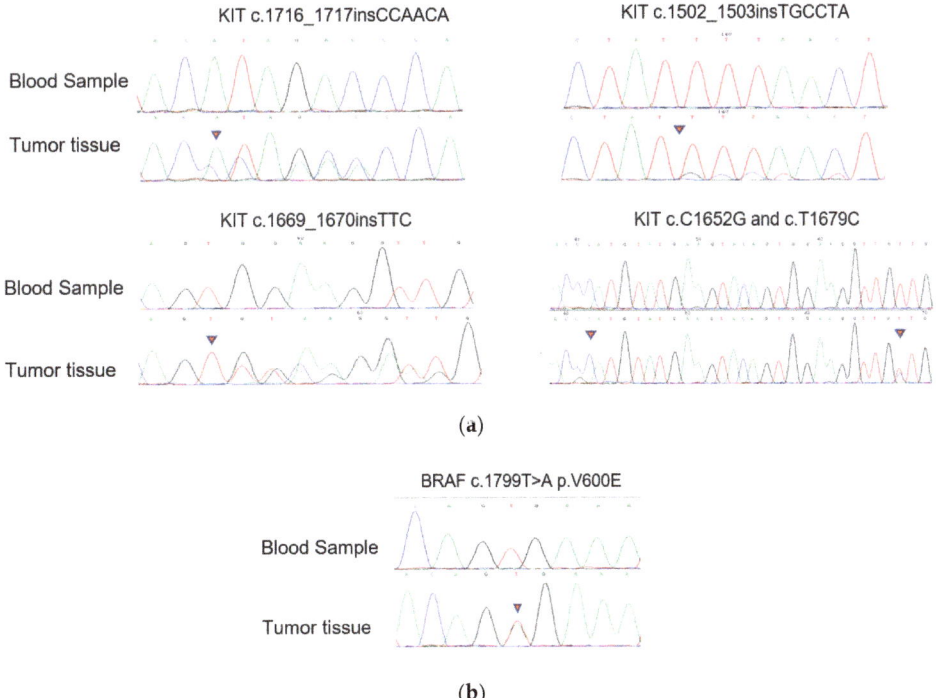

Figure 4. Mutation alleles based on Sanger sequencing. (**a**) Validation of KIT novel mutations using PCR-based Sanger sequencing; (**b**) validation of BRAF mutations using PCR-based Sanger sequencing.

3.3. KIT/PDGFRA Wild-Type (WT) Small GISTs

KIT/PDGFRA WT GISTs had no mutations in the hotspot regions of *KRAS* (codons 12/13/59/61/117/146), *PIK3CA* (codons 542/545/1047), *NRAS* (codons 12/13/59/61/117/146), or *AKT1* (codon 17). Nevertheless, we discovered four cases harboring BRAF mutations (V600E) among these KIT/PDGFRA WT GISTs using WES. Surprisingly, 18.4% (7/38) of the samples in the expanded FFPE samples were found to harbor the BRAF mutation (V600E), which was verified by Sanger sequencing (Figure 4b). Seven patients with the V600E mutation had micro-GISTs, and the remaining patients had mini-GISTs. These tumors had a spindle morphology, and immunohistochemistry was positive for CD117, CD34, and DOG1 but weakly positive or negative for Ki67.

3.4. Suspicious Oncogenic Mutations in Small GISTs

We screened samples for other known oncogenic driver genes in KIT/PDGFRA/BRAF WT tumors to identify whether other potential elements influenced tumorigenesis (P14). We filtered two oncogenes with somatic mutations that had been reported to be related to malignant tumors (Table 3). A common mutation site in SIRT6 (c. A956C) and a suspected mutation in GDF5 (c.A630T) were detected by WES.

Table 3. Probable driver mutations of rare genes in wild-type GISTs.

Gene	Size (cm)	Nucleotide Change (c.Notation)	Amino Acid Change (p.Notation)	SIFT	Polyphen2_HVAR	Malignancy Potential
SIRT6	2 ×1.5	c.A956C	p.K319T	0.007,D	0.987,D	Low
GDF5	2 ×1.5	c.A630T	p.Q210H	0.248,T	0.395,B	Low

SIFT: sorting intolerant from tolerant; Polyphen2_HVAR: polymorphism phenotyping v2 based on HumanVar database.

4. Discussion

In this study, 74 small GISTs were collected for mutational analysis using WES and targeted Sanger sequencing. The mean age of the patients was 56 years, lower than the predominant median age at diagnosis of 65 years [18]. Risk assessment was conducted according to the modified NIH classification criteria standard, by considering the tumor size, primary sites, mitotic index, and tumor rupture. One case in this study was evaluated as high-risk, with a size of 1.5 cm, and three cases were classified as intermediate risk with sizes of 1.2×1.1 cm, 1.8×1.3 cm, and 2×1.6 cm. All other cases were assessed as very low or low risk. Therefore, even if the lesion was less than 2 cm, there was still the possibility of a medium-to-high risk. However, the cutoff size of small GISTs for endoscopic resection remains controversial. Fang et al. investigated the clinical course of small GISTs and demonstrated that a cutoff value of 1.4 cm is appropriate for treatment [19], and Wang et al. proposed that a tumor diameter of 1.45 cm should be the optimal cutoff value for resection, which were consistent with our other retrospective study [20] which identified that a smaller tumor diameter cutoff (1.48 cm) might have better efficacy in differentiating risk grades. Furthermore, a single-institution retrospective study of 69 patients with EUS-suspected GISTs showed that GISTs > 9.5 mm in diameter are associated with significant progression and that 23% of these patients show significant changes in size after more than 3 years of onset [21]. Currently, intensive monitoring with EUS is recommended for most small GISTs, while this is considered an economic and psychological burden for patients [22]. For the radical treatment of small GISTs, ESD and EFTR are relatively safe and effective treatment modalities that can significantly improve patient prognosis [12,22]. With the development of endoscopy, it is also feasible to conduct the genotype diagnosis of tumor cells via EUS-based biopsy in the early stage of GISTs [23,24]. Therefore, whether the current criteria for risk classification can be used to comprehensively evaluate or predict the prognosis of small GISTs needs to be further explored, and more scientific management of small stromal tumors needs further revision.

C-KIT and PDGFRA play vital roles in the occurrence and progression of GISTs [25]. Our study strongly indicated that the oncogenic mutation frequency in small GISTs might be underestimated, since the total mutation rate (96% vs. 74%) was much higher than expected, which suggested that oncogenic mutations are early molecular events in patients with GISTs. Among the 74 small GIST samples in this study, sequencing results revealed that the C-KIT mutation was predominant (76%, 56/74), and exon 11 of KIT was found to be a hotspot that accounted for 65% of the mutations (48/74). Moreover, the mutations occurring at exons 9 and 17 comprised 6.8% and 1.4% of all mutations, respectively. *PDGFRA* mutations occurring at exons 18 and 12 accounted for 5% of all mutations. The mutation comprising a substitution at position 842 in the A-loop of an aspartic acid (D) with a valine (V) in exon 18 confers primary resistance to imatinib and sunitinib but sensitivity to avapritinib [26,27]. Somatic mutations in *C-KIT* are usually found in exon 11, which might confer sensitivity to imatinib [1,2,28]. The second most common mutational hotspot in *KIT* is exon 9, which might confer resistance to imatinib, the first-line targeted therapy for GISTs. The molecular mechanisms underlying oncogenic mutations, such as KIT mutations concerning the Ras-ERK and PI3-kinase pathways, are therapeutic targets of GISTs [29,30].

Notably, we found that 11 of 74 cases (15%) (Figure 3) harbored malignant BRAF-V600E mutations, which had not been detected in previous studies of small GISTs. These results contradict the previous studies which reported the mutation rate of BRAF ranges from 1~4% for large GISTs [31], suggesting that BRAF-mutated tumors might represent a low-risk subtype of small gastric GISTs. A previous study reported that 54.8% of BRAF-mutated GISTs, which were classified as intermediate or high risk [32], were located in the small bowel or colorectum, whereas stomach-derived tumors tended to have a low risk. BRAF mutants generally activate MEK/MAPK and regulate the downstream factor ETV1, thereby promoting ICC proliferation and transformation into a tumor. Activating BRAF mutations are also frequently detected in some malignant carcinomas and tumors such as melanomas, promoting proliferation and drug resistance through the constitutive activation of the MAPK pathway [33]. Ran et al. demonstrated that the BRAF-V600E mutation could promote ICC hyperplasia in adult mouse models. However, this was insufficient to drive the malignant transformation of GIST unless it was coupled with other dysfunctions in tumor-associated genes, such as TP53 loss [34]. Another study showed that BRAF mutations along with TP53 disruption could drive smooth-muscle-cell-derived GISTs, rather than those derived from ICCs [35]. In addition to TP53, the loss of TP16, another tumor-suppressive gene, promotes the development of and leads to poor outcomes for GISTs with BRAF mutations [36]. Therefore, considering the high prevalence of gastric and small intestinal GISTs (60% and 20%, respectively), "secondary hits", such as epigenetic regulation, likely participate in the progression of small GISTs to malignant tumors. For WT GISTs, we analyzed probable oncogenic mutations, namely in SIRT6 and GDF5, which are thought to play roles in the development of ICC hyperplasia or small GISTs. SIRT6 has been identified in patients with colon adenocarcinoma and is related to the promotion of DNA repair in cells with DNA damage [37]. Mutations in GDF5 are usually associated with skeletal developmental deficiency [38], which was also predicted to be disease-causing via the SIFT algorithm and Polyphen2_HVAR.

5. Conclusions

In this study, we demonstrated that genetic alterations are prevalent in small gastric GISTs, suggesting an underestimated risk of these small GISTs. Despite the high frequency of the BRAF-V600E mutation, these small gastric stromal tumors might be benign and represent a low-risk subtype of GISTs. Molecular analysis will be helpful to facilitate personalized medicine and settle disputes related to treatment for small GISTs.

Supplementary Materials: The following supporting information can be downloaded at: https://www.mdpi.com/article/10.3390/cancers14236008/s1, Table S1: Clinicopathological characteristics and mutation information of 74 patients with small GISTs. The risk classification was according to the modified NIH criteria.

Author Contributions: J.G. contributed to sequencing analysis and supervised the study; Q.G. performed the majority of sample collection, analyzed sequencing results, and wrote the manuscript, F.Y. provided input for this paper and took part in the design of the outline; S.W., N.G. and X.L. performed partial tumor endoscopic resection; J.S. assisted in collecting clinical samples; P.F. was responsible for the revision of the manuscript for important intellectual content; S.S. and Y.L. designed and supervised the study; and Y.L. revised the manuscript. All authors have read and agreed to the published version of the manuscript.

Funding: This study received funding from the following: the National Natural Science Foundation of China (Grant No. 81900601), the National Natural Science Foundation of China (Grant No. 81872446), the youth talent project of Xingliao Yingcai program (Grant No. XLYC1807071), the University Innovation Team and Innovative Talent Support Program of Liaoning Province (Grant No. LR2019073), and the Shenyang Young and Middle-aged Science and Technology Innovation Talent Support Program (Grant No. RC200438).

Institutional Review Board Statement: Tumor tissues for sequencing and clinical information collected in the study were reviewed and approved by the Ethics Review Committee of Shengjing Hospital of China Medical University (No: 2022PS049K).

Informed Consent Statement: To protect the privacy of the patients, data related to patients cannot be made available for public access, but all sequencing results from this manuscript are saved by the Ethics Committee of Shengjing Hospital and are available from the corresponding author (sunsy@sj-hospital.org) upon reasonable request approved by the Ethics Committee.

Data Availability Statement: Data of this study can be available from the corresponding author (sunsy@sj-hospital.org) upon reasonable request approved by the Ethics Committee.

Acknowledgments: We thank Si-yu Sun, the co-corresponding author of this article, for his support and guidance during this study. We also thank all other doctors who participated in this study.

Conflicts of Interest: We claim that there are no potential competing interests.

References

1. Blay, J.-Y.; Kang, Y.-K.; Nishida, T.; von Mehren, M. Gastrointestinal Stromal Tumours. *Nat. Rev. Dis. Prim.* **2021**, *7*, 22. [CrossRef] [PubMed]
2. Joensuu, H.; Hohenberger, P.; Corless, C.L. Gastrointestinal Stromal Tumour. *Lancet* **2013**, *382*, 973–983. [CrossRef]
3. Ma, G.L.; Murphy, J.D.; Martinez, M.E.; Sicklick, J.K. Epidemiology of Gastrointestinal Stromal Tumors in the Era of Histology Codes: Results of a Population-Based Study. *Cancer Epidemiol. Biomark. Prev.* **2015**, *24*, 298–302. [CrossRef]
4. Nishida, T.; Goto, O.; Raut, C.P.; Yahagi, N. Diagnostic and Treatment Strategy for Small Gastrointestinal Stromal Tumors: Small Gastrointestinal Stromal Tumors. *Cancer* **2016**, *122*, 3110–3118. [CrossRef] [PubMed]
5. Li, J.; Ye, Y.; Wang, J.; Zhang, B.; Qin, S.; Shi, Y.; He, Y.; Liang, X.; Liu, X.; Zhou, Y.; et al. Chinese Consensus Guidelines for Diagnosis and Management of Gastrointestinal Stromal Tumor. *Chin. J. Cancer Res.* **2017**, *29*, 281–293. [CrossRef] [PubMed]
6. von Mehren, M.; Randall, R.L.; Benjamin, R.S.; Boles, S.; Bui, M.M.; Ganjoo, K.N.; George, S.; Gonzalez, R.J.; Heslin, M.J.; Kane, J.M.; et al. Soft Tissue Sarcoma, Version 2.2018, NCCN Clinical Practice Guidelines in Oncology. *J. Natl. Compr. Cancer Netw.* **2018**, *16*, 536–563. [CrossRef]
7. Poveda, A.; García del Muro, X.; López-Guerrero, J.A.; Cubedo, R.; Martínez, V.; Romero, I.; Serrano, C.; Valverde, C.; Martín-Broto, J. GEIS Guidelines for Gastrointestinal Sarcomas (GIST). *Cancer Treat. Rev.* **2017**, *55*, 107–119. [CrossRef]
8. Joensuu, H. Risk Stratification of Patients Diagnosed with Gastrointestinal Stromal Tumor. *Hum. Pathol.* **2008**, *39*, 1411–1419. [CrossRef]
9. Miettinen, M.; Lasota, J. Gastrointestinal Stromal Tumors: Pathology and Prognosis at Different Sites. *Semin. Diagn. Pathol.* **2006**, *23*, 70–83. [CrossRef]
10. Coe, T.M.; Fero, K.E.; Fanta, P.T.; Mallory, R.J.; Tang, C.-M.; Murphy, J.D.; Sicklick, J.K. Population-Based Epidemiology and Mortality of Small Malignant Gastrointestinal Stromal Tumors in the USA. *J. Gastrointest. Surg.* **2016**, *20*, 1132–1140. [CrossRef]
11. Kawanowa, K.; Sakuma, Y.; Sakurai, S.; Hishima, T.; Iwasaki, Y.; Saito, K.; Hosoya, Y.; Nakajima, T.; Funata, N. High Incidence of Microscopic Gastrointestinal Stromal Tumors in the Stomach. *Hum. Pathol.* **2006**, *37*, 1527–1535. [CrossRef] [PubMed]

12. Zhu, L.; Khan, S.; Hui, Y.; Zhao, J.; Li, B.; Ma, S.; Guo, J.; Chen, X.; Wang, B. Treatment Recommendations for Small Gastric Gastrointestinal Stromal Tumors: Positive Endoscopic Resection. *Scand. J. Gastroenterol.* **2019**, *54*, 297–302. [CrossRef] [PubMed]
13. Rossi, S.; Gasparotto, D.; Toffolatti, L.; Pastrello, C.; Gallina, G.; Marzotto, A.; Sartor, C.; Barbareschi, M.; Cantaloni, C.; Messerini, L.; et al. Molecular and Clinicopathologic Characterization of Gastrointestinal Stromal Tumors (GISTs) of Small Size. *Am. J. Surg. Pathol.* **2010**, *34*, 1480–1491. [CrossRef]
14. Feng, X.; Yang, Z.; Zhang, P.; Chen, T.; Qiu, H.; Zhou, Z.; Li, G.; Tao, K.; Wang, H.; Li, Y. Which Size Is the Best Cutoff for Primary Small Gastric Gastrointestinal Stromal Tumor? *J. Gastrointest. Oncol.* **2020**, *11*, 402–410. [CrossRef]
15. Tran, T.; Davila, J.A.; El-Serag, H.B. The Epidemiology of Malignant Gastrointestinal Stromal Tumors: An Analysis of 1,458 Cases from 1992 to 2000. *Am. J. Gastroenterol.* **2005**, *100*, 162–168. [CrossRef] [PubMed]
16. Agaimy, A.; Blaszyk, H.; Dietmaier, W. Minute Gastric Sclerosing Stromal Tumors (GIST Tumorlets) Are Common in Adults and Frequently Show c-KIT Mutations. *Am. J. Surg. Pathol.* **2007**, *31*, 8. [CrossRef] [PubMed]
17. Søreide, K. Cancer Biology of Small Gastrointestinal Stromal Tumors (<2 cm): What Is the Risk of Malignancy? *Eur. J. Surg. Oncol.* **2017**, *43*, 1344–1349. [CrossRef] [PubMed]
18. Basse, C.; Italiano, A.; Penel, N.; Mir, O.; Chemin, C.; Toulmonde, M.; Duffaud, F.; Le Cesne, A.; Chevreau, C.; Maynou, C.; et al. Sarcomas in Patients over 90: Natural History and Treatment-A Nationwide Study over 6 Years. *Int. J. Cancer* **2019**, *145*, 2135–2143. [CrossRef]
19. Fang, Y.-J.; Cheng, T.-Y.; Sun, M.-S.; Yang, C.-S.; Chen, J.-H.; Liao, W.-C.; Wang, H.-P. Suggested Cutoff Tumor Size for Management of Small EUS-Suspected Gastric Gastrointestinal Stromal Tumors. *J. Formos. Med. Assoc.* **2012**, *111*, 88–93. [CrossRef]
20. Ge, Q.-C.; Wu, Y.-F.; Liu, Z.-M.; Wang, Z.; Wang, S.; Liu, X.; Ge, N.; Guo, J.-T.; Sun, S.-Y. Efficacy of Endoscopic Ultrasound in the Evaluation of Small Gastrointestinal Stromal Tumors. *World J. Gastroenterol.* **2022**, *28*, 5457–5468. [CrossRef]
21. Gao, Z.; Wang, C.; Xue, Q.; Wang, J.; Shen, Z.; Jiang, K.; Shen, K.; Liang, B.; Yang, X.; Xie, Q.; et al. The Cut-off Value of Tumor Size and Appropriate Timing of Follow-up for Management of Minimal EUS-Suspected Gastric Gastrointestinal Stromal Tumors. *BMC Gastroenterol.* **2017**, *17*, 8. [CrossRef] [PubMed]
22. Wang, M.; Xue, A.; Yuan, W.; Gao, X.; Fu, M.; Fang, Y.; Wang, L.; Shu, P.; Li, H.; Hou, Y.; et al. Clinicopathological Features and Prognosis of Small Gastric Gastrointestinal Stromal Tumors (GISTs). *J. Gastrointest. Surg.* **2019**, *23*, 2136–2143. [CrossRef] [PubMed]
23. Kuwatani, M.; Sakamoto, N. Evolution and a Promising Role of EUS-FNA in Gene and Future Analyses. *Endosc. Ultrasound* **2020**, *9*, 151–153. [CrossRef] [PubMed]
24. Nagai, K.; Sofuni, A.; Tsuchiya, T.; Kono, S.; Ishii, K.; Tanaka, R.; Tonozuka, R.; Mukai, S.; Yamamoto, K.; Matsunami, Y.; et al. Efficacy of the Franseen Needle for Diagnosing Gastrointestinal Submucosal Lesions Including Small Tumors. *Endosc. Ultrasound* **2021**, *10*, 424–430. [CrossRef] [PubMed]
25. Boye, K.; Berner, J.-M.; Hompland, I.; Bruland, Ø.S.; Stoldt, S.; Sundby Hall, K.; Bjerkehagen, B.; Hølmebakk, T. Genotype and Risk of Tumour Rupture in Gastrointestinal Stromal Tumour. *Br. J. Surg.* **2018**, *105*, e169–e175. [CrossRef]
26. Rizzo, A.; Pantaleo, M.A.; Astolfi, A.; Indio, V.; Nannini, M. The Identity of PDGFRA D842V-Mutant Gastrointestinal Stromal Tumors (GIST). *Cancers* **2021**, *13*, 705. [CrossRef]
27. Heinrich, M.C.; Jones, R.L.; von Mehren, M.; Schöffski, P.; Serrano, C.; Kang, Y.-K.; Cassier, P.A.; Mir, O.; Eskens, F.; Tap, W.D.; et al. Avapritinib in Advanced PDGFRA D842V-Mutant Gastrointestinal Stromal Tumour (NAVIGATOR): A Multicentre, Open-Label, Phase 1 Trial. *Lancet Oncol.* **2020**, *21*, 935–946. [CrossRef]
28. Abbaspour Babaei, M.; Kamalidehghan, B.; Saleem, M.; Zaman Huri, H.; Ahmadipour, F. Receptor Tyrosine Kinase (c-Kit) In Drug Des. Dev. Ther. **2016**, *10*, 2443–2459. [CrossRef]
29. Duan, Y.; Haybaeck, J.; Yang, Z. Therapeutic Potential of PI3K/AKT/MTOR Pathway in Gastrointestinal Stromal Tumors: Rationale and Progress. *Cancers* **2020**, *12*, 2972. [CrossRef]
30. Gupta, A.; Singh, J.; García-Valverde, A.; Serrano, C.; Flynn, D.L.; Smith, B.D. Ripretinib and MEK Inhibitors Synergize to Induce Apoptosis in Preclinical Models of GIST and Systemic Mastocytosis. *Mol. Cancer Ther.* **2021**, *20*, 1234–1245. [CrossRef]
31. Haefliger, S.; Marston, K.; Juskevicius, D.; Meyer-Schaller, N.; Forster, A.; Nicolet, S.; Komminoth, P.; Stauffer, E.; Cathomas, G.; Hoeller, S.; et al. Molecular Profile of Gastrointestinal Stromal Tumors in Sixty-Eight Patients from a Single Swiss Institution. *Pathobiology* **2020**, *87*, 171–178. [CrossRef] [PubMed]
32. Huss, S.; Pasternack, H.; Ihle, M.A.; Merkelbach-Bruse, S.; Heitkötter, B.; Hartmann, W.; Trautmann, M.; Gevensleben, H.; Büttner, R.; Schildhaus, H.-U.; et al. Clinicopathological and Molecular Features of a Large Cohort of Gastrointestinal Stromal Tumors (GISTs) and Review of the Literature: BRAF Mutations in KIT/PDGFRA Wild-Type GISTs Are Rare Events. *Hum. Pathol.* **2017**, *62*, 206–214. [CrossRef]
33. Alqathama, A. BRAF in Malignant Melanoma Progression and Metastasis: Potentials and Challenges. *Am. J. Cancer Res.* **2020**, *10*, 1103–1114. [PubMed]
34. Ran, L.; Murphy, D.; Sher, J.; Cao, Z.; Wang, S.; Walczak, E.; Guan, Y.; Xie, Y.; Shukla, S.; Zhan, Y.; et al. ETV1-Positive Cells Give Rise to BRAF V600E-Mutant Gastrointestinal Stromal Tumors. *Cancer Res.* **2017**, *77*, 3758–3765. [CrossRef] [PubMed]
35. Kondo, J.; Huh, W.J.; Franklin, J.L.; Heinrich, M.C.; Rubin, B.P.; Coffey, R.J. A Smooth Muscle-derived, BRAF-driven Mouse Model of Gastrointestinal Stromal Tumor (GIST): Evidence for an Alternative GIST Cell-of-origin. *J. Pathol.* **2020**, *252*, 441–450. [CrossRef] [PubMed]

36. Shi, S.; Wang, X.; Xia, Q.; Rao, Q.; Shen, Q.; Ye, S.; Li, R.; Shi, Q.; Lu, Z.; Ma, H.; et al. P16 Overexpression in BRAF -Mutated Gastrointestinal Stromal Tumors. *Expert Rev. Mol. Diagn.* **2017**, *17*, 195–201. [CrossRef]
37. Geng, A.; Tang, H.; Huang, J.; Qian, Z.; Qin, N.; Yao, Y.; Xu, Z.; Chen, H.; Lan, L.; Xie, H.; et al. The Deacetylase SIRT6 Promotes the Repair of UV-Induced DNA Damage by Targeting DDB2. *Nucleic Acids Res.* **2020**, *48*, 9181–9194. [CrossRef]
38. Kiapour, A.M.; Cao, J.; Young, M.; Capellini, T.D. The Role of Gdf5 Regulatory Regions in Development of Hip Morphology. *PLoS ONE* **2018**, *13*, e0202785. [CrossRef]

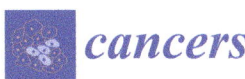

Review

MicroRNAs in the Pathogenesis, Prognostication and Prediction of Treatment Resistance in Soft Tissue Sarcomas

Andrea York Tiang Teo [1], Vivian Yujing Lim [2] and Valerie Shiwen Yang [2,3,4,*]

1. Yong Loo Lin School of Medicine, National University of Singapore, Singapore 117597, Singapore
2. Institute of Molecular and Cell Biology, A*STAR, Singapore 138673, Singapore
3. Division of Medical Oncology, National Cancer Centre Singapore, Singapore 169610, Singapore
4. Oncology Academic Clinical Program, Duke-NUS Medical School, Singapore 169857, Singapore
* Correspondence: yangswv@imcb.a-star.edu

Simple Summary: Soft tissue sarcoma is a rare entity that accounts for 1% of adult cancers but represents 20% of paediatric solid tumours. Overall prognosis in advanced disease remains poor. MicroRNAs (miRNAs) are short non-coding RNAs that target mRNAs and control gene expression and may exert both oncogenic and tumour suppressor functions in cancers. The deregulation of miRNAs in soft tissue sarcomas may be exploited in the development of miRNA-based strategies for the prognostication of disease outcomes, identification of treatment resistance and new-generation therapeutics.

Abstract: Soft tissue sarcomas are highly aggressive malignant neoplasms of mesenchymal origin, accounting for less than 1% of adult cancers, but comprising over 20% of paediatric solid tumours. In locally advanced, unresectable, or metastatic disease, outcomes from even the first line of systemic treatment are invariably poor. MicroRNAs (miRNAs), which are short non-coding RNA molecules, target and modulate multiple dysregulated target genes and/or signalling pathways within cancer cells. Accordingly, miRNAs demonstrate great promise for their utility in diagnosing, prognosticating and improving treatment for soft tissue sarcomas. This review aims to provide an updated discussion on the known roles of specific miRNAs in the pathogenesis of sarcomas, and their potential use in prognosticating outcomes and prediction of therapeutic resistance.

Keywords: soft tissue sarcomas; microRNA; prognostic biomarkers; predictive biomarkers; treatment resistance

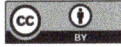

1. Introduction

Sarcomas are malignant neoplasms of mesenchymal origin with over 70 histologic subtypes and may be broadly divided into two categories: soft tissue sarcomas (thought to arise from the muscle, fat, nerve/nerve sheath, blood vessels or other connective tissue) and bone sarcomas (Figure 1) [1]. They account for 1% of adult cancers, and nearly 21% of all paediatric solid malignant cancers, with soft tissue sarcomas comprising nearly 90% of sarcomas [2]. Soft tissue sarcomas may arise anywhere in the body, but most originate in the extremities, the abdomen, or the head and neck [3,4]. While no formal etiology has yet been defined, multiple gene rearrangements have been associated with an increased risk of certain soft tissue sarcoma subtypes, such as in Ewing's sarcoma (EWSR1–FLI-1 fusion), myxoid liposarcoma (TLS–CHOP fusion), alveolar rhabdomyosarcoma (PAX3–FHKR fusion) and synovial sarcoma (SSX–SYT fusion) [5].

Traditionally, soft tissue sarcomas are managed by wide excisional surgery for localized disease. Surgery may also be used as a palliative procedure in metastatic disease [6]. With the exception of gastrointestinal stromal tumours (GIST), adjuvant treatment is not standard, even in R_0 resections. Radiotherapy and chemotherapy are typically reserved for advanced disease; radiotherapy is usually provided in high-risk tumours that are large, deep and/or high grade [7], while adjuvant systemic treatment is controversial, but may be considered on a case-by-case basis [8]. While a meta-analysis of randomized trials found a statistically significant—albeit marginal—advantage of adjuvant chemotherapy in terms of both recurrence-free survival and overall survival [9], a large phase III randomised controlled trial subsequently demonstrated that adjuvant chemotherapy in resected soft tissue sarcoma failed to show improved survival [10]. Increasingly, novel targeted therapies are also used in the management of soft tissue sarcomas following better understanding of the molecular pathogenesis and genomic profiles of some soft tissue sarcomas, but this applies only to a minority of subtypes [8]. The median survival in soft tissue sarcoma patients with metastatic disease is one year [11–13]. Even in patients with localized disease, up to 50% develop metastases and die despite undergoing definitive therapy [5,14], thus highlighting the need for earlier diagnosis, appropriate management and novel treatment approaches in soft tissue sarcomas.

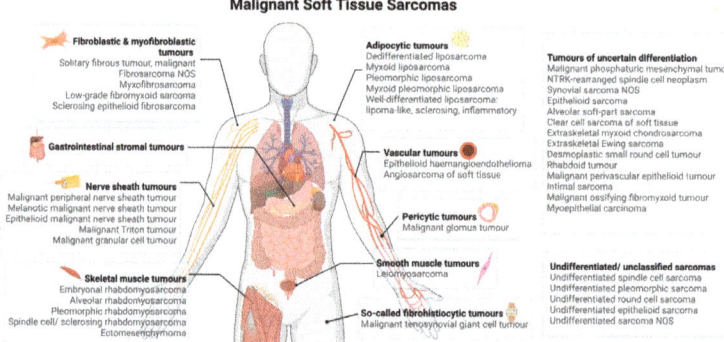

Figure 1. Types of soft tissue sarcomas based on the 2020 WHO classification [15].

MicroRNAs (miRNAs) are short non-coding RNAs of 19–25 nucleotides that regulate post-transcriptional gene expression. Mature miRNAs bind to complementary sites on target mRNAs, usually at the 3′ UTR, thereby suppressing mRNA translation or causing degradation of the mRNA transcript [16]. Because of their ability to target multiple different mRNAs, miRNAs are able to modulate almost any biological pathway. Accordingly, miRNAs are important regulators of various cancer-related processes, such as differentiation, proliferation, metastasis and apoptosis [17], and are therefore attractive targets for miRNA-based therapies. They have been found to be generally downregulated in tumours [18] but can exert both oncogenic and tumour suppressor functions in cancers. Although miRNAs comprise ~0.01% of the total RNA mass in a given sample, advances in strategies to detect and target miRNAs have greatly improved, thus making miRNAs attractive biomarkers in the early diagnosis, staging and monitoring of cancer progression [19], as well as targets for drug development [20].

The role of miRNAs in the diagnosis of soft tissue sarcomas has been proposed and discussed elsewhere [21,22]; however, the use of miRNA as biomarkers for predicting patient outcomes and therapeutic resistance in soft tissue sarcomas is less defined. In this review, we will first summarise the known roles of specific miRNAs in the pathogenesis of sarcomas, then discuss their potential use in prognosticating outcomes and prediction of therapeutic resistance.

2. MicroRNAs in the Pathogenesis of Soft Tissue Sarcomas

miRNAs mediate soft tissue sarcoma progression by influencing various pathogenic processes, thereby acting as oncogenes or tumour suppressors. As the clinical behaviours underlying pathogenesis and management of soft tissue sarcomas differ between subtypes, the following discussion will review the roles of relevant miRNAs within each soft tissue sarcoma subtype. Table 1 summarises the key miRNAs known to be involved in the regulation of various soft tissue sarcoma subtypes.

Table 1. Differential expression of miRNAs and their roles in cancer development in soft tissue sarcomas.

Soft Tissue Sarcoma	Effect on Cancer Development	microRNA
GIST	Inhibit	miR-494 [23,24] miR-218 [25–27] miR-221/222 [28–30] miR-17 [30] miR-20a [30] miR-4510 [31] miR-152 [32] miR-133b [33] miR-518a-5p [34] miR-137 [35]
	Promote	miR-374b [36] miR-196a [37]
Liposarcoma	Inhibit	miR-143 [38,39] miR-486 [40] miR-145 [38,41] miR-451 [39,41] miR-193b [42,43] miR-133a [44] miR-195 [45]
	Promote	miR-155 [39,46–48] miR-26a-2 [38,49,50] miR-135b [51] miR-25-3p [52] miR-92a-3p [52] miR-3613-3p [53]
Rhabdomyosarcoma	Inhibit	miR-206 [54–61] miR-1 [55,56,62,63] miR-29 [56,64,65] miR-26a [66,67] miR-7 [68,69] miR-324-5p [69] miR-378 family [70] miR-133a [62] miR-133b [63] miR-450b-5p [71] miR-203 [72] miR-411-5p [73] miR-221/222 [74] miR-214 [75] miR-101 [76] miR-874 [77] miR-410-3p [78]
	Promote	miR-27a [79,80] miR-486-5p [74]
Malignant peripheral nerve sheath tumour	Inhibit	miR-204 [81] miR-30d [82] miR-30a [83] miR-200b [83] miR-34a [84]
	Promote	miR-21 [85] miR-801 [86] miR-214 [86]
Leiomyosarcoma	Inhibit	miR-1246 [87] miR-191-5p [87] miR-34a [88] miR-152 [89]
	Promote	miR-181b [90] miR-320a [91]
Synovial sarcoma	Inhibit	miR-494-3p [92] miR-126 [93]
	Promote	Let-7e [94] miR-99b [94] miR-92b-3p [95] miR-214 [96] miR-9 [97] miR-17 [98]
Fibrosarcoma	Inhibit	miR-29 [99] miR-197 [100]
	Promote	miR-520c [101] miR-373 [101]
Angiosarcoma	Inhibit	miR-497-5p [102] miR-210 [103] miR-340 [104]
	Promote	-

2.1. Gastrointestinal Stromal Tumour

Gastrointestinal stromal tumour (GIST) is the most common mesenchymal tumour specific to the gastrointestinal tract and is commonly characterized by activating mutations in the KIT or PDGFRA receptor tyrosine kinases [105]. KIT is an oncogene which has a gain-of-function mutation in approximately 70% of GISTs [106,107]. Several miRNAs are shown to inhibit the progression of GIST via the regulation of KIT (Figure 2).

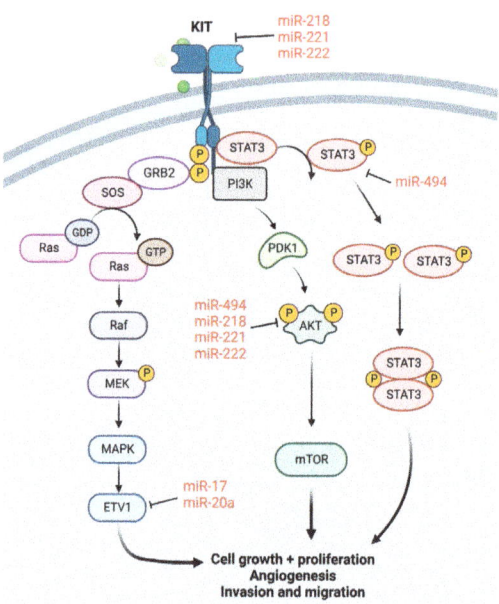

Figure 2. miRNAs regulating KIT and downstream pathways in GIST.

Downregulation of miR-494 has been observed in GIST cell lines, and miR-494 overexpression in GIST cells triggered apoptosis and inhibited cell growth [23,24]. miR-494 was found to regulate the expression of KIT and other molecules in its downstream signaling cascade, including phospho-AKT and phospho-STAT3 [23]. miR-494 was also shown to target survivin, with downregulation of survivin leading to G2-M phase arrest and apoptosis, along with inhibition of cell proliferation and colony formation [24]. Analysis of survivin/KIT interaction showed that survivin regulated KIT expression at the transcription level, thus exerting effects on the PI3K-AKT pathway in GIST as well [24]. Another miRNA found to be markedly decreased in GIST tissues is miR-218 [25,26], with ectopic overexpression in GIST cells via chitosan-tocopherol nanoparticle or liposome delivery demonstrating decreased cell proliferation and increased apoptosis [25,27]. KIT was identified as a target of miR-218 in both studies [25,27]. The miR-221/222 cluster, dysregulated in many malignancies [108–110], is also downregulated in GIST [28–30]. KIT-positive GISTs showed significant repression of miR-221/222 as compared to normal tissues and KIT-negative GISTs [28]. The role of miR-221/222 in the modulation of KIT and the PI3K/AKT pathway in GIST was confirmed by Ihle et al. who demonstrated that transient transfection of miR-221/222 reduced GIST cell viability and induced apoptosis by inhibition of KIT expression and its downstream signalling cascade [29]. This was corroborated by Gits et al. who showed the direct regulation of KIT by miR-222 in GIST [30].

Other miRNAs that are downregulated in GIST include miR-17, miR-20a, miR-4510, miR-133b, miR-152, miR-518-5p and miR-137 [30–34]. These miRNAs play a role in controlling tumour proliferation, migration and invasion, and in inducing apoptosis. miR-17 and miR-20a act by targeting ETV1 [30], a transcription factor that supports tumorigenesis and is universally highly expressed in GISTs [111]. miR-4510 demonstrated its tumour suppressor effects by targeting and inhibiting apolipoprotein C-II (ApoC2) expression, and also decreased the activity of AKT, ERK1/2, MMP2 and MMP9 [31]. miR-152 was found to target and suppress the expression of cathepsin L (CTSL) [32], a lysosomal cysteine protease correlated with metastatic aggressiveness and poor patient prognosis [112]. Epithelial mesenchymal transition (EMT) was another key process in cancer progression regulated by miR-137, which was reported to target Twist1 and increase the expression of epithelial markers E-cadherin and cytokeratin while decreasing the expression of mesenchymal markers N-cadherin and vimentin in GIST cells. As with the other aforementioned miRNAs, miR-137 also decreased GIST cell migration, activated G1 cell cycle arrest, and induced cell apoptosis [35].

On the contrary, oncogenic miRNAs promote the development of GIST. miR-374b was highly expressed in GIST tissues, and its expression increased the mRNA and protein levels of various molecules in the PI3K/AKT cell survival pathway in GIST cells [36]. miR-374b was also found to promote cell viability, migration, invasion and cell cycle progression in GIST cells, along with inhibition of apoptosis [36]. It was further reported that miR-196a expression is overexpressed in high-risk GIST samples as compared to the low- or intermediate-risk GIST tissues, with the upregulation of miR-196a associated with GIST malignancy [37].

2.2. Liposarcoma

Liposarcoma is one of the most common soft tissue sarcomas, and may be classified into four subtypes based on its pathological and molecular genetic characteristics: pleomorphic (PLPS), myxoid/round cell (MLPS/RLPS), dedifferentiated (DDLPS) and well-differentiated (WDLPS). The round cell component in MLPS/RLPS is thought to be associated with metastasis and poorer prognosis [113]. The regulation of liposarcoma by miRNAs occurs through various mechanisms (Figure 3).

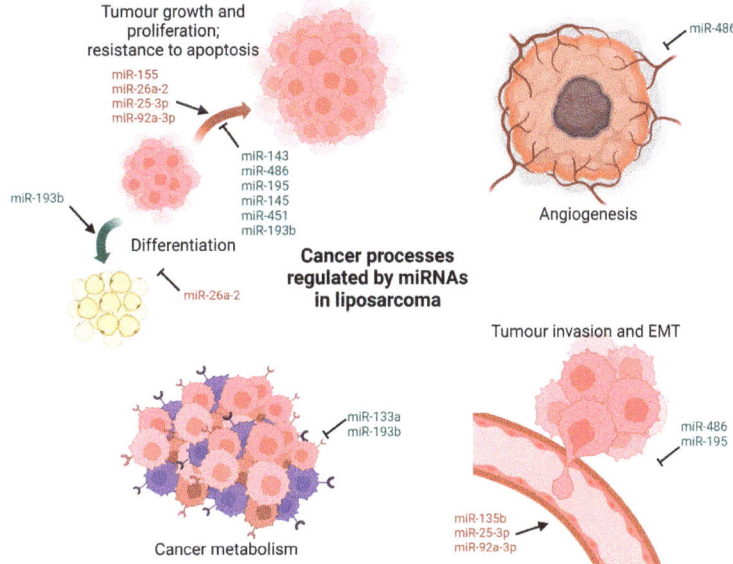

Figure 3. microRNAs involved in the regulation of liposarcoma.

miR-155 is known to act as an oncogene in multiple malignant tumours [114]. It has been found to be the most over-expressed miRNA identified in DDLPS tumour samples and cell lines [46] and is also over-expressed in PLPS and MLPS/RLPS [39,47]. miR-155 was further shown to promote tumour cell growth in DDLPS by targeting casein kinase 1α (CK1α), thereby enhancing β-catenin signalling and cyclin D1 expression [46]. miR-26a-2 has also been found to be overexpressed in WDLPS, DDLPS and MLPS/RLPS [38,49]. Overexpression of miR-26a-2 in LPS cell lines improved sarcoma cell growth and survival, including faster cell proliferation and migration, enhanced clonogenicity, suppressed adipocyte differentiation and/or resistance to apoptosis. Overexpression of RCBTB1, a direct target of miR-26a-2, made LPS cells more susceptible to apoptosis [49]. HOXA5 has also been demonstrated to be a target of miR-26a-2, with the downregulation of HOXA5 inhibiting the apoptotic response in LPS cells [50].

Other miRNAs which are overexpressed in LPS and play a role in invasion and metastasis include miR-135b, miR-25-3p and miR-92a-3p [51–53]. miR-135b is highly expressed in the round cell component of MLPS/RLPS and has been found to promote MLPS/RLPS cell invasion in vitro and metastasis in vivo by targeting the expression of thrombospondin 2 (THBS2). Decreased THBS2 expression increases the amount of matrix metalloproteinase 2 (MMP2) thereby modulating the extracellular matrix structure, resulting in a morphological change of the tumour [51]. A study on the extracellular vesicles secreted by LPS cells showed that they contained miR-25-3p and miR-92a-3p, though they were downregulated within the liposarcoma tumour itself. The secretion of miR-25-3p and miR-92a-3p then initiated the release of proinflammatory cytokine IL-6 from tumour-associated macrophages, in turn enhancing LPS cell proliferation, invasion and metastasis [52]. More recently, miR-1246, miR-4532, miR-4454, miR-619-5p and miR-6126 have been identified to be highly expressed in human DDLPS cell lines and exosomes and are believed to promote tumour progression [115].

On the contrary, certain miRNAs have been found to inhibit the progression of LPS through suppression of proliferation and induction of apoptosis. miR-143 is downregulated in both WDLPS and DDLPS tumours and cell lines [38,39]. Restoring miR-143 expression in DDLPS cells decreased the expression of BCL2, topoisomerase 2A, protein regulator of cytokinesis 1 (PRC1), and polo-like kinase 1 (PLK1). It was further shown that treatment of LPS cells with a PLK1 inhibitor potently arrested cytokinesis in the G2–M phase and induced apoptosis [38]. miR-486 expression was also found to be repressed in MLPS tissues, with the restoration of miR-486 expression resulting in repressed MLPS cell growth [40]. Plasminogen activator inhibitor-1 (PAI-1), shown to promote tumour invasion and angiogenesis [116], was identified as a target of miR-486. Accordingly, knockdown of PAI-1 inhibited the growth of MLPS cells [40]. Another miRNA that inhibits LPS cell growth and migration in vitro and suppresses tumour growth in vivo is miR-195. Oxysterol-binding protein (OSBP) was demonstrated as a direct target of miR-195, with the overexpression of OSBP reversing the effects of miR-195 on LPS cell growth, migration and apoptosis [45]. miR-145 and miR-451 expression have also been found to be reduced in human LPS samples of all subtypes [38,39,41], with the reintroduction of miR-145 and miR-451 in LPS cell lines resulting in impaired cell cycle progression and cellular proliferation and increased cellular apoptosis [41].

Some miRNAs may also regulate LPS progression by interfering with tumour cell metabolism and introducing oxidative stress. miR-133a, significantly underexpressed in DDLPS tissues, has been found to modulate DDLPS cell metabolism, with enforced expression of miR-133a resulting in decreased glycolysis and increased oxidative phosphorylation. This was coupled with impaired cell proliferation and cell cycle progression [44]. miR-193b is found to be underexpressed in DDLPS, with exogenous reintroduction of miR-193b resulting in LPS cell apoptosis [42]. miR-193b targets CRK-like proto-oncogene (CRKL) and focal adhesion kinase (FAK); in vivo studies to introduce miR-193b mimetics and an FAK inhibitor resulted in inhibited LPS xenograft growth in both cases. In addition, miR-193b also induced oxidative stress in LPS cells by targeting an antioxidant, methionine sulfoxide reductase A (MsrA) [42]. Further studies revealed that miR-193b also directly targets PDGFRβ, SMAD4, and YAP1 [43]. Inhibition of PDGFRβ attenuates the differentiation and proliferation of LPS cells, while knockdown of SMAD4 promotes adipogenic differentiation. Direct inhibition of YAP1 reduces the activity of Wnt/β-catenin signalling. Subsequent introduction of a PDGFR inhibitor and a Wnt/β-catenin inhibitor demonstrated reduced cell viability and increased apoptosis in DDLPS and WDLPS cells [43].

2.3. Rhabdomyosarcoma

Rhabdomyosarcoma (RMS) is the most common soft tissue sarcoma in paediatric patients and young adults. RMS can be classified into two major histological subtypes: embryonal rhabdomyosarcoma (ERMS) and alveolar rhabdomyosarcoma (ARMS). RMS may be further classified based on clinical outcome into fusion-positive RMS or fusion-negative RMS based on the presence or absence of either PAX3-FOXO1 or PAX7-FOXO1 gene fusions. As these gene fusions are absent in ERMS, ERMS patients are all fusion-negative, while majority of ARMS patients are fusion positive [117–119]. Fusion-positive RMS tends to have a worse prognosis and overall survival than fusion-negative RMS, thus ARMS is associated with poorer prognosis [120–122].

In recent studies, miRNAs which have been identified to play a role in skeletal muscle proliferation and differentiation such as miR-1, miR-133, miR-206 and miR-29 [123,124], have been investigated for their roles in RMS. miR-206 plays an important role in the regulation of RMS, with multiple studies demonstrating downregulation of miR-206 in RMS tissues and cell lines as compared to human myotubes and skeletal muscle [54–61]. Exogenously increasing miR-206 levels in RMS has been shown to promote myogenic differentiation and block tumour growth in xenografted mice by switching the global mRNA expression profile to one that resembles mature muscle [54]. This was corroborated by a separate study showing that the activation of miR-206 resulted in a genetic switch in RMS cells from a proliferative growth phase to differentiation [57]. In ERMS, the following regulation pathway of miR-206 was uncovered: PAX3/7-FOXO1 induced oxidative stress response factor HO-1 expression, which in turn resulted in miR-206 repression. HO-1 inhibition showed reduced RMS tumour growth and vascularisation in vivo, accompanied by the induction of miR-206 [60]. miR-206 then exerts its anti-tumorigenic effects by targeting and suppressing the Met receptor tyrosine kinase (c-Met), which is overexpressed in both ARMS and ERMS [125], and has been implicated in RMS pathogenesis [54,55]. SMYD1 silencing, which occurs with low levels of miR-206 in RMS, impairs differentiation of all subtypes of RMS. On the contrary, silencing of G6PD, a direct target of miR-206, successfully suppressed RMS cell proliferation and growth [59]. Furthermore, ectopic expression of miR-206 in a ERMS fusion-negative RMS cell line showed significant downregulation of PAX3 protein expression, but this was not observed in ARMS fusion-positive RMS cells as the formation of a fusion transcript between PAX3 and FOXO1 enabled the cells to evade miRNA-mediated regulation of PAX3 [56]. In addition, PAX7 downregulation was shown to be essential for miR-206-induced cell cycle exit and myogenic differentiation in fusion-negative RMS but not in fusion-positive RMS. Genetic deletion of miR-206 in a mouse model of fusion-negative RMS promoted tumor development [58]. Interestingly, while there is much evidence to show that miR-206 is downregulated in RMS tumours and cell lines, analysis of plasma samples of RMS patients has found significantly increased levels of miR-206 as compared to healthy individuals and patients with non-RMS tumours [67,126]. This may be because RMS forms within skeletal muscle, and miR-206 is a muscle-specific miRNA, thus elevated levels of this miRNA may be found in RMS patient serum.

Another notable miRNA in RMS regulation is miR-1 [54,55,63]. Besides downregulating PAX3 expression in ERMS [56], miR-1 was also found to suppress c-Met expression in RMS [55]. miR-1 was shown to encourage myogenic differentiation in RMS cells, and ectopic increase in miR-1 expression resulted in growth inhibition of RMS cells, likely due to G1-S cell cycle arrest [62]. Furthermore, overexpression of miR-1 and miR-133b also resulted in autophagic cell death through the silencing of polypyrimidine tract-binding protein 1 (PTBP1), a positive regulator of cancer-specific energy metabolism [63]. PAX3-FOXO1, which could upregulate the expression of a key kinase involved in glycolysis and the Warburg effect through increased expression of PTBP1, was targeted and repressed by miR-133b [63]. Overexpression of miR-133a in ERMS cells resulted in cell cycle arrest, suggesting its role as a tumour suppressor [62].

Several miRNAs share similar targets in the regulation of RMS. miR-29 is a key miRNA that is epigenetically silenced in RMS tissues and cell lines [56,64,65]. It has been reported that the downregulation of miR-29 occurs via an activated NF-κB YY1 pathway, in which NF-κB acts through Ying Yang 1 (YY1) [64]. miR-29 was found to target and repress the expression of cell cycle regulators cyclin D2 and E2F7, resulting in partial G1 arrest and decreased cell proliferation in RMS [56]. In addition, miR-29 also targets GEFT, which is associated with poor prognosis in patients with RMS [127]. Repression of GEFT activity by miR-29 weakened the effect of GEFT on the migration, invasion and apoptosis of RMS cells [65] while restoration of miR-29 in mice inhibited tumour growth and stimulated differentiation [64,65]. GEFT translation and expression were also found to be inhibited by miR-874, an miRNA downregulated in RMS tissues. Overexpression of miR-874 in RMS cells inhibited proliferation, invasion and migration in RMS cells and also induced apoptosis, while GEFT restoration partially reversed the anti-tumour effects of miR-874 [77]. miR-26a has also been found to be downregulated in RMS tumours and cell lines. Expression levels of miR-26a were further demonstrated to be inversely related to EZH2 [66], a histone methyltransferase overexpressed in various aggressive cancers [128,129]. Circulating levels of miR-26a in RMS patient plasma were also reduced, and miR-26a plasma levels were associated with fusion status, with PAX3/7-FOXO1-positive RMS samples displaying lower levels of miR-26a compared to fusion-negative samples [67]. Separately, EZH2 was found to downregulate miR-101 in ERMS cells via a negative feedback loop, and overexpression of miR-101 was able to reduce ERMS tumorigenic potential, impairing colony formation and cell cycle progression [76].

Other miRNAs which are downregulated in RMS cell lines and tissue samples have also demonstrated anti-tumour effects in RMS by inducing apoptosis and myogenic differentiation, as well as impairing cell proliferation, invasion and metastasis. In miR-7 transfected RMS cells, miR-7 acts via its target mitochondrial proteins solute carrier family 25 member 37 (SLC25A37) and translocase of inner mitochondrial membrane 50 (TIMM50) to promote apoptosis and necroptosis [68], and also impair tumour invasion and lung metastasis [69]. In addition, miR-7 and miR-324-5p regulate pro-oncogenic protein ITGA9, and overexpression of the two miRNAs reduced tumour growth in orthotopic mice tumour models [69]. Insulin-like growth factor receptor 1 (IGF1R), a key signalling molecule in RMS, was shown to be a target of miR-378a-3p. Upregulation of miR-378a-5p expression resulted in apoptosis, decreased cell viability and G2 phase cell cycle arrest in RMS cells, along with upregulation of myogenic proteins such as MyoD and MyHC, demonstrating a shift towards myogenic differentiation [70]. Similarly, miR-450b-5p, suppressed in RMS by TGF-β1 through a pathway mediated by Smad3 and Smad4, exerted anti-tumour effects in tumour implants and cells by arresting RMS growth and upregulating MyoD expression [71]. An autoregulatory loop between TGF-β1/miR-411-5p/SPRY4 and MAPK in RMS has also been established, in which it is suggested that miR-411-5p inhibits SPRY4 to activate MAPK, promoting apoptosis and myogenic differentiation in RMS cells [73]. miR-203 was also reported to be downregulated by promoter hypermethylation in RMS tumour samples and cell lines. Restoration of miR-203 expression in RMS cells was able to inhibit their migration and proliferation. Furthermore, miR-203 promoted myogenic differentiation by inhibiting the Notch and JAK1/STAT1/STAT3 pathways via its target proteins p63 and leukaemia inhibitory factor receptor [72]. miR-214 reintroduction into RMS cells was able to inhibit tumour cell growth, promote apoptosis and induce myogenic differentiation. Proto-oncogene N-ras was reported as a conserved target of miR-214 in its suppression of xenograft tumour growth [75]. Lastly, exogenous expression of miR-410-3p was shown to inhibit EMT in RMS, with the inhibition of RMS cell invasion, migration and proliferation [78].

In contrast, miR-27a and miR-486-5p were discovered to be upregulated in the more aggressive fusion-positive RMS samples and cell lines [74,79]. miR-27a was further found to enhance cell cycle progression by targeting the retinoic acid alpha receptor (RARA) and retinoic X receptor alpha (RXRA), resulting in increased RMS cell proliferation [79]. Regulation of miR-27a via a HDAC3–SMARCA4–miR-27a–PAX3-FOXO1 circuit further demonstrated the ability of miR-27a to destabilize PAX3-FOXO1 mRNA in ARMS cells [80].

2.4. Malignant Peripheral Nerve Sheath Tumour

Malignant peripheral nerve sheath tumour (MPNST) is an aggressive soft tissue sarcoma arising from peripheral nerves or deep neurofibromas. It has a poor prognosis due to its propensity for metastasis and local recurrence. MPNSTs may occur sporadically, but around half of MPNST cases arise in patients with the autosomal dominant genetic disorder neurofibromatosis type 1 (NF1) [130,131]. Most NF1-related tumours demonstrate abnormal Ras signalling pathways, with various genes involved in the Ras pathway deregulated in MPNSTs [132].

miR-204 was found to be downregulated in both NF1 and non-NF1 MPNST tissues and cell lines [81]. Restoration of miR-204 levels resulted in reduced cellular proliferation, migration and invasion in vitro, and decreased tumour growth and invasion in vivo. It was further found that miR-204 modulated Ras signalling and carcinogenesis progression in MPNSTs via direct inhibition of HMGA2 [81]. Members of the miR-30 family have also been reported to be downregulated in MPNSTs. The transcription of miR-30d is inhibited by high levels of enhancer of zeste homolog 2 (EZH2) in MPNST, thereby leading to enhanced expression of karyopherin beta 1 (KPNB1), a direct target of miR-30d. Exogenous regulation of the EZH2–miR-30d–KPNB1 signalling pathway was able to induce MPNST cell apoptosis in vitro and suppress tumorigenesis in vivo [82]. A further study showed that miR-30a demonstrated similar regulation of expression in MPNSTs via the EZH2–miR-30a–KPNB1 signalling pathway [83]. MiR-200b was found to be suppressed by EZH2, resulting in EMT in MPNST cells, often thought to be one of the initial steps in metastasis [83]. Finally, miR-34a expression is downregulated in MPNSTs relative to neurofibromas due to p53 inactivation, with exogenously increased expression of miR-34a demonstrating increased apoptotic cell death [84].

Likewise, certain miRNAs in MPNSTs are upregulated. miR-21 expression levels in MPNST clinical samples were significantly higher compared to NF samples [85], congruent to its high levels of expression in multiple other types of cancers and soft tissue tumours [133]. Inhibition of miR-21 in MPNST cell lines showed suppressed cell growth and upregulated levels of its target protein, programmed cell death protein 4 (PDCD4), which is known to act as a tumour suppressor gene and is upregulated during apoptosis [134]. It was further found that miR-21 inhibition decreased caspase activity, suggesting that miR-21 plays a crucial role in modulating programmed cell death in MPNSTs [85].

2.5. Leiomyosarcoma

Leiomyosarcomas (LMS) are highly aggressive malignancies of smooth muscle tissues which account for approximately 10% of all STS [135]. Uterine leiomyosarcomas (UMLS) account for the single largest site-specific group of LMS and is also the most common subtype of uterine sarcomas [135,136].

There are statistically significant differences in the expression of multiple miRNAs between LMS and smooth muscle samples [137], endometrial stromal sarcomas [138] and undifferentiated pleomorphic sarcomas [91], pointing towards a unique miRNA signature which could be used for the detection and diagnosis of LMS. In LMS, high levels of miR-181b were observed in both ULMS and soft tissue LMS, though to a greater extent in ULMS [90]. On the contrary, miR-152 down regulation was observed in LMS samples [89]. Transfection of miR-152 into LMS cells resulted in decreased proliferation, increased apoptosis and S-phase cell cycle arrest. This was coupled with downregulation of proto-oncogenes MET and KIT mRNA and protein expression, which in turn was associated with a transient down-regulation of the PI3K/AKT pathway [89]. In addition, overexpression of maternal embryonic leucine zipper kinase (MELK), an oncogenic kinase [139,140], in ULMS showed significant downregulation of miR-34a expression. The IL-6 receptor was identified as the target gene of miR-34a, such that decreased miR-34a could induce the activation of the JAK2/STAT3 pathway and a consequent anti-apoptotic mechanism [88].

2.6. Synovial Sarcoma

Synovial sarcoma is a high-grade mesenchymal neoplasm that accounts for 10% to 20% of all soft tissue sarcomas in adolescents and young adults [141,142].

Downregulation of miR-494-3p and miR-126 was discovered in synovial sarcoma tumours [92,93]. Re-expression of miR-494-3p in synovial sarcoma cells was associated with a decrease in cell proliferation and migration, along with apoptosis induction. CXCR4, involved in tumour development and metastatic spread in a variety of cancers [143,144], as well as synovial sarcoma cell migration and invasion [145], has been identified as a potential target of miR-494-3p [92]. The long non-coding RNA HOTAIR was shown to regulate the expression of miR-126 in synovial sarcoma, and miR-126 in turn targeted SDF-1, a protein that modulates EMT, migration and proliferation in synovial sarcoma [93].

Likewise, oncogenic miRNAs involved in the potentiation of synovial sarcoma were also reported. Overexpression of let-7e microRNA and miR-99b in synovial sarcoma were found, and the downregulation of the two miRNAs using miRNA inhibitors resulted in the suppression of cell proliferation, accompanied by an increased expression of their putative targets, high mobility group (HMGA2) and SMARCA5 [94], both of which are associated with the development of tumours [146–149]. miR-214 also played a role in synovial sarcoma development by enhancing cytokine expression, though there was no evidence to suggest that it could induce cellular growth, migration or invasion [96]. In addition, miR-9 was found to induce EMT in synovial sarcoma cell via its target protein CDH1, thereby activating associated MAPK/ERK and Wnt/β-catenin signalling pathways and eliciting pro-tumorigenic effects and inhibiting apoptosis [97]. miR-17, expressed and upregulated in synovial sarcoma, was shown to target p21 [98], a tumour suppressor shown to induce growth arrest and differentiation in cancers [150]. Knockdown of miR-17 in turn showed significantly decreased cell growth [98].

2.7. Fibrosarcoma

Fibrosarcomas are defined as a malignant neoplasm composed of fibroblasts with variable collagen production [151]. miR-197-3p is downregulated in human fibrosarcoma cells [100]; restoration of miR-197-3p levels inhibits fibrosarcoma cell viability, colony forming and migration ability, and triggers G2-M phase cell cycle arrest and autophagy. Ras-related nuclear protein (RAN) which is overexpressed in various cancers [152–154], has been identified as a direct target of miR-197-3p. Exogenous expression of miR-197-3p resulted in the suppression of RAN and the consequent attenuation of fibrosarcoma cell proliferation and migration [100]. The miR-29 family (miR-29s) has also been found to be under expressed in human fibrosarcoma cells [99]. It was further discovered that MMP2, a pro-tumorigenic pro-angiogenic enzyme commonly overexpressed in metastatic cancer [155,156], is a direct target of miR-29s. Ectopic expression of miR-29s resulted in reduced MMP2 enzyme activity and inhibition of fibrosarcoma cell invasion [99]. Conversely, miR-520c and miR-373, overexpressed in fibrosarcoma cells, directly target mTOR and SIRT1, which are negative regulators of MMP9 expression. An ectopic increase in miR-520c and miR-373 levels therefore demonstrated a resultant increase in MMP9 activity, enhancing cell migration and growth [101].

2.8. Angiosarcoma

Angiosarcomas are vascular sarcomas of endothelial cell origin [157]. Three microRNAs, miR-497-5p, miR-210 and miR-340 act as tumour suppressors and are downregulated in angiosarcomas [102–104]. Theintroduction of miR-497-5p mimics in vitro inhibited cell proliferation, cell cycle progression, and invasion by downregulating MMP9 and cell cycle related proteins cyclin D1 and p53. miR-497-5p was also found to target and repress the calcium-activated potassium channel KCa3.1, such that the use of a KCa3.1 inhibitor or miR-497-5p mimics in an in vivo angiosarcoma xenograft inhibited tumour growth [102]. miR-210 was shown to target E2F transcription factor 3 and ephrin A3, in which knockdown of the two proteins resulted in angiosarcoma cell number reduction [103]. Finally, overexpression of miR-340, an established tumour-suppressor in multiple cancers [158–160], demonstrated growth inhibition and reduced invasion in angiosarcoma cells. Sirtuin 7 (SIRT7) was identified as a target gene of miR-340, with silencing of SIRT7 resulting in the inhibition of angiosarcoma cell proliferation and invasion [104].

3. MicroRNAs in Prognostication of Soft Tissue Sarcomas

Recent studies have also reported the correlations between miRNA expression and metastatic risk, tumour grade, overall survival and recurrence-free survival, indicating the possible utility of miRNA-guided prognostication of soft tissue sarcomas. A summary of the miRNAs involved in the prognostication of soft tissue sarcomas is found in Table 2.

Table 2. miRNAs that prognosticate for poor survival and metastasis in soft tissue sarcoma.

GIST	Poor patient survival	miR-494 (downregulation) [24] miR-133b (downregulation) [33] miR-1915 (downregulation) [161] miR-196a (overexpression) [37] let-7e (downregulation) [162]
	Increased metastatic risk	miR-494 (downregulation) [24] miR-133b (downregulation) [33] miR-1915 (downregulation) [161] miR-186 (downregulation) [163] miR-196a (overexpression) [37] miR-215-5p (downregulation) [164]
Liposarcoma	Poor patient survival	miR-26a-2 (overexpression) [49] miR-135b (overexpression) [51] miR-155 (overexpression) [39]
	Increased metastatic risk	miR-135b (overexpression) [51]
Rhabdomyosarcoma	Poor patient survival	miR-206 (downregulation) [61] miR-26a (downregulation) [67]
	Increased metastatic risk	miR-206 (downregulation) [61] miR-486-5p (overexpression) [74]
Leiomyosarcoma	Poor patient survival	miR-181b (downregulation) [90]
	Increased metastatic risk	miR-15a (overexpression) [138] miR-92a (overexpression) [138] miR-31 (downregulation) [138]
Synovial sarcoma	Poor patient survival	miR-214 (overexpression) [96]
	Increased metastatic risk	miR-494-3p (downregulation) [92]

3.1. Gastrointestinal Stromal Tumour

In GIST, smaller tumour size and a lower mitotic rate correspond with lower metastatic risk [165]. Negative correlations between miR-494 expression and tumour size, mitotic index, grade and survival were found. Kaplan–Meier analysis revealed that patients expressing weak levels of miR-494 had poorer overall survival [24]. miR-133b, downregulated in GIST, has been found to target and suppress the expression of fascin-1 directly. Elevated levels of fascin-1 expression were significantly correlated with shorter disease-free survival, and several pathological features associated with a more aggressive phenotype and metastasis, such as tumour size, mitotic counts, risk grade, blood vessel invasion and mucosal ulceration [33]. In addition, low expression of miR-1915 has been correlated with metastasis, shorter disease-free survival and overall survival using Kaplan-Meier analysis [161]. Low miR-186 levels in GIST are also associated with metastatic recurrence and a poor prognosis, with the inhibition of miR-186 resulting in the upregulation of a set of genes implicated in cancer metastasis [163]. Furthermore, under-expression of let-7e miRNA and the overexpression of its target genes were associated with poorer relapse-free survival [162]. miR-215-5p expression and the risk grade of GIST were also negatively correlated [164]. In contrast, overexpression of miR-196a in GIST was associated with a high-risk grade, a greater propensity for metastasis and poor survival [37].

3.2. Liposarcoma

Kaplan Meier survival analysis revealed that overexpression of miR-26a-2 was significantly correlated with poor patient survival in WDLPS, DDLPS and MLPS [49]. The expression levels of miR-135b and THBS2 were associated with a higher risk of metastasis, and accordingly correlated significantly with a poorer prognosis in MLPS/RLPS patients [51]. Furthermore, miR-155 has been found as an indicator of unfavourable prognosis in LPS, with higher miR-155 expression levels associated with a worse overall survival rate and relapse-free survival [39].

3.3. Rhabdomyosarcoma

In RMS, certain miRNAs are differentially expressed between fusion-negative RMS and fusion-positive RMS (RMS with either PAX3-FOXO1 or PAX7-FOXO1 fusion oncogenes) and therefore point toward varied clinical outcomes. Low miR-206 expression was correlated with poor overall survival and was an independent predictor of shorter survival in metastatic ERMS and fusion-negative ARMS. Low miR-206 expression also significantly correlated with high SIOP stage and the presence of metastases at diagnosis [61]. Lower levels of circulating miR-26a were found to be present in patients with fusion-positive RMS as compared to fusion-negative RMS, and patients with progressive disease and poorer overall and progression-free survival showed lower levels of miR-26a as well [67]. Furthermore, the PAX3-FOXO1 fusion protein, present in fusion-positive RMS, repressed miR-221/222 that exerts anti-tumorigenic effects on RMS through the negative regulation of cyclin D2, CDK6 and ERBB3. In contrast, PAX3-FOXO1 transcriptionally upregulates miR-486-5p expression and promotes fusion-positive RMS proliferation, invasion and colony formation [74].

3.4. Leiomyosarcoma

In LMS, miR-181b-5p was associated with recurrence-free survival, and high miR-181b levels were found to be an independent predictor of recurrence-free survival regardless of LMS subtype and tumour size [90]. Furthermore, a comparison between primary and metastatic ULMS lesions showed relative overexpression of miR-15a and miR-92a in metastatic ULMS, while miR-31 was relatively overexpressed in primary lesions instead [138]. These three miRNAs control the expression of six different genes that are part of the Wnt signalling pathway, including the Frizzled-6 precursor (FZD6) gene, which was found to be of higher levels in metastatic ULMS samples. Subsequent siRNA silencing of Frizzled-6 inhibited cellular invasion and impaired MMP2 activity in ULMS cells [138].

3.5. Synovial Sarcoma

In metastatic tumour samples of synovial sarcoma, downregulation of miR-494-3p and increased expression of its potential target CXCR4 were more pronounced than in non-metastatic tumours and healthy tissues [92]. High expression levels of miR-214 in synovial sarcoma tumours were also correlated with poor prognosis and shorter overall survival [96]. Interestingly, the correlation between serum miR-92b-3p levels and tumour size was observed to be statistically significant, thus suggesting that serum miR-92b-3p levels could reflect tumour burden in synovial sarcoma patients [95].

4. MicroRNAs in Treatment Resistance

miRNAs have also been shown to play a role in influencing the resistance of soft tissue sarcomas to various forms of treatment (Figure 4). Reversal of miRNA expression in resistant tumours has the ability to modulate tumour progression, demonstrating the potential utility of miRNA-based therapy in the treatment of soft tissue sarcomas.

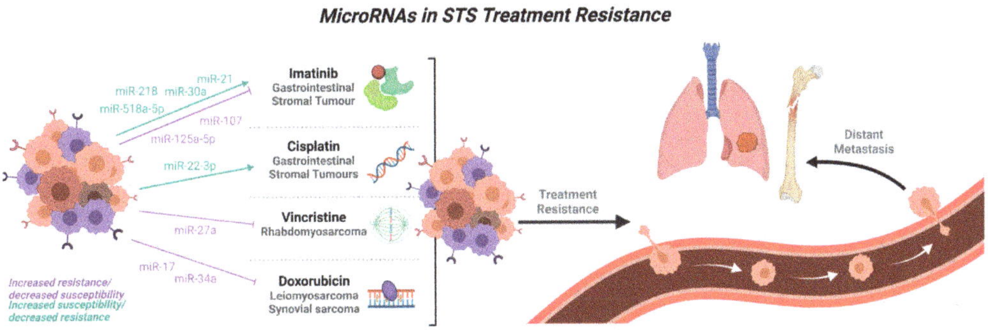

Figure 4. Known microRNAs implicated in treatment resistance of soft tissue sarcomas.

Imatinib, a tyrosine kinase inhibitor, works by inhibiting KIT activation, thereby blocking the activation of the downstream MAP kinase and PI3K-AKT cell survival pathways. Due to the prevalence of GISTs harbouring activating mutations in KIT, clinical management of metastatic or recurrent GIST usually involves the use of a tyrosine kinase inhibitor such as imatinib mesylate [166]. However, a number of GISTs may progress during or after treatment with imatinib, posing a challenge to clinicians [167]. Recent studies show that miRNAs play a role in modulating imatinib resistance in GIST, which could be useful in guiding clinical management of imatinib-resistant GISTs, or even using miRNAs as a novel therapeutic tool in the treatment of GIST.

miR-218 expression was found to be decreased in imatinib-resistant cell lines, but subsequent ectopic overexpression of miR-218 in imatinib-resistant cells under the effect of imatinib mesylate resulted in significantly decreased cell viability and increased apoptosis. It was further suggested that the PI3K/AKT signalling pathways could play a role in this mechanism [26]. Similarly, miR-21 increased the susceptibility of GIST cells to imatinib, with miR-21-transfected GIST cells demonstrating increased growth inhibition and apoptosis in response to imatinib treatment compared to controls [168]. miR-518a-5p, downregulated in imatinib-resistant GISTs, was able to reduce imatinib-resistant GIST cell proliferation and increase apoptosis when introduced exogenously. It is suggested that modulation of PIK3C2A, the direct target of miR-518a-5p, affects the cellular response of GIST to imatinib mesylate, thereby causing resistance [34]. Lower levels of miR-30a were also detected in GIST cells with lower sensitivity to imatinib treatment, with imatinib treatment further reducing miR-30a levels in GIST cells. miR-30a was found to increase susceptibility to imatinib via Beclin-1 knockdown, which increased imatinib sensitivity in GIST cells. These results were confirmed in mouse tumour models [169]. miR-130a suppression by the long non-coding RNA HOTAIR increased autophagy and promoted imatinib-resistance in GIST, through its target autophagy-related protein 2 homolog B (ATG2B) [170]. Interestingly, GISTs with lower miR-320a expression showed significantly shorter time to imatinib resistance, though the mechanism through which this was mediated was not indicated in the study [171].

In contrast, overexpression of miR-125a-5p and miR-107 was associated with imatinib resistance in GIST specimens. It was further shown that expression of the miR-125a-5p target PTPN18 was suppressed in imatinib-resistant GIST samples, and that the silencing of PTPN18 expression increased cell viability in GIST882 cells with a homozygous KIT mutation subsequent to imatinib treatment. However, miR-125a-5p expression did not modulate imatinib sensitivity in GIST48 cells with double KIT mutations [161]. It was also observed that higher expression levels of phosphorylated FAK (pFAK), a downstream target of PTPN18, were present in a GIST cell line with acquired imatinib resistance as compared to its imatinib-sensitive parental cells. High FAK and pFAK levels were also associated with KIT mutation status in clinical GIST samples. Treatment with a FAK inhibitor showed that it could reverse the imatinib-resistance effect due to miR-125a-5p overexpression and cause reduced cell viability and increased apoptosis with imatinib treatment [172].

The use of miRNAs as potential biomarkers of imatinib resistance in GIST was studied by Kou et al. who found that serum miR-518e-5p could discriminate imatinib-resistant GIST patients from healthy controls and imatinib-sensitive GIST patients [173]. This could have potential implications in the way detection and diagnosis of imatinib resistance is made, thereby influencing clinical management.

In ARMS, the PAX3-FOXO1 fusion oncogene regulates chemotherapy and radiotherapy tolerance [120]. Repression of the oncogenic miR-27a was found to play a role in PAX3-FOXO1 mRNA destabilization and increased susceptibility of RMS models to the chemotherapy drug vincristine. This downregulation of miR-27a could be achieved through the use of the histone deacetylase inhibitor entinostat, which repressed the activity of the chromatin remodeling enzyme SMARCA4 by inhibiting HDAC3 expression, thereby downregulating miR-27a [80].

Higher levels of MELK were associated with doxorubicin chemoresistance in ULMS cells. MELK overexpression in ULMS could induce M2 macrophage polarization via the miR-34a/JAK2/STAT3 pathway, contributing to doxorubicin chemoresistance in the tumour microenvironment [88]. In synovial sarcoma, miR-17 was able to confer doxorubicin resistance by reversing the effects of doxorubicin in p21 expression [98].

A summary of the miRNAs implicated in treatment resistance in soft tissue sarcomas may be found in Table 3.

Table 3. miRNAs implicated in treatment resistance in soft tissue sarcomas.

Type of Treatment	Soft Tissue Sarcoma	microRNA Involvement
Imatinib	GIST	miR-218 [26] miR-518a-5p [34] miR-130a [170] miR-320a [171] miR-21 [168] miR-30a [169] miR-125a-5p [161,172] miR-107 [161] miR-518e-5p [173]
Vincristine	Rhabdomyosarcoma	miR-27a [80]
Doxorubicin resistance	Leiomyosarcoma	miR-34a [88]
	Synovial sarcoma	miR-17 [98]

5. Conclusions and Future Directions

The exciting field of miRNA research has seen miRNA-based technology entering pre-clinical and clinical settings as diagnostic and therapeutic tools for various diseases in recent years. At present, several miRNA-targeted therapeutics for cancer have reached clinical development, including the use of an miR-34 mimic (MRX34) encapsulated in lipid nanoparticles for the treatment of multiple solid tumours and an miR-16 mimic for the treatment of lung cancer [174]. However, important challenges to the clinical use of miRNA-based therapies remain. The ability of miRNAs to target multiple different mRNAs is a double-edged sword—while a single miRNA can regulate multiple cancer-related pathways, off-target effects in healthy cells remain a significant concern. Thus, identification of miRNAs specific to cancer cells, and directed delivery of miRNAs to target sites to eliminate this risk is crucial. Furthermore, the delivery of miRNAs is in itself one of the biggest hurdles for miRNA advancement into the clinical setting. Delivery associated toxicity, immune response, and difficulties in transfection and biodistribution are but some of the barriers facing safe and efficient miRNA delivery [175]. Therefore, the need for rigorous evaluation of toxicity and target engagement is required to avoid early failure in clinical trials.

In this review, three key areas in which miRNAs may be utilised in the management of soft tissue sarcomas have been discussed: (i) prognostication, (ii) prediction of treatment resistance, and (iii) therapeutics. The use of miRNAs in the prognostication of soft tissue sarcomas could guide clinical management by identifying patients who have higher metastatic risk and thus require closer surveillance or a lower threshold for adjuvant treatment. Studying miRNA expression in patient serum could also serve as a biomarker for the earlier detection of disease relapse. Distinguishing which cancers are more amenable to treatment options based on their miRNA signature could also increase the overall efficacy of soft tissue sarcoma therapy. Furthermore, the prediction of treatment resistance to specific agents can potentially guide systemic treatment choices in advanced soft tissue sarcomas. Finally, miRNA-based therapies offer an appealing approach to cancer treatment because a single miRNA can regulate multiple target genes and/or signalling pathways within cancer cells. While few miRNA-based strategies have reached clinical routine, continuous advancements in this field offer great promise for their utility in diagnosing, prognosticating and improving treatment outcomes for soft tissue sarcomas.

Author Contributions: Conceptualization, V.S.Y.; writing—original draft preparation, A.Y.T.T.; writing—review and editing, V.Y.L. and V.S.Y.; visualization, A.Y.T.T.; supervision, V.S.Y. All authors have read and agreed to the published version of the manuscript.

Funding: This research received no external funding.

Acknowledgments: The corresponding author is supported by the SingHealth Duke-NUS Academic Medical Centre and Oncology ACP, as well as the National Medical Research Council Transition Award. The authors are responsible for the content and writing of this paper. The final version of the paper has been seen and approved by all authors. The figures in this paper were created with BioRender.com.

Conflicts of Interest: The authors declare no conflict of interest.

References

1. Demetri, G.D.; Antonia, S.; Benjamin, R.S.; Bui, M.M.; Casper, E.S.; Conrad, E.U.; DeLaney, T.F.; Ganjoo, K.N.; Heslin, M.J.; Hutchinson, R.J. Soft tissue sarcoma. *J. Natl. Compr. Cancer Netw.* **2010**, *8*, 630–674. [CrossRef] [PubMed]
2. Burningham, Z.; Hashibe, M.; Spector, L.; Schiffman, J.D. The Epidemiology of Sarcoma. *Clin. Sarcoma Res.* **2012**, *2*, 14. [CrossRef]
3. DeVita, V.T.; Hellman, S.; Rosenberg, S.A. *Cancer, Principles and Practice of Oncology*; Lippincott: New York, NY, USA, 1982; Volume 1.
4. Clark, M.A.; Fisher, C.; Judson, I.; Thomas, J.M. Soft-tissue sarcomas in adults. *N. Engl. J. Med.* **2005**, *353*, 701–711. [CrossRef] [PubMed]
5. Cormier, J.N.; Pollock, R.E. Soft tissue sarcomas. *CA: A Cancer J. Clin.* **2004**, *54*, 94–109. [CrossRef]
6. Grimer, R.; Judson, I.; Peake, D.; Seddon, B. Guidelines for the management of soft tissue sarcomas. *Sarcoma* **2010**, *2010*, 506182. [CrossRef]
7. Alektiar, K.M.; Velasco, J.; Zelefsky, M.J.; Woodruff, J.M.; Lewis, J.J.; Brennan, M.F. Adjuvant radiotherapy for margin-positive high-grade soft tissue sarcoma of the extremity. *Int. J. Radiat. Oncol. Biol. Phys.* **2000**, *48*, 1051–1058. [CrossRef] [PubMed]
8. Linch, M.; Miah, A.B.; Thway, K.; Judson, I.R.; Benson, C. Systemic treatment of soft-tissue sarcoma—Gold standard and novel therapies. *Nat. Rev. Clin. Oncol.* **2014**, *11*, 187–202. [CrossRef] [PubMed]
9. Pervaiz, N.; Colterjohn, N.; Farrokhyar, F.; Tozer, R.; Figueredo, A.; Ghert, M. A systematic meta-analysis of randomized controlled trials of adjuvant chemotherapy for localized resectable soft-tissue sarcoma. *Cancer* **2008**, *113*, 573–581. [CrossRef]
10. Woll, P.J.; Reichardt, P.; Le Cesne, A.; Bonvalot, S.; Azzarelli, A.; Hoekstra, H.J.; Leahy, M.; Van Coevorden, F.; Verweij, J.; Hogendoorn, P.C.W.; et al. Adjuvant chemotherapy with doxorubicin, ifosfamide, and lenograstim for resected soft-tissue sarcoma (EORTC 62931): A multicentre randomised controlled trial. *Lancet Oncol.* **2012**, *13*, 1045–1054. [CrossRef]
11. Demetri, G.D.; Le Cesne, A.; Chawla, S.P.; Brodowicz, T.; Maki, R.G.; Bach, B.A.; Smethurst, D.P.; Bray, S.; Hei, Y.-j.; Blay, J.-Y. First-line treatment of metastatic or locally advanced unresectable soft tissue sarcomas with conatumumab in combination with doxorubicin or doxorubicin alone: A Phase I/II open-label and double-blind study. *Eur. J. Cancer* **2012**, *48*, 547–563. [CrossRef]
12. Tap, W.D.; Papai, Z.; Van Tine, B.A.; Attia, S.; Ganjoo, K.N.; Jones, R.L.; Schuetze, S.; Reed, D.; Chawla, S.P.; Riedel, R.F.; et al. Doxorubicin plus evofosfamide versus doxorubicin alone in locally advanced, unresectable or metastatic soft-tissue sarcoma (TH CR-406/SARC021): An international, multicentre, open-label, randomised phase 3 trial. *Lancet Oncol.* **2017**, *18*, 1089–1103. [CrossRef]
13. Judson, I.; Verweij, J.; Gelderblom, H.; Hartmann, J.T.; Schöffski, P.; Blay, J.Y.; Kerst, J.M.; Sufliarsky, J.; Whelan, J.; Hohenberger, P.; et al. Doxorubicin alone versus intensified doxorubicin plus ifosfamide for first-line treatment of advanced or metastatic soft-tissue sarcoma: A randomised controlled phase 3 trial. *Lancet Oncol.* **2014**, *15*, 415–423. [CrossRef] [PubMed]

14. Howlader, N.; Noone, A.M.; Krapcho, M.; Miller, D.; Brest, A.; Yu, M.; Ruhl, J.; Tatalovich, Z.; Mariotto, A.; Lewis, D.R.; et al. SEER Cancer Statistics Review, 1975–2017; Based on November 2019 SEER data submission, posted to the SEER web site; National Cancer Institute: Bethesda, MD, USA, April 2020.
15. Sbaraglia, M.; Bellan, E.; Dei Tos, A.P. The 2020 WHO Classification of Soft Tissue Tumours: News and perspectives. *Pathologica* **2021**, *113*, 70–84. [CrossRef] [PubMed]
16. Leva, G.D.; Garofalo, M.; Croce, C.M. MicroRNAs in Cancer. *Annu. Rev. Pathol. Mech. Dis.* **2014**, *9*, 287–314. [CrossRef] [PubMed]
17. Garzon, R.; Calin, G.A.; Croce, C.M. MicroRNAs in Cancer. *Annu. Rev. Med.* **2009**, *60*, 167–179. [CrossRef]
18. Lu, J.; Getz, G.; Miska, E.A.; Alvarez-Saavedra, E.; Lamb, J.; Peck, D.; Sweet-Cordero, A.; Ebert, B.L.; Mak, R.H.; Ferrando, A.A.; et al. MicroRNA expression profiles classify human cancers. *Nature* **2005**, *435*, 834–838. [CrossRef]
19. Xue, T.; Liang, W.; Li, Y.; Sun, Y.; Xiang, Y.; Zhang, Y.; Dai, Z.; Duo, Y.; Wu, L.; Qi, K.; et al. Ultrasensitive detection of miRNA with an antimonene-based surface plasmon resonance sensor. *Nat. Commun.* **2019**, *10*, 28. [CrossRef]
20. Ling, H.; Fabbri, M.; Calin, G.A. MicroRNAs and other non-coding RNAs as targets for anticancer drug development. *Nat. Rev. Drug Discov.* **2013**, *12*, 847–865. [CrossRef]
21. Asano, N.; Matsuzaki, J.; Ichikawa, M.; Kawauchi, J.; Takizawa, S.; Aoki, Y.; Sakamoto, H.; Yoshida, A.; Kobayashi, E.; Tanzawa, Y.; et al. A serum microRNA classifier for the diagnosis of sarcomas of various histological subtypes. *Nat. Commun.* **2019**, *10*, 1299. [CrossRef]
22. Smolle, M.A.; Leithner, A.; Posch, F.; Szkandera, J.; Liegl-Atzwanger, B.; Pichler, M. MicroRNAs in Different Histologies of Soft Tissue Sarcoma: A Comprehensive Review. *Int. J. Mol. Sci.* **2017**, *18*, 1960. [CrossRef]
23. Kim, W.K.; Park, M.; Kim, Y.-K.; Tae, Y.K.; Yang, H.-K.; Lee, J.M.; Kim, H. MicroRNA-494 downregulates KIT and inhibits gastrointestinal stromal tumor cell proliferation. *Clin. Cancer Res.* **2011**, *17*, 7584–7594. [CrossRef] [PubMed]
24. Yun, S.; Kim, W.K.; Kwon, Y.; Jang, M.; Bauer, S.; Kim, H. Survivin is a novel transcription regulator of KIT and is downregulated by miRNA-494 in gastrointestinal stromal tumors. *Int. J. Cancer* **2018**, *142*, 2080–2093. [CrossRef] [PubMed]
25. Fan, R.; Zhong, J.; Zheng, S.; Wang, Z.; Xu, Y.; Li, S.; Zhou, J.; Yuan, F. MicroRNA-218 inhibits gastrointestinal stromal tumor cell and invasion by targeting KIT. *Tumor Biol.* **2014**, *35*, 4209–4217. [CrossRef]
26. Fan, R.; Zhong, J.; Zheng, S.; Wang, Z.; Xu, Y.; Li, S.; Zhou, J.; Yuan, F. microRNA-218 increase the sensitivity of gastrointestinal stromal tumor to imatinib through PI3K/AKT pathway. *Clin. Exp. Med.* **2015**, *15*, 137–144. [CrossRef] [PubMed]
27. Tu, L.; Wang, M.; Zhao, W.-Y.; Zhang, Z.-Z.; Tang, D.-F.; Zhang, Y.-Q.; Cao, H.; Zhang, Z.-G. miRNA-218-loaded carboxymethyl chitosan-Tocopherol nanoparticle to suppress the proliferation of gastrointestinal stromal tumor growth. *Mater. Sci. Eng. C* **2017**, *72*, 177–184. [CrossRef] [PubMed]
28. Koelz, M.; Lense, J.; Wrba, F.; Scheffler, M.; Dienes, H.P.; Odenthal, M. Down-regulation of miR-221 and miR-222 correlates with pronounced Kit expression in gastrointestinal stromal tumors. *Int. J. Oncol.* **2011**, *38*, 503–511. [CrossRef]
29. Ihle, M.A.; Trautmann, M.; Kuenstlinger, H.; Huss, S.; Heydt, C.; Fassunke, J.; Wardelmann, E.; Bauer, S.; Schildhaus, H.-U.; Buettner, R. miRNA-221 and miRNA-222 induce apoptosis via the KIT/AKT signalling pathway in gastrointestinal stromal tumours. *Mol. Oncol.* **2015**, *9*, 1421–1433. [CrossRef] [PubMed]
30. Gits, C.M.; van Kuijk, P.F.; Jonkers, M.B.; Boersma, A.W.; Van Ijcken, W.; Wozniak, A.; Sciot, R.; Rutkowski, P.; Schöffski, P.; Taguchi, T. MiR-17-92 and miR-221/222 cluster members target KIT and ETV1 in human gastrointestinal stromal tumours. *Br. J. Cancer* **2013**, *109*, 1625–1635. [CrossRef] [PubMed]
31. Chen, Y.; Qin, C.; Cui, X.; Geng, W.; Xian, G.; Wang, Z. miR-4510 acts as a tumor suppressor in gastrointestinal stromal tumor by targeting APOC2. *J. Cell Physiol.* **2020**, *235*, 5711–5721. [CrossRef]
32. Lu, H.-J.; Yan, J.; Jin, P.-Y.; Zheng, G.-H.; Qin, S.-M.; Wu, D.-M.; Lu, J.; Zheng, Y.-L. MicroRNA-152 inhibits tumor cell growth while inducing apoptosis via the transcriptional repression of cathepsin L in gastrointestinal stromal tumor. *Cancer Biomark.* **2018**, *21*, 711–722. [CrossRef]
33. Yamamoto, H.; Kohashi, K.; Fujita, A.; Oda, Y. Fascin-1 overexpression and miR-133b downregulation in the progression of gastrointestinal stromal tumor. *Mod. Pathol.* **2013**, *26*, 563–571. [CrossRef] [PubMed]
34. Shi, Y.; Gao, X.; Hu, Q.; Li, X.; Xu, J.; Lu, S.; Liu, Y.; Xu, C.; Jiang, D.; Lin, J. PIK3C2A is a gene-specific target of microRNA-518a-5p in imatinib mesylate-resistant gastrointestinal stromal tumor. *Lab. Investig.* **2016**, *96*, 652–660. [CrossRef] [PubMed]
35. Liu, S.; Cui, J.; Liao, G.; Zhang, Y.; Ye, K.; Lu, T.; Qi, J.; Wan, G. MiR-137 regulates epithelial-mesenchymal transition in gastrointestinal stromal tumor. *Tumor Biol.* **2014**, *35*, 9131–9138. [CrossRef] [PubMed]
36. Long, Z.-W.; Wu, J.-H.; Cai-Hong, Y.-N.W.; Zhou, Y. MiR-374b promotes proliferation and inhibits apoptosis of human GIST cells by inhibiting PTEN through activation of the PI3K/Akt pathway. *Mol. Cells* **2018**, *41*, 532. [PubMed]
37. Niinuma, T.; Suzuki, H.; Nojima, M.; Nosho, K.; Yamamoto, H.; Takamaru, H.; Yamamoto, E.; Maruyama, R.; Nobuoka, T.; Miyazaki, Y. Upregulation of miR-196a and HOTAIR drive malignant character in gastrointestinal stromal tumors. *Cancer Res.* **2012**, *72*, 1126–1136. [CrossRef]
38. Ugras, S.; Brill, E.; Jacobsen, A.; Hafner, M.; Socci, N.D.; DeCarolis, P.L.; Khanin, R.; O'Connor, R.; Mihailovic, A.; Taylor, B.S. Small RNA sequencing and functional characterization reveals MicroRNA-143 tumor suppressor activity in liposarcoma. *Cancer Res.* **2011**, *71*, 5659–5669. [CrossRef]
39. Kapodistrias, N.; Mavridis, K.; Batistatou, A.; Gogou, P.; Karavasilis, V.; Sainis, I.; Briasoulis, E.; Scorilas, A. Assessing the clinical value of microRNAs in formalin-fixed paraffin-embedded liposarcoma tissues: Overexpressed miR-155 is an indicator of poor prognosis. *Oncotarget* **2017**, *8*, 6896. [CrossRef]

40. Borjigin, N.; Ohno, S.; Wu, W.; Tanaka, M.; Suzuki, R.; Fujita, K.; Takanashi, M.; Oikawa, K.; Goto, T.; Motoi, T. TLS-CHOP represses miR-486 expression, inducing upregulation of a metastasis regulator PAI-1 in human myxoid liposarcoma. *Biochem. Biophys. Res. Commun.* 2012, 427, 355–360. [CrossRef]
41. Gits, C.M.; van Kuijk, P.F.; Jonkers, M.B.; Boersma, A.W.; Smid, M.; van Ijcken, W.F.; Coindre, J.M.; Chibon, F.; Verhoef, C.; Mathijssen, R.H. MicroRNA expression profiles distinguish liposarcoma subtypes and implicate miR-145 and miR-451 as tumor suppressors. *Int. J. Cancer* 2014, 135, 348–361. [CrossRef]
42. Mazzu, Y.Z.; Hu, Y.; Soni, R.K.; Mojica, K.M.; Qin, L.-X.; Agius, P.; Waxman, Z.M.; Mihailovic, A.; Socci, N.D.; Hendrickson, R.C. miR-193b–Regulated Signaling Networks Serve as Tumor Suppressors in Liposarcoma and Promote Adipogenesis in Adipose-Derived Stem Cells. *Cancer Res.* 2017, 77, 5728–5740. [CrossRef]
43. Mazzu, Y.Z.; Hu, Y.; Shen, Y.; Tuschl, T.; Singer, S. miR-193b regulates tumorigenesis in liposarcoma cells via PDGFR, TGFβ, and Wnt signaling. *Sci. Rep.* 2019, 9, 3197. [CrossRef] [PubMed]
44. Peter, Y.Y.; Lopez, G.; Braggio, D.; Koller, D.; Bill, K.L.J.; Prudner, B.C.; Zewdu, A.; Chen, J.L.; Iwenofu, O.H.; Lev, D. miR-133a function in the pathogenesis of dedifferentiated liposarcoma. *Cancer Cell Int.* 2018, 18, 89.
45. Cao, Y.; Li, L.; Han, L.; Zheng, J.; Lv, C. miR-195 Serves as a Tumor Suppressor in the Progression of Liposarcoma by Targeting OSBP. *OncoTargets Ther.* 2020, 13, 6465. [CrossRef] [PubMed]
46. Zhang, P.; Bill, K.; Liu, J.; Young, E.; Peng, T.; Bolshakov, S.; Hoffman, A.; Song, Y.; Demicco, E.G.; Terrada, D.L. MiR-155 is a liposarcoma oncogene that targets casein kinase-1α and enhances β-catenin signaling. *Cancer Res.* 2012, 72, 1751–1762. [CrossRef] [PubMed]
47. Vincenzi, B.; Iuliani, M.; Zoccoli, A.; Pantano, F.; Fioramonti, M.; De Lisi, D.; Frezza, A.M.; Rabitti, C.; Perrone, G.; Muda, A.O. Deregulation of dicer and mir-155 expression in liposarcoma. *Oncotarget* 2015, 6, 10586. [CrossRef]
48. Boro, A.; Bauer, D.; Born, W.; Fuchs, B. Plasma levels of miRNA-155 as a powerful diagnostic marker for dedifferentiated liposarcoma. *Am. J. Cancer Res.* 2016, 6, 544.
49. Lee, D.; Amanat, S.; Goff, C.; Weiss, L.; Said, J.; Doan, N.; Sato-Otsubo, A.; Ogawa, S.; Forscher, C.; Koeffler, H. Overexpression of miR-26a-2 in human liposarcoma is correlated with poor patient survival. *Oncogenesis* 2013, 2, e47. [CrossRef]
50. Lee, D.H.; Forscher, C.; Di Vizio, D.; Koeffler, H.P. Induction of p53-independent apoptosis by ectopic expression of HOXA5 in human liposarcomas. *Sci. Rep.* 2015, 5, 12580. [CrossRef]
51. Nezu, Y.; Hagiwara, K.; Yamamoto, Y.; Fujiwara, T.; Matsuo, K.; Yoshida, A.; Kawai, A.; Saito, T.; Ochiya, T. miR-135b, a key regulator of malignancy, is linked to poor prognosis in human myxoid liposarcoma. *Oncogene* 2016, 35, 6177–6188. [CrossRef]
52. Casadei, L.; Calore, F.; Creighton, C.J.; Guescini, M.; Batte, K.; Iwenofu, O.H.; Zewdu, A.; Braggio, D.A.; Bill, K.L.; Fadda, P. Exosome-derived miR-25-3p and miR-92a-3p stimulate liposarcoma progression. *Cancer Res.* 2017, 77, 3846–3856. [CrossRef]
53. Fricke, A.; Cimniak, A.; Ullrich, P.; Becherer, C.; Bickert, C.; Pfeifer, D.; Heinz, J.; Stark, G.; Bannasch, H.; Braig, D. Whole blood miRNA expression analysis reveals miR-3613-3p as a potential biomarker for dedifferentiated liposarcoma. *Cancer Biomark.* 2018, 22, 199–207. [CrossRef] [PubMed]
54. Taulli, R.; Bersani, F.; Foglizzo, V.; Linari, A.; Vigna, E.; Ladanyi, M.; Tuschl, T.; Ponzetto, C. The muscle-specific microRNA miR-206 blocks human rhabdomyosarcoma growth in xenotransplanted mice by promoting myogenic differentiation. *J. Clin. Investig.* 2009, 119, 2366–2378. [CrossRef]
55. Yan, D.; Da Dong, X.; Chen, X.; Wang, L.; Lu, C.; Wang, J.; Qu, J.; Tu, L. MicroRNA-1/206 targets c-Met and inhibits rhabdomyosarcoma development. *J. Biol. Chem.* 2009, 284, 29596–29604. [CrossRef] [PubMed]
56. Li, L.; Sarver, A.L.; Alamgir, S.; Subramanian, S. Downregulation of microRNAs miR-1,-206 and-29 stabilizes PAX3 and CCND2 expression in rhabdomyosarcoma. *Lab. Investig.* 2012, 92, 571–583. [CrossRef]
57. MacQuarrie, K.L.; Yao, Z.; Young, J.M.; Cao, Y.; Tapscott, S.J. miR-206 integrates multiple components of differentiation pathways to control the transition from growth to differentiation in rhabdomyosarcoma cells. *Skelet. Muscle* 2012, 2, 7. [CrossRef]
58. Hanna, J.; Garcia, M.; Go, J.; Finkelstein, D.; Kodali, K.; Pagala, V.; Wang, X.; Peng, J.; Hatley, M. PAX7 is a required target for microRNA-206-induced differentiation of fusion-negative rhabdomyosarcoma. *Cell Death Dis.* 2016, 7, e2256. [CrossRef] [PubMed]
59. Coda, D.M.; Lingua, M.F.; Morena, D.; Foglizzo, V.; Bersani, F.; Ala, U.; Ponzetto, C.; Taulli, R. SMYD1 and G6PD modulation are critical events for miR-206-mediated differentiation of rhabdomyosarcoma. *Cell Cycle* 2015, 14, 1389–1402. [CrossRef]
60. Ciesla, M.; Marona, P.; Kozakowska, M.; Jez, M.; Seczynska, M.; Loboda, A.; Bukowska-Strakova, K.; Szade, A.; Walawender, M.; Kusior, M. Heme oxygenase-1 controls an HDAC4-miR-206 pathway of oxidative stress in rhabdomyosarcoma. *Cancer Res.* 2016, 76, 5707–5718. [CrossRef]
61. Missiaglia, E.; Shepherd, C.J.; Patel, S.; Thway, K.; Pierron, G.; Pritchard-Jones, K.; Renard, M.; Sciot, R.; Rao, P.; Oberlin, O.; et al. MicroRNA-206 expression levels correlate with clinical behaviour of rhabdomyosarcomas. *Br. J. Cancer* 2010, 102, 1769–1777. [CrossRef]
62. Rao, P.K.; Missiaglia, E.; Shields, L.; Hyde, G.; Yuan, B.; Shepherd, C.J.; Shipley, J.; Lodish, H.F. Distinct roles for miR-1 and miR-133a in the proliferation and differentiation of rhabdomyosarcoma cells. *FASEB J.* 2010, 24, 3427–3437. [CrossRef]
63. Sugito, N.; Taniguchi, K.; Kuranaga, Y.; Ohishi, M.; Soga, T.; Ito, Y.; Miyachi, M.; Kikuchi, K.; Hosoi, H.; Akao, Y. Cancer-specific energy metabolism in rhabdomyosarcoma cells is regulated by microRNA. *Nucleic Acid Ther.* 2017, 27, 365–377. [CrossRef] [PubMed]

64. Wang, H.; Garzon, R.; Sun, H.; Ladner, K.J.; Singh, R.; Dahlman, J.; Cheng, A.; Hall, B.M.; Qualman, S.J.; Chandler, D.S. NF-κB–YY1–miR-29 regulatory circuitry in skeletal myogenesis and rhabdomyosarcoma. *Cancer Cell* **2008**, *14*, 369–381. [CrossRef] [PubMed]
65. Wang, Y.; Zhang, L.; Pang, Y.; Song, L.; Shang, H.; Li, Z.; Liu, Q.; Zhang, Y.; Wang, X.; Li, Q. MicroRNA-29 family inhibits rhabdomyosarcoma formation and progression by regulating GEFT function. *Am. J. Transl. Res.* **2020**, *12*, 1136. [PubMed]
66. Ciarapica, R.; Russo, G.; Verginelli, F.; Raimondi, L.; Donfrancesco, A.; Rota, R.; Giordano, A. Deregulated expression of miR-26a and EZH2 in rhabdomyosarcoma. *Cell Cycle* **2009**, *8*, 172–175. [CrossRef]
67. Tombolan, L.; Millino, C.; Pacchioni, B.; Cattelan, M.; Zin, A.; Bonvini, P.; Bisogno, G. Circulating miR-26a as potential prognostic biomarkers in pediatric rhabdomyosarcoma. *Front. Genet.* **2020**, *11*, 606274. [CrossRef]
68. Yang, L.; Kong, D.; He, M.; Gong, J.; Nie, Y.; Tai, S.; Teng, C.-B. MiR-7 mediates mitochondrial impairment to trigger apoptosis and necroptosis in Rhabdomyosarcoma. *Biochim. Biophys. Acta (BBA)-Mol. Cell Res.* **2020**, *1867*, 118826. [CrossRef]
69. Molist, C.; Navarro, N.; Giralt, I.; Zarzosa, P.; Gallo-Oller, G.; Pons, G.; Magdaleno, A.; Moreno, L.; Guillén, G.; Hladun, R. miRNA-7 and miRNA-324-5p regulate alpha9-Integrin expression and exert anti-oncogenic effects in rhabdomyosarcoma. *Cancer Lett.* **2020**, *477*, 49–59. [CrossRef]
70. Megiorni, F.; Cialfi, S.; McDowell, H.P.; Felsani, A.; Camero, S.; Guffanti, A.; Pizer, B.; Clerico, A.; De Grazia, A.; Pizzuti, A. Deep Sequencing the microRNA profile in rhabdomyosarcoma reveals down-regulation of miR-378 family members. *BMC Cancer* **2014**, *14*, 880. [CrossRef]
71. Sun, M.; Li, J.; Guo, L.; Xiao, L.; Dong, L.; Wang, F.; Huang, F.; Cao, D.; Qin, T.; Yin, X. TGF-β1 suppression of microRNA-450b-5p expression: A novel mechanism for blocking myogenic differentiation of rhabdomyosarcoma. *Oncogene* **2014**, *33*, 2075–2086. [CrossRef]
72. Diao, Y.; Guo, X.; Jiang, L.; Wang, G.; Zhang, C.; Wan, J.; Jin, Y.; Wu, Z. miR-203, a tumor suppressor frequently down-regulated by promoter hypermethylation in rhabdomyosarcoma. *J. Biol. Chem.* **2014**, *289*, 529–539. [CrossRef]
73. Sun, M.; Huang, F.; Yu, D.; Zhang, Y.; Xu, H.; Zhang, L.; Li, L.; Dong, L.; Guo, L.; Wang, S. Autoregulatory loop between TGF-β1/miR-411-5p/SPRY4 and MAPK pathway in rhabdomyosarcoma modulates proliferation and differentiation. *Cell Death Dis.* **2015**, *6*, e1859. [CrossRef] [PubMed]
74. Hanna, J.A.; Garcia, M.R.; Lardennois, A.; Leavey, P.J.; Maglic, D.; Fagnan, A.; Go, J.C.; Roach, J.; Wang, Y.-D.; Finkelstein, D.; et al. PAX3-FOXO1 drives miR-486-5p and represses miR-221 contributing to pathogenesis of alveolar rhabdomyosarcoma. *Oncogene* **2018**, *37*, 1991–2007. [CrossRef] [PubMed]
75. Huang, H.-J.; Liu, J.; Hua, H.; Li, S.-E.; Zhao, J.; Yue, S.; Yu, T.-T.; Jin, Y.-C.; Cheng, S.Y. MiR-214 and N-ras regulatory loop suppresses rhabdomyosarcoma cell growth and xenograft tumorigenesis. *Oncotarget* **2014**, *5*, 2161. [CrossRef] [PubMed]
76. Vella, S.; Pomella, S.; Leoncini, P.P.; Colletti, M.; Conti, B.; Marquez, V.E.; Strillacci, A.; Roma, J.; Gallego, S.; Milano, G.M. MicroRNA-101 is repressed by EZH2 and its restoration inhibits tumorigenic features in embryonal rhabdomyosarcoma. *Clin. Epigenetics* **2015**, *7*, 82. [CrossRef] [PubMed]
77. Shang, H.; Liu, Y.; Li, Z.; Liu, Q.; Cui, W.; Zhang, L.; Pang, Y.; Liu, C.; Li, F. MicroRNA-874 functions as a tumor suppressor in rhabdomyosarcoma by directly targeting GEFT. *Am. J. Cancer Res.* **2019**, *9*, 668.
78. Zhang, L.; Pang, Y.; Cui, X.; Jia, W.; Cui, W.; Liu, Y.; Liu, C.; Li, F. MicroRNA-410-3p upregulation suppresses proliferation, invasion and migration, and promotes apoptosis in rhabdomyosarcoma cells. *Oncol. Lett.* **2019**, *18*, 936–943. [CrossRef]
79. Tombolan, L.; Zampini, M.; Casara, S.; Boldrin, E.; Zin, A.; Bisogno, G.; Rosolen, A.; De Pittà, C.; Lanfranchi, G. MicroRNA-27a contributes to rhabdomyosarcoma cell proliferation by suppressing RARA and RXRA. *PLoS ONE* **2015**, *10*, e0125171. [CrossRef]
80. Bharathy, N.; Berlow, N.E.; Wang, E.; Abraham, J.; Settelmeyer, T.P.; Hooper, J.E.; Svalina, M.N.; Ishikawa, Y.; Zientek, K.; Bajwa, Z. The HDAC3–SMARCA4–miR-27a axis promotes expression of the PAX3: FOXO1 fusion oncogene in rhabdomyosarcoma. *Sci. Signal.* **2018**, *11*, eaau7632. [CrossRef]
81. Gong, M.; Ma, J.; Li, M.; Zhou, M.; Hock, J.M.; Yu, X. MicroRNA-204 critically regulates carcinogenesis in malignant peripheral nerve sheath tumors. *Neuro-oncology* **2012**, *14*, 1007–1017. [CrossRef]
82. Zhang, P.; Garnett, J.; Creighton, C.J.; Al Sannaa, G.A.; Igram, D.R.; Lazar, A.; Liu, X.; Liu, C.; Pollock, R.E. EZH2–miR-30d–KPNB1 pathway regulates malignant peripheral nerve sheath tumour cell survival and tumourigenesis. *J. Pathol.* **2014**, *232*, 308–318. [CrossRef]
83. Zhang, P.; Yang, X.; Ma, X.; Ingram, D.R.; Lazar, A.J.; Torres, K.E.; Pollock, R.E. Antitumor effects of pharmacological EZH2 inhibition on malignant peripheral nerve sheath tumor through the miR-30a and KPNB1 pathway. *Mol. Cancer* **2015**, *14*, 55. [CrossRef] [PubMed]
84. Subramanian, S.; Thayanithy, V.; West, R.B.; Lee, C.H.; Beck, A.H.; Zhu, S.; Downs-Kelly, E.; Montgomery, K.; Goldblum, J.R.; Hogendoorn, P.C. Genome-wide transcriptome analyses reveal p53 inactivation mediated loss of miR-34a expression in malignant peripheral nerve sheath tumours. *J. Pathol. A J. Pathol. Soc. Great Br. Irel.* **2010**, *220*, 58–70. [CrossRef] [PubMed]
85. Itani, S.; Kunisada, T.; Morimoto, Y.; Yoshida, A.; Sasaki, T.; Ito, S.; Ouchida, M.; Sugihara, S.; Shimizu, K.; Ozaki, T. MicroRNA-21 correlates with tumorigenesis in malignant peripheral nerve sheath tumor (MPNST) via programmed cell death protein 4 (PDCD4). *J. Cancer Res. Clin. Oncol.* **2012**, *138*, 1501–1509. [CrossRef] [PubMed]
86. Weng, Y.; Chen, Y.; Chen, J.; Liu, Y.; Bao, T. Identification of serum microRNAs in genome-wide serum microRNA expression profiles as novel noninvasive biomarkers for malignant peripheral nerve sheath tumor diagnosis. *Med. Oncol.* **2013**, *30*, 531. [CrossRef] [PubMed]

87. Yokoi, A.; Matsuzaki, J.; Yamamoto, Y.; Tate, K.; Yoneoka, Y.; Shimizu, H.; Uehara, T.; Ishikawa, M.; Takizawa, S.; Aoki, Y. Serum microRNA profile enables preoperative diagnosis of uterine leiomyosarcoma. *Cancer Sci.* **2019**, *110*, 3718. [CrossRef]
88. Zhang, Z.; Sun, C.; Li, C.; Jiao, X.; Griffin, B.B.; Dongol, S.; Wu, H.; Zhang, C.; Cao, W.; Dong, R.; et al. Upregulated MELK Leads to Doxorubicin Chemoresistance and M2 Macrophage Polarization via the miR-34a/JAK2/STAT3 Pathway in Uterine Leiomyosarcoma. *Front. Oncol.* **2020**, *10*, 453. [CrossRef]
89. Pazzaglia, L.; Novello, C.; Conti, A.; Pollino, S.; Picci, P.; Benassi, M.S. miR-152 down-regulation is associated with MET up-regulation in leiomyosarcoma and undifferentiated pleomorphic sarcoma. *Cell Oncol.* **2017**, *40*, 77–88. [CrossRef]
90. Abeshouse, A.; Anderson, M.L.; Armenia, J.; Auman, J.T.; Bailey, M.H.; Baker, L.; Balasundaram, M.; Balu, S.; Behera, M.; Benz, C.; et al. Comprehensive and Integrated Genomic Characterization of Adult Soft Tissue Sarcomas. *Cell* **2017**, *171*, 950–965.e28. [CrossRef]
91. Guled, M.; Pazzaglia, L.; Borze, I.; Mosakhani, N.; Novello, C.; Benassi, M.S.; Knuutila, S. Differentiating soft tissue leiomyosarcoma and undifferentiated pleomorphic sarcoma: A miRNA analysis. *Genes Chromosomes Cancer* **2014**, *53*, 693–702. [CrossRef]
92. Pazzaglia, L.; Pollino, S.; Vitale, M.; Bientinesi, E.; Benini, S.; Ferrari, C.; Palmerini, E.; Gambarotti, M.; Picci, P.; Benassi, M.S. miR-494.3 p expression in synovial sarcoma: Role of CXCR4 as a potential target gene. *Int. J. Oncol.* **2019**, *54*, 361–369.
93. Feng, Q.; Wang, D.; Guo, P.; Zhang, Z.; Feng, J. Long non-coding RNA HOTAIR promotes the progression of synovial sarcoma through microRNA-126/stromal cell-derived factor-1 regulation. *Oncol. Lett.* **2021**, *21*, 444. [CrossRef] [PubMed]
94. Hisaoka, M.; Matsuyama, A.; Nagao, Y.; Luan, L.; Kuroda, T.; Akiyama, H.; Kondo, S.; Hashimoto, H. Identification of altered MicroRNA expression patterns in synovial sarcoma. *Genes Chromosomes Cancer* **2011**, *50*, 137–145. [CrossRef] [PubMed]
95. Uotani, K.; Fujiwara, T.; Yoshida, A.; Iwata, S.; Morita, T.; Kiyono, M.; Yokoo, S.; Kunisada, T.; Takeda, K.; Hasei, J. Circulating MicroRNA-92b-3p as a novel biomarker for monitoring of synovial sarcoma. *Sci. Rep.* **2017**, *7*, 14634. [CrossRef] [PubMed]
96. Tanaka, M.; Homme, M.; Yamazaki, Y.; Ae, K.; Matsumoto, S.; Subramanian, S.; Nakamura, T. Cooperation between SS18-SSX1 and miR-214 in synovial sarcoma development and progression. *Cancers* **2020**, *12*, 324. [CrossRef] [PubMed]
97. Xu, X.-Z.; Li, X.-A.; Luo, Y.; Liu, J.-F.; Wu, H.-W.; Huang, G. MiR-9 promotes synovial sarcoma cell migration and invasion by directly targeting CDH1. *Int. J. Biochem. Cell Biol.* **2019**, *112*, 61–71. [CrossRef] [PubMed]
98. Minami, Y.; Kohsaka, S.; Tsuda, M.; Yachi, K.; Hatori, N.; Tanino, M.; Kimura, T.; Nishihara, H.; Minami, A.; Iwasaki, N. SS 18-SSX-regulated miR-17 promotes tumor growth of synovial sarcoma by inhibiting p21 WAF 1/CIP 1. *Cancer Sci.* **2014**, *105*, 1152–1159. [CrossRef]
99. Kim, J.H.; Jeon, S.; Shin, B.A. MicroRNA-29 family suppresses the invasion of HT1080 human fibrosarcoma cells by regulating matrix metalloproteinase 2 expression. *Chonnam Med. J.* **2017**, *53*, 161. [CrossRef]
100. Jain, N.; Das, B.; Mallick, B. Restoration of microRNA-197 expression suppresses oncogenicity in fibrosarcoma through negative regulation of RAN. *IUBMB Life* **2020**, *72*, 1034–1044. [CrossRef]
101. Liu, P.; Wilson, M.J. miR-520c and miR-373 upregulate MMP9 expression by targeting mTOR and SIRT1, and activate the Ras/Raf/MEK/Erk signaling pathway and NF-κB factor in human fibrosarcoma cells. *J. Cell Physiol.* **2012**, *227*, 867–876. [CrossRef]
102. Chen, Y.; Kuang, D.; Zhao, X.; Chen, D.; Wang, X.; Yang, Q.; Wan, J.; Zhu, Y.; Wang, Y.; Zhang, S. miR-497-5p inhibits cell proliferation and invasion by targeting KCa3. 1 in angiosarcoma. *Oncotarget* **2016**, *7*, 58148. [CrossRef]
103. Nakashima, S.; Jinnin, M.; Kanemaru, H.; Kajihara, I.; Igata, T.; Okamoto, S.; Tazaki, Y.; Harada, M.; Masuguchi, S.; Fukushima, S. The role of miR-210, E2F3 and ephrin A3 in angiosarcoma cell proliferation. *Eur. J. Dermatol.* **2017**, *27*, 464–471. [CrossRef] [PubMed]
104. Wang, X.; Song, Y. MicroRNA-340 inhibits the growth and invasion of angiosarcoma cells by targeting SIRT7. *Biomed. Pharmacother.* **2018**, *103*, 1061–1068. [CrossRef] [PubMed]
105. Corless, C.L.; Fletcher, J.A.; Heinrich, M.C. Biology of gastrointestinal stromal tumors. *J. Clin. Oncol.* **2004**, *22*, 3813–3825. [CrossRef]
106. Miettinen, M.; Lasota, J. Gastrointestinal stromal tumors-definition, clinical, histological, immunohistochemical, and molecular genetic features and differential diagnosis. *Virchows Arch.* **2001**, *438*, 1–12. [CrossRef]
107. Liegl, B.; Kepten, I.; Le, C.; Zhu, M.; Demetri, G.D.; Heinrich, M.C.; Fletcher, C.D.; Corless, C.L.; Fletcher, J.A. Heterogeneity of kinase inhibitor resistance mechanisms in GIST. *J. Pathol.* **2008**, *216*, 64–74. [CrossRef]
108. Miller, T.E.; Ghoshal, K.; Ramaswamy, B.; Roy, S.; Datta, J.; Shapiro, C.L.; Jacob, S.; Majumder, S. MicroRNA-221/222 confers tamoxifen resistance in breast cancer by targeting p27Kip1. *J. Biol. Chem.* **2008**, *283*, 29897–29903. [CrossRef]
109. Zhang, C.-Z.; Zhang, J.-X.; Zhang, A.-L.; Shi, Z.-D.; Han, L.; Jia, Z.-F.; Yang, W.-D.; Wang, G.-X.; Jiang, T.; You, Y.-P. MiR-221 and miR-222 target PUMA to induce cell survival in glioblastoma. *Mol. Cancer* **2010**, *9*, 229. [CrossRef] [PubMed]
110. Le Sage, C.; Nagel, R.; Egan, D.A.; Schrier, M.; Mesman, E.; Mangiola, A.; Anile, C.; Maira, G.; Mercatelli, N.; Ciafrè, S.A. Regulation of the p27Kip1 tumor suppressor by miR-221 and miR-222 promotes cancer cell proliferation. *EMBO J.* **2007**, *26*, 3699–3708. [CrossRef]
111. Chi, P.; Chen, Y.; Zhang, L.; Guo, X.; Wongvipat, J.; Shamu, T.; Fletcher, J.A.; Dewell, S.; Maki, R.G.; Zheng, D.; et al. ETV1 is a lineage survival factor that cooperates with KIT in gastrointestinal stromal tumours. *Nature* **2010**, *467*, 849–853. [CrossRef]
112. Sudhan, D.R.; Siemann, D.W. Cathepsin L targeting in cancer treatment. *Pharmacol. Ther.* **2015**, *155*, 105–116. [CrossRef]

113. Moreau, L.C.; Turcotte, R.; Ferguson, P.; Wunder, J.; Clarkson, P.; Masri, B.; Isler, M.; Dion, N.; Werier, J.; Ghert, M.; et al. Myxoid\round cell liposarcoma (MRCLS) revisited: An analysis of 418 primarily managed cases. *Ann. Surg. Oncol.* **2012**, *19*, 1081–1088. [CrossRef] [PubMed]
114. Faraoni, I.; Antonetti, F.R.; Cardone, J.; Bonmassar, E. miR-155 gene: A typical multifunctional microRNA. *Biochim. Biophys Acta* **2009**, *1792*, 497–505. [CrossRef] [PubMed]
115. Kohama, I.; Asano, N.; Matsuzaki, J.; Yamamoto, Y.; Yamamoto, T.; Takahashi, R.-U.; Kobayashi, E.; Takizawa, S.; Sakamoto, H.; Kato, K. Comprehensive serum and tissue microRNA profiling in dedifferentiated liposarcoma. *Oncol. Lett.* **2021**, *22*, 623. [CrossRef] [PubMed]
116. Bajou, K.; Maillard, C.; Jost, M.; Lijnen, R.H.; Gils, A.; Declerck, P.; Carmeliet, P.; Foidart, J.-M.; Noel, A. Host-derived plasminogen activator inhibitor-1 (PAI-1) concentration is critical for in vivo tumoral angiogenesis and growth. *Oncogene* **2004**, *23*, 6986–6990. [CrossRef] [PubMed]
117. Shapiro, D.N.; Sublett, J.E.; Li, B.; Downing, J.R.; Naeve, C.W. Fusion of PAX3 to a member of the forkhead family of transcription factors in human alveolar rhabdomyosarcoma. *Cancer Res.* **1993**, *53*, 5108–5112. [PubMed]
118. Galili, N.; Davis, R.J.; Fredericks, W.J.; Mukhopadhyay, S.; Rauscher, F.J., 3rd; Emanuel, B.S.; Rovera, G.; Barr, F.G. Fusion of a fork head domain gene to PAX3 in the solid tumour alveolar rhabdomyosarcoma. *Nat. Genet.* **1993**, *5*, 230–235. [CrossRef] [PubMed]
119. Davis, R.J.; D'Cruz, C.M.; Lovell, M.A.; Biegel, J.A.; Barr, F.G. Fusion of PAX7 to FKHR by the variant t(1;13)(p36;q14) translocation in alveolar rhabdomyosarcoma. *Cancer Res.* **1994**, *54*, 2869–2872.
120. Missiaglia, E.; Williamson, D.; Chisholm, J.; Wirapati, P.; Pierron, G.; Petel, F.; Concordet, J.P.; Thway, K.; Oberlin, O.; Pritchard-Jones, K.; et al. PAX3/FOXO1 fusion gene status is the key prognostic molecular marker in rhabdomyosarcoma and significantly improves current risk stratification. *J. Clin. Oncol.* **2012**, *30*, 1670–1677. [CrossRef]
121. Skapek, S.X.; Anderson, J.; Barr, F.G.; Bridge, J.A.; Gastier-Foster, J.M.; Parham, D.M.; Rudzinski, E.R.; Triche, T.; Hawkins, D.S. PAX-FOXO1 fusion status drives unfavorable outcome for children with rhabdomyosarcoma: A children's oncology group report. *Pediatr. Blood Cancer* **2013**, *60*, 1411–1417. [CrossRef]
122. Sorensen, P.H.; Lynch, J.C.; Qualman, S.J.; Tirabosco, R.; Lim, J.F.; Maurer, H.M.; Bridge, J.A.; Crist, W.M.; Triche, T.J.; Barr, F.G. PAX3-FKHR and PAX7-FKHR gene fusions are prognostic indicators in alveolar rhabdomyosarcoma: A report from the children's oncology group. *J. Clin. Oncol.* **2002**, *20*, 2672–2679. [CrossRef]
123. Chen, J.-F.; Mandel, E.M.; Thomson, J.M.; Wu, Q.; Callis, T.E.; Hammond, S.M.; Conlon, F.L.; Wang, D.-Z. The role of microRNA-1 and microRNA-133 in skeletal muscle proliferation and differentiation. *Nat. Genet.* **2006**, *38*, 228–233. [CrossRef] [PubMed]
124. Winbanks, C.E.; Wang, B.; Beyer, C.; Koh, P.; White, L.; Kantharidis, P.; Gregorevic, P. TGF-β regulates miR-206 and miR-29 to control myogenic differentiation through regulation of HDAC4. *J. Biol. Chem.* **2011**, *286*, 13805–13814. [CrossRef] [PubMed]
125. Taulli, R.; Scuoppo, C.; Bersani, F.; Accornero, P.; Forni, P.E.; Miretti, S.; Grinza, A.; Allegra, P.; Schmitt-Ney, M.; Crepaldi, T. Validation of met as a therapeutic target in alveolar and embryonal rhabdomyosarcoma. *Cancer Res.* **2006**, *66*, 4742–4749. [CrossRef] [PubMed]
126. Miyachi, M.; Tsuchiya, K.; Yoshida, H.; Yagyu, S.; Kikuchi, K.; Misawa, A.; Iehara, T.; Hosoi, H. Circulating muscle-specific microRNA, miR-206, as a potential diagnostic marker for rhabdomyosarcoma. *Biochem. Biophys. Res. Commun.* **2010**, *400*, 89–93. [CrossRef]
127. Sun, C.; Liu, C.; Li, S.; Li, H.; Wang, Y.; Xie, Y.; Li, B.; Cui, X.; Chen, Y.; Zhang, W.; et al. Overexpression of GEFT, a Rho family guanine nucleotide exchange factor, predicts poor prognosis in patients with rhabdomyosarcoma. *Int. J. Clin. Exp. Pathol.* **2014**, *7*, 1606–1615.
128. Varambally, S.; Dhanasekaran, S.M.; Zhou, M.; Barrette, T.R.; Kumar-Sinha, C.; Sanda, M.G.; Ghosh, D.; Pienta, K.J.; Sewalt, R.G.; Otte, A.P. The polycomb group protein EZH2 is involved in progression of prostate cancer. *Nature* **2002**, *419*, 624–629. [CrossRef]
129. Kim, K.H.; Roberts, C.W. Targeting EZH2 in cancer. *Nat. Med.* **2016**, *22*, 128–134. [CrossRef]
130. Ducatman, B.S.; Scheithauer, B.W.; Piepgras, D.G.; Reiman, H.M.; Ilstrup, D.M. Malignant peripheral nerve sheath tumors. A clinicopathologic study of 120 cases. *Cancer* **1986**, *57*, 2006–2021. [CrossRef]
131. Grobmyer, S.R.; Reith, J.D.; Shahlaee, A.; Bush, C.H.; Hochwald, S.N. Malignant peripheral nerve sheath tumor: Molecular pathogenesis and current management considerations. *J. Surg. Oncol.* **2008**, *97*, 340–349. [CrossRef]
132. Widemann, B.C. Current status of sporadic and neurofibromatosis type 1-associated malignant peripheral nerve sheath tumors. *Curr. Oncol. Rep.* **2009**, *11*, 322–328. [CrossRef]
133. Pfeffer, S.R.; Yang, C.H.; Pfeffer, L.M. The role of miR-21 in cancer. *Drug Dev. Res.* **2015**, *76*, 270–277. [CrossRef] [PubMed]
134. Lankat-Buttgereit, B.; Göke, R. The tumour suppressor Pdcd4: Recent advances in the elucidation of function and regulation. *Biol. Cell* **2009**, *101*, 309–317. [CrossRef] [PubMed]
135. George, S.; Serrano, C.; Hensley, M.L.; Ray-Coquard, I. Soft Tissue and Uterine Leiomyosarcoma. *J. Clin. Oncol.* **2018**, *36*, 144–150. [CrossRef]
136. Brooks, S.E.; Zhan, M.; Cote, T.; Baquet, C.R. Surveillance, epidemiology, and end results analysis of 2677 cases of uterine sarcoma 1989–1999. *Gynecol. Oncol.* **2004**, *93*, 204–208. [CrossRef]
137. Benna, C.; Rajendran, S.; Rastrelli, M.; Mocellin, S. miRNA deregulation targets specific pathways in leiomyosarcoma development: An in silico analysis. *J. Transl. Med.* **2019**, *17*, 153. [CrossRef] [PubMed]
138. Ravid, Y.; Formanski, M.; Smith, Y.; Reich, R.; Davidson, B. Uterine leiomyosarcoma and endometrial stromal sarcoma have unique miRNA signatures. *Gynecol. Oncol.* **2016**, *140*, 512–517. [CrossRef] [PubMed]

139. Lin, M.-L.; Park, J.-H.; Nishidate, T.; Nakamura, Y.; Katagiri, T. Involvement of maternal embryonic leucine zipper kinase (MELK) in mammary carcinogenesis through interaction with Bcl-G, a pro-apoptotic member of the Bcl-2 family. *Breast Cancer Res.* **2007**, *9*, R17. [CrossRef]
140. Kuner, R.; Fälth, M.; Pressinotti, N.C.; Brase, J.C.; Puig, S.B.; Metzger, J.; Gade, S.; Schäfer, G.; Bartsch, G.; Steiner, E. The maternal embryonic leucine zipper kinase (MELK) is upregulated in high-grade prostate cancer. *J. Mol. Med.* **2013**, *91*, 237–248. [CrossRef]
141. Kransdorf, M.J. Malignant soft-tissue tumors in a large referral population: Distribution of diagnoses by age, sex, and location. *AJR Am. J. Roentgenol.* **1995**, *164*, 129–134. [CrossRef]
142. Ladanyi, M.; Antonescu, C.R.; Leung, D.H.; Woodruff, J.M.; Kawai, A.; Healey, J.H.; Brennan, M.F.; Bridge, J.A.; Neff, J.R.; Barr, F.G.; et al. Impact of SYT-SSX fusion type on the clinical behavior of synovial sarcoma: A multi-institutional retrospective study of 243 patients. *Cancer Res.* **2002**, *62*, 135–140.
143. Schimanski, C.C.; Schwald, S.; Simiantonaki, N.; Jayasinghe, C.; Gönner, U.; Wilsberg, V.; Junginger, T.; Berger, M.R.; Galle, P.R.; Moehler, M. Effect of chemokine receptors CXCR4 and CCR7 on the metastatic behavior of human colorectal cancer. *Clin. Cancer Res.* **2005**, *11*, 1743–1750. [CrossRef] [PubMed]
144. Zeelenberg, I.S.; Ruuls-Van Stalle, L.; Roos, E. The chemokine receptor CXCR4 is required for outgrowth of colon carcinoma micrometastases. *Cancer Res.* **2003**, *63*, 3833–3839. [PubMed]
145. Li, Y.-J.; Dai, Y.-L.; Zhang, W.-B.; Li, S.-J.; Tu, C.-Q. Clinicopathological and prognostic significance of chemokine receptor CXCR4 in patients with bone and soft tissue sarcoma: A meta-analysis. *Clin. Exp. Med.* **2017**, *17*, 59–69. [CrossRef] [PubMed]
146. Kumar, M.S.; Armenteros-Monterroso, E.; East, P.; Chakravorty, P.; Matthews, N.; Winslow, M.M.; Downward, J. HMGA2 functions as a competing endogenous RNA to promote lung cancer progression. *Nature* **2014**, *505*, 212–217. [CrossRef]
147. Park, S.-M.; Shell, S.; Radjabi, A.R.; Schickel, R.; Feig, C.; Boyerinas, B.; Dinulescu, D.M.; Lengyel, E.; Peter, M.E. Let-7 prevents early cancer progression by suppressing expression of the embryonic gene HMGA2. *Cell Cycle* **2007**, *6*, 2585–2590. [CrossRef]
148. Jin, Q.; Mao, X.; Li, B.; Guan, S.; Yao, F.; Jin, F. Overexpression of SMARCA5 correlates with cell proliferation and migration in breast cancer. *Tumor Biol.* **2015**, *36*, 1895–1902. [CrossRef]
149. Kong, Z.; Wan, X.; Zhang, Y.; Zhang, P.; Zhang, Y.; Zhang, X.; Qi, X.; Wu, H.; Huang, J.; Li, Y. Androgen-responsive circular RNA circSMARCA5 is up-regulated and promotes cell proliferation in prostate cancer. *Biochem. Biophys. Res. Commun.* **2017**, *493*, 1217–1223. [CrossRef]
150. Abbas, T.; Dutta, A. p21 in cancer: Intricate networks and multiple activities. *Nat. Rev. Cancer* **2009**, *9*, 400–414. [CrossRef]
151. Folpe, A.L. Fibrosarcoma: A review and update. *Histopathology* **2014**, *64*, 12–25. [CrossRef]
152. Abe, H.; Kamai, T.; Shirataki, H.; Oyama, T.; Arai, K.; Yoshida, K.I. High expression of Ran GTPase is associated with local invasion and metastasis of human clear cell renal cell carcinoma. *Int. J. Cancer* **2008**, *122*, 2391–2397. [CrossRef]
153. Kurisetty, V.; Johnston, P.G.; Johnston, N.; Erwin, P.; Crowe, P.; Fernig, D.; Campbell, F.C.; Anderson, I.; Rudland, P.; El-Tanani, M. RAN GTPase is an effector of the invasive/metastatic phenotype induced by osteopontin. *Oncogene* **2008**, *27*, 7139–7149. [CrossRef] [PubMed]
154. Barrès, V.; Ouellet, V.; Lafontaine, J.; Tonin, P.N.; Provencher, D.M.; Mes-Masson, A.-M. An essential role for Ran GTPase in epithelial ovarian cancer cell survival. *Mol. Cancer* **2010**, *9*, 272. [CrossRef] [PubMed]
155. Jezierska, A.; Motyl, T. Matrix metalloproteinase-2 involvement in breast cancer progression: A mini-review. *Med. Sci. Monit.* **2009**, *15*, RA32–RA40. [PubMed]
156. Ellenrieder, V.; Alber, B.; Lacher, U.; Hendler, S.F.; Menke, A.; Boeck, W.; Wagner, M.; Wilda, M.; Friess, H.; Büchler, M. Role of MT-MMPs and MMP-2 in pancreatic cancer progression. *Int. J. Cancer* **2000**, *85*, 14–20. [CrossRef]
157. Young, R.J.; Brown, N.J.; Reed, M.W.; Hughes, D.; Woll, P.J. Angiosarcoma. *Lancet Oncol.* **2010**, *11*, 983–991. [CrossRef]
158. Zhou, X.; Wei, M.; Wang, W. MicroRNA-340 suppresses osteosarcoma tumor growth and metastasis by directly targeting ROCK1. *Biochem. Biophys. Res. Commun.* **2013**, *437*, 653–658. [CrossRef]
159. Sun, Y.; Zhao, X.; Zhou, Y.; Hu, Y. miR-124, miR-137 and miR-340 regulate colorectal cancer growth via inhibition of the Warburg effect. *Oncol. Rep.* **2012**, *28*, 1346–1352. [CrossRef]
160. Fernandez, S.; Risolino, M.; Mandia, N.; Talotta, F.; Soini, Y.; Incoronato, M.; Condorelli, G.; Banfi, S.; Verde, P. miR-340 inhibits tumor cell proliferation and induces apoptosis by targeting multiple negative regulators of p27 in non-small cell lung cancer. *Oncogene* **2015**, *34*, 3240–3250. [CrossRef]
161. Akcakaya, P.; Caramuta, S.; Åhlen, J.; Ghaderi, M.; Berglund, E.; Östman, A.; Bränström, R.; Larsson, C.; Lui, W. microRNA expression signatures of gastrointestinal stromal tumours: Associations with imatinib resistance and patient outcome. *Br. J. Cancer* **2014**, *111*, 2091–2102. [CrossRef]
162. Fernandez-Serra, A.; Moura, D.S.; Sanchez-Izquierdo, M.D.; Calabuig-Fariñas, S.; Lopez-Alvarez, M.; Martínez-Martínez, A.; Carrasco-Garcia, I.; Ramírez-Calvo, M.; Blanco-Alcaina, E.; López-Reig, R. Prognostic Impact of let-7e MicroRNA and Its Target Genes in Localized High-Risk Intestinal GIST: A Spanish Group for Research on Sarcoma (GEIS) Study. *Cancers* **2020**, *12*, 2979. [CrossRef]
163. Niinuma, T.; Kai, M.; Kitajima, H.; Yamamoto, E.; Harada, T.; Maruyama, R.; Nobuoka, T.; Nishida, T.; Kanda, T.; Hasegawa, T. Downregulation of miR-186 is associated with metastatic recurrence of gastrointestinal stromal tumors. *Oncol. Lett.* **2017**, *14*, 5703–5710. [CrossRef] [PubMed]

164. Gyvyte, U.; Juzenas, S.; Salteniene, V.; Kupcinskas, J.; Poskiene, L.; Kucinskas, L.; Jarmalaite, S.; Stuopelyte, K.; Steponaitiene, R.; Hemmrich-Stanisak, G. MiRNA profiling of gastrointestinal stromal tumors by next-generation sequencing. *Oncotarget* **2017**, *8*, 37225. [CrossRef] [PubMed]
165. Miettinen, M.; Lasota, J. Gastrointestinal stromal tumors: Pathology and prognosis at different sites. *Semin. Diagn. Pathol.* **2006**, *23*, 70–83. [CrossRef] [PubMed]
166. Akahoshi, K.; Oya, M.; Koga, T.; Shiratsuchi, Y. Current clinical management of gastrointestinal stromal tumor. *World J. Gastroenterol.* **2018**, *24*, 2806–2817. [CrossRef]
167. Søreide, K.; Sandvik, O.M.; Søreide, J.A.; Giljaca, V.; Jureckova, A.; Bulusu, V.R. Global epidemiology of gastrointestinal stromal tumours (GIST): A systematic review of population-based cohort studies. *Cancer Epidemiol.* **2016**, *40*, 39–46. [CrossRef]
168. Cao, C.; Niu, H.; Kang, S.; Cong, C.; Kang, S. miRNA-21 sensitizes gastrointestinal stromal tumors (GISTs) cells to Imatinib via targeting B-cell lymphoma 2 (Bcl-2). *Eur. Rev. Med. Pharm. Sci.* **2016**, *20*, 3574–3581.
169. Chen, W.; Li, Z.; Liu, H.; Jiang, S.; Wang, G.; Sun, L.; Li, J.; Wang, X.; Yu, S.; Huang, J. MicroRNA-30a targets BECLIN-1 to inactivate autophagy and sensitizes gastrointestinal stromal tumor cells to imatinib. *Cell Death Dis.* **2020**, *11*, 198. [CrossRef]
170. Zhang, J.; Chen, K.; Tang, Y.; Luan, X.; Zheng, X.; Lu, X.; Mao, J.; Hu, L.; Zhang, S.; Zhang, X. LncRNA-HOTAIR activates autophagy and promotes the imatinib resistance of gastrointestinal stromal tumor cells through a mechanism involving the miR-130a/ATG2B pathway. *Cell Death Dis.* **2021**, *12*, 367. [CrossRef]
171. Gao, X.; Shen, K.; Wang, C.; Ling, J.; Wang, H.; Fang, Y.; Shi, Y.; Hou, Y.; Qin, J.; Sun, Y. MiR-320a downregulation is associated with imatinib resistance in gastrointestinal stromal tumors. *Acta Biochim. Biophys Sin.* **2014**, *46*, 72–75. [CrossRef]
172. Huang, W.-K.; Akçakaya, P.; Gangaev, A.; Lee, L.; Zeljic, K.; Hajeri, P.; Berglund, E.; Ghaderi, M.; Åhlén, J.; Bränström, R. miR-125a-5p regulation increases phosphorylation of FAK that contributes to imatinib resistance in gastrointestinal stromal tumors. *Exp. Cell Res.* **2018**, *371*, 287–296. [CrossRef]
173. Kou, Y.; Yang, R.; Wang, Q. Serum miR-518e-5p is a potential biomarker for secondary imatinib-resistant gastrointestinal stromal tumor. *J. Biosci.* **2018**, *43*, 1015–1023. [CrossRef] [PubMed]
174. Rupaimoole, R.; Slack, F.J. MicroRNA therapeutics: Towards a new era for the management of cancer and other diseases. *Nat. Rev. Drug Discov.* **2017**, *16*, 203–222. [CrossRef] [PubMed]
175. Orellana, E.A.; Kasinski, A.L. MicroRNAs in Cancer: A Historical Perspective on the Path from Discovery to Therapy. *Cancers* **2015**, *7*, 1388–1405. [CrossRef] [PubMed]

Disclaimer/Publisher's Note: The statements, opinions and data contained in all publications are solely those of the individual author(s) and contributor(s) and not of MDPI and/or the editor(s). MDPI and/or the editor(s) disclaim responsibility for any injury to people or property resulting from any ideas, methods, instructions or products referred to in the content.

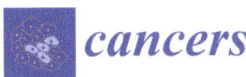

Communication

Electronic Patient Reported Outcome (ePRO) Measures in Patients with Soft Tissue Sarcoma (STS) Receiving Palliative Treatment

Silvia Hofer [1,*], Leopold Hentschel [2], Stephan Richter [3], Veronika Blum [4], Michael Kramer [5], Bernd Kasper [6], Christoph Riese [7] and Markus K. Schuler [3]

1. Department of Neurology, University Hospital Zurich, 8091 Zurich, Switzerland
2. Division of Psycho-Oncology, NCT/UCC, University Hospital Carl Gustav Carus, Technical University of Dresden, 01307 Dresden, Germany
3. Clinic and Polyclinic for Internal Medicine I, Sarcoma Center, NCT/UCC, University Hospital Carl Gustav Carus, Technical University of Dresden, 01307 Dresden, Germany
4. Department of Internal Medicine, Cantonal Hospital Lucerne, 6002 Lucerne, Switzerland
5. AvenCell Europe GmbH Dresden, 01307 Dresden, Germany
6. Sarcoma Unit, Mannheim Cancer Center (MCC), Mannheim University Medical Center, University of Heidelberg, 68167 Mannheim, Germany
7. DTB Gesellschaft für digitale Therapiebegleitung mbH, 07745 Jena, Germany
* Correspondence: silvia.hofer@usz.ch; Tel.: +41-43-2531569

Simple Summary: Therapeutic options for advanced soft tissue sarcoma (STS) are limited. Health-related quality of life (HRQoL), along with traditional outcome parameters such as tumor control and toxicity, is one of the most important endpoints for palliative STS treatment. The PazoQoL prospective, randomized, controlled, multicenter study (EudraCT number 2017-003382-10, ClinicalTrials.gov Identifier NCT0373575) was designed to assess the impact of treatment on HRQoL and patient-reported outcomes. Although the study had to be terminated early due to the pandemic, some valuable results were collected on the continuous recording of symptoms over a 9-week period and on patient satisfaction with therapy. Our findings could be translated into clinical practice without much effort and outside of a trial.

Abstract: The PazoQoL prospective, randomized, controlled, multicenter study was designed to continuously assess global health related quality of life (HRQoL) during treatment with pazopanib or physician-preferred chemotherapy over a 9-week period. The questionnaires were completed by the patients at home with great reliability during this time period. Continuous electronic patient reported outcome (ePRO) enabled early detection of the onset of deterioration and timely initiation of countermeasures. The Cancer Therapy Satisfaction Questionnaire (CTSQ) showed high interindividual variability and decline over a 9-week period, whereas the Time Trade-off (TTO) proved to be an efficient method for assessing individual benefit from cancer therapy. In our cohort, the TTO clearly demonstrated that the prolongation of life and the side effect profile of continued therapy were not as satisfactory as expected by patients when starting a new therapy. Although the study had to be stopped early due to the pandemic, our findings could translate into clinical practice without much effort and outside of a trial.

Keywords: soft tissue sarcoma; electronic patient reported outcome; health related quality of life; randomized controlled trial; palliative treatment

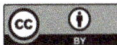

1. Introduction

Patient-reported outcome (PRO) measures with the aim to capture health-related quality of life (HRQoL) from a patient's perspective and without the interpretation of caregivers are key outcome instruments in contemporary clinical trials for cancer treatment [1,2]. The value added from electronic and mobile PRO, hereafter called "ePRO", includes real-time monitoring, support of therapy-management, lower administrative burden, fewer missing data, and the possibility for immediate interactions [3,4]. Nevertheless, ePRO has not yet been implemented into routine daily practice in soft tissue sarcoma (STS) and oncologists in general demonstrate little familiarity and lack standardization of PROs [5,6].

Palliative treatment strategies should aim not only to prolong survival but, more importantly, to control and relieve symptoms, limit disease- and treatment-related morbidity, and preserve the performance of activities of daily living as far as possible. This is particularly important for palliative STS therapies, which offer only modest survival benefits.

HRQoL in general is a multidimensional construct that takes into account the impact of a person's health status on their life and can identify unmet needs during treatment and in the follow-up period. It has been previously shown that HRQoL at baseline is a prognostic factor for clinical outcome in various cancers [7,8]. Because HRQoL is based on patient perceptions, relies on self-reflection, and is influenced by impairments, functional status, and social background, all of these measures are useful in discussions with the treating physician as part of shared decision making.

The PRO questionnaires currently in use, largely lack patients' views of their expectations and satisfaction with therapy. However, such questionnaires have been developed and validated for different types of cancer, especially for patients receiving intravenous or oral cancer drugs [9,10].

The delicate balance between longer survival and disadvantages of palliative therapy can be captured by the "Time Trade-off" (TTO) method. Two simple and straightforward questions help in the decision-making process for continuing or stopping an ongoing treatment. Patients are asked to rate their preference for quantity versus quality of life, i.e., how much additional survival time a further line of cancer treatment would be worth to them [11,12]. Previous studies that addressed this issue showed that oncologists value prolongation of survival time more than quality of life (QoL) [13]. To date, TTO has rarely been used in sarcoma trials.

Here, we present results of the PazoQoL trial, a randomized, controlled trial (RCT) on QoL in patients with non-adipocyte STS under palliative treatment. The trial was designed by the German Interdisciplinary Sarcoma Group (GISG-11; EudraCT number 2017-003382-10, ClinicalTrials.gov Identifier NCT0373575).

2. Materials and Methods

The multi-center, longitudinal PazoQoL study allowed patients with several STS subtypes to be included. After progression of one or more lines of systemic STS therapies, patients could be randomized in a 1:1 fashion and allocated to in-label use of the oral agent pazopanib, a selective, multitargeted receptor tyrosine kinase inhibitor of vascular endothelial growth factor receptor 1–3 (VEGFR-1–3), PDGFR-a, PDGFR-b, and KIT or systemic treatment according to investigator's choice. According to the study plan, 150 patients should have been recruited, 75 in each arm.

HRQoL as well as other secondary outcome measures, were recorded continuously, i.e., over the first 9 weeks of a new palliative treatment at the times indicated in the protocol (8 in total, Figure 1).

The primary objective of the RCT was the comparison of global HRQoL under treatment with pazopanib or physician-preferred chemotherapy (ChT) after 9 weeks.

Secondary objectives included QoL three times in cycle 1 and cycle 3 (corresponding to weeks 1, 2, 3 and 7, 8, 9, respectively). Other objectives assessed cross-group evaluation of pain, fatigue, and categories such as physical, mental, cognitive, and emotional wellbeing, as well as anorexia/cachexia, both markers of HRQoL. Special attention was paid to parameters of satisfaction with care.

HRQoL was measured applying the EORTC QLQ-C30, a well-validated, extensively used instrument, consisting of 30 items to obtain different domains including five functional scales, symptom scales as well as global QoL. Higher scores (ranging from 0–100) represent higher functioning and global HRQoL, while also describing higher symptom burden [14].

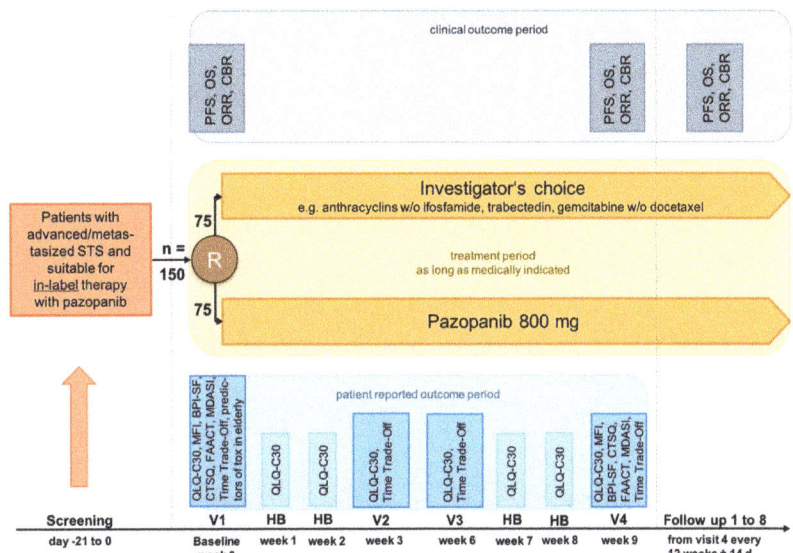

Figure 1. PazoQoL study design. STS, soft tissue sarcoma; V1–4, visit 1–4; HB, home based patient reported outcome measures; PFS, progression free survival; OS, overall survival; ORR, objective remission rate; CBR, clinical benefit rate; QLQ C30, EORTC QoL questionnaire; BPI-SF, brief pain inventory; CTSQ, Cancer therapy satisfaction questionnaire; FAACT, functional assessment of anorexia/cachexia therapy; MDASI, M.D. Anderson symptom inventory; MFI, multidimensional fatigue inventory.

The Cancer Therapy Satisfaction Questionnaire (CTSQ) was used to record satisfaction with therapy (Table 1). The calculation results in a score ranging from 0 to 100 for each domain, with a higher score associated with the best outcome on each domain [9,10].

Table 1. Cancer therapy satisfaction questionnaire (CTSQ) domains. https://docplayer.net/51309772-Administration-and-scoring-guide-for-the-cancer-therapy-satisfaction-questionnaire-ctsq.html (accessed on 12 February 2023).

CTSQ Domains	Content of Items
Expectations of therapy	Return to normal life. Get rid of cancer. Prevent cancer from coming back. Stop cancer from spreading. Help you to live longer
Feeling about side effects	Cancer therapy (CT) limited daily activities. Upset about side effects. Taking CT as difficult as expected. Were side effects as expected
Satisfaction with therapy	Worth taking even with side effects. Think about stopping CT. How worthwhile was CT. Benefits meet expectations. Satisfaction with form of CT, Satisfaction with recent CT. Would you take the CT again

All participants received tablet-computers with all questionnaires in electronic form to be completed at home. The IT solution Digital Health Management from Compliance Solutions GmbH was used to record and evaluate the patient responses. The tablets with

SIM cards (mobile internet) were made available to the respective patients for 9 weeks each to document the diaries.

The questionnaires had to be started by the clinic staff, who trained the patients in their use. After completion of a 9-week patient diary phase, data had to be exported by the clinic staff and then deleted from the device before the tablet had been given to another patient. Access to other functions of the tablets had been blocked for patients.

The PazoQoL study was approved by the Ethics Committee of the State of Berlin (State Office for Health and Social Affairs) and bears the number 17/0390—EK 15 and by the Ethics Committee Northwestern and Central Switzerland (EKNZ) Project ID 2019-00386.

3. Results

The PazoQoL trial was terminated early due to low enrollment during the COVID pandemic and no further funding provided thereafter. Ultimately, only 11 patients could be randomized and 10 of them evaluated (Consort diagram, Figure 2). However, key elements could be exploited despite the small number of patients.

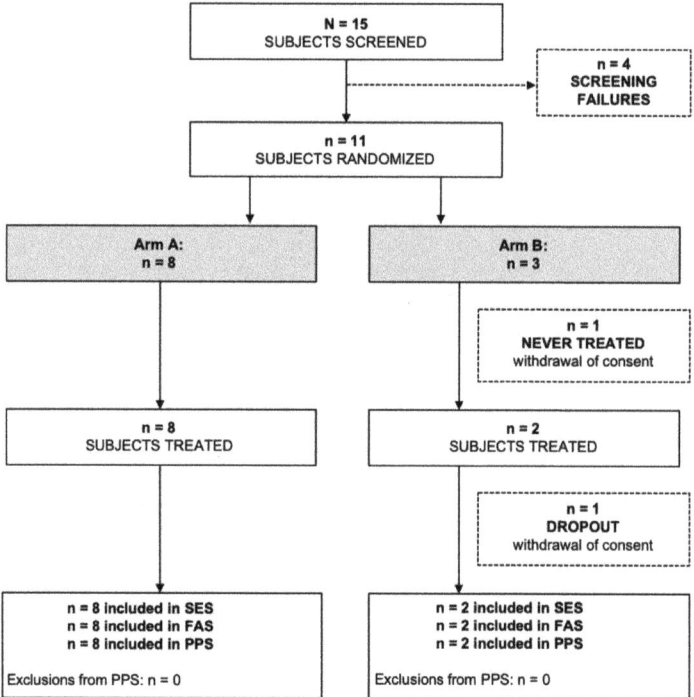

Figure 2. Consort diagram. Arm A, pazopanib; Arm B, physician-preferred chemotherapy; SES, safety evaluation set; FAS, full analysis set; PPS, per protocol set.

The PazoQoL study was able to demonstrate that a 9-week application of ePRO appears to be sufficient to evaluate therapies for advanced STS in terms of HRQoL and treatment satisfaction.

For the EORTC QLQ30 questionnaire, 92% of the data were complete, and for the TTO and CTSQ questionnaires, the respective rate was 89%. The relatively short assessment period of 9 weeks was therefore associated with a high patient adherence rate.

ePRO enabled tracking of short-term changes of symptoms that varied significantly from patient to patient and over time and therefore did not reflect a general trend (Examples, Figure 3).

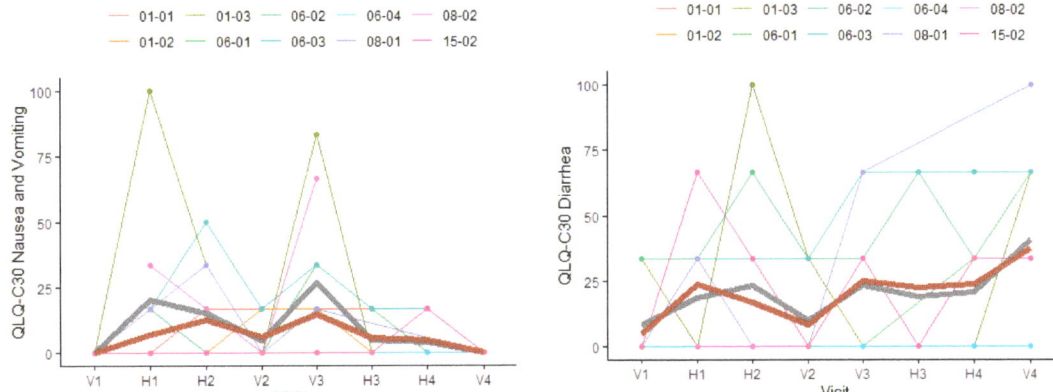

Figure 3. Examples of short-term fluctuations in symptoms.

(a) Ten individual and mean data for nausea and vomiting, EORTC QLQ-C30 questionnaire. Total mean plotted bold in grey (n = 10), pazopanib arm mean plotted bold in red (n = 8), V1–4, symptoms recorded at regular visits 1–4, H1–4, home based ePRO data (Figure 3 left).

(b) Ten individual and mean data for diarrhea, EORTC QLQ-C30 questionnaire. Total mean plotted bold in grey (n = 10), pazopanib arm mean plotted bold in red (n = 8), V1–4, symptoms recorded at regular visits 1–4, H1–4, home based ePRO data (Figure 3 right).

Close monitoring and continuous ePROs facilitated early detection of incipient deterioration and timely initiation of countermeasures.

The Cancer Therapy Satisfaction Questionnaire (CTSQ) has shown high interindividual variability and a decline over time (Table 2).

Table 2. Results Cancer Therapy Satisfaction Questionnaire (CTSQ). Given numbers are mean/SD and (min–max); EoT, end of treatment; Score ranging from 0–100 for each domain, with a higher score associated with the best outcome.

Domains		All Patients, n = 10	Pazopanib Arm, n = 8
Expectations of therapy	Baseline	43.89/28.7 (0–95)	37.86/29.56 (0–95)
	EoT	36.25/31.48 (0–100)	35.71/33.96 (0–100)
Feelings about side effects	Baseline	43.06/22.41 (12.5–75)	41.96/25.19 (12.5–75)
	EoT	37.50/29.32 (0–87.5)	30.36/22.94 (0–62.5)
Satisfaction with therapy	Baseline	17.00/4.21 (10–23)	16.43/4.35 (10–23)
	EoT	15.00/6.21 (8–25)	13.57/5.09 (8–22)

The "Time Trade-off" (TTO), an efficient method for evaluating the individual benefit of cancer therapy, yielded the following results: the additional lifetime, a patient would like to gain if he or she is willing to undergo further treatment, increased significantly over time. At the beginning of therapy, it was a median of 24 months; at the end of the study, it was a median of 72 months. When asked how much additional survival time a patient would sacrifice to be symptom-free with continued therapy, the responses were as follows: they would sacrifice a median of 0 months of their lives to be symptom-free (Table 3). However, there were individual patients who would sacrifice some time to be symptom-free. One patient as an example would sacrifice 15 months at visit 1 (baseline) and 12 months at visit 4 (EoT), another patient would sacrifice 1 month at visit 4 after not sacrificing any time at baseline.

Table 3. Results Time Trade-off (TTO). Given are median (SD), EoT, end of treatment ChT, chemotherapy.

Parameter		All Patients, n = 10
Extra time for ChT (months)	Baseline	24 (12–72)
	EoT	72 (54.5–72)
Time for being symptom-free (months)	Baseline	0 (0–0)
	EoT	0 (0–0.25)

4. Discussion

PazoQoL has shed light on various aspects for the implementation of ePRO from research to routine and provides recommendations for its use in palliative STS therapy, where individual patient perspectives and preferences are of the utmost interest.

In our study, home-based use of ePRO enabled symptom capture in real time and independent of scheduled visits. A recently published RCT [15] with continuous home measurements was also able to provide a more detailed HRQoL profile and thus, better capture symptom fluctuations.

Satisfaction and expectations with treatment are closely related to decision making and treatment adherence. For this reason, we applied the Cancer Therapy Satisfaction Questionnaire (CTSQ) in our study. To our knowledge, this questionnaire has not been previously used to assess palliative STS therapies. High interindividual variability and decline over time have been observed. Therefore, we consider these personalized statements to be highly relevant and support their implementation in daily clinical practice.

Of particular interest is the TTO, an efficient method of assessing the individual and subjective benefit of a cancer therapy. The results of our cohort clearly indicate that the life extension and side effect profile of continuing therapy were not as satisfactory as expected by patients at the start of a new therapy. Our findings are particularly noteworthy because a detailed and informative discussion with the treating physician took place as a standard procedure in every patient before the start of a next line of therapy. The discrepancy in the different perceptions of the doctor and his patient is a phenomenon that is generally underestimated [13]. Attention to this should be increased and the patient should be given the opportunity to express his concerns in more detail, e.g., to rule out depression as a reason for his current statement.

In order to keep patients' motivation high to complete the ePRO questionnaires, its application should not exceed a certain time frame, 10–15 min per session might be appropriate (expert opinion). A careful selection of questions covering relevant domains is therefore required. For daily clinical practice, we suggest using a generic and well-established instrument (e.g., the EORTC QLQ-C30 questionnaire) to capture a wide range of symptoms and HRQoL topics and to compare the results with data from ongoing and completed studies. The average time spent completing the QLQ-C30 was reported to be 9 and 7 min before and during treatment, respectively. In our cohort, this time requirement was even lower, at 5.5 and 4 min, respectively. To assess satisfaction with treatment, we suggest including a brief "satisfaction and expectations" questionnaire and the two "Time Trade-off" questions, which take an additional 7–10 min to complete in total (Table 4.).

There will be some costs associated with implementing ePRO in daily clinical practice [16], but these costs are disproportionate to the drug costs that are expected to be recovered as a result. It is noteworthy that regulatory authorities are now paying greater attention to PRO data in their drug approval decisions, in fact, recommendations have already been issued by the U.S. Food and Drug Administration (FDA) and the European Medicines Agency (EMA) [17,18]. One could also imagine that the cost of ePRO could be borne by the pharmaceutical industry in terms of quality of care.

Our RCT is subject to several limitations. Only a small fraction of the planned patients could be recruited due to reasons already mentioned and thus, a majority of the secondary endpoints could neither be reliably evaluated nor could a comparison be made between the two study arms. Nevertheless, our study clearly demonstrates that satisfaction with palliative treatment is a valuable endpoint that can be readily implemented in clinical practice as a suitable tool for shared decision making.

Table 4. Proposal for ePRO in daily clinical practice for advanced STS. CTSQ, Cancer Therapy Satisfaction Questionnaire, QoL, quality of life, STS, soft tissue sarcoma.

	Captures	Questions	Time Spent
EORTC QLQ-C30	Physical, psychological & social functions	30	4–5 min
CTSQ	Satisfaction with therapy	16	5–10 min
Time Trade-off	QoL	2	2 min

5. Conclusions

For daily clinical practice, electronic tools need to be developed further to provide patients with regular reminders and incentives, such as information about their disease, strategies to cope with symptoms, or to enable a prompt way to contact the care team. Data security is a challenge that needs to be harmonized. Since electronic health care systems are being developed worldwide, it is only a matter of time before the infrastructure for ePRO will be widely available and only the contents of choice need to be filled in.

HRQoL, along with traditional outcome parameters such as tumor control and toxicity, is one of the most important endpoints for palliative STS therapies.

Author Contributions: Conceptualization, M.K.S. and L.H.; methodology, M.K.S.; software, Compliance Solutions, GmbH, Stuttgart; formal analysis, M.K., M.K.S. and S.H.; investigation, M.K.S., S.R., V.B. and S.H.; resources, M.K.S. and S.H.; data curation, M.K.S., M.K. and S.H.; writing—original draft preparation, S.H. and M.K.S.; writing—review and editing, S.H., M.K.S., M.K., L.H., C.R., S.R., V.B. and B.K.; funding acquisition, M.K.S., SAKK (Swiss Group for Clinical Cancer Research). All authors have read and agreed to the published version of the manuscript.

Funding: This research received external funding by an unrestricted grant from Novartis Pharma GmbH, Germany (Grant number CPZP034BDE17T). The Swiss Group for Clinical Cancer Research (SAKK) received financial support from the Swiss State Secretariat for Education, Research and Innovation (SERI) and Swiss Cancer Research Foundation.

Institutional Review Board Statement: The PazoQoL study was approved by the Ethics Committee of the State of Berlin (State Office for Health and Social Affairs) and bears the number 17/0390—EK 15 and by the Ethics Committee Northwestern and Central Switzerland (EKNZ) Project ID 2019-00386. The study was conducted in accordance with the Declaration of Helsinki.

Informed Consent Statement: Written informed consent was obtained from all subjects involved in the study.

Data Availability Statement: The data underlying this article will be shared on reasonable request to the last author M.K.S.

Acknowledgments: We would like to thank Marinela Augustin, Universitätsklinik der Paracelsus Medizinischen Privatuniversität Nürnberg, Nürnberg Germany for patient recruitment, the Swiss Group for Clinical Cancer Research (SAKK) for support in initiating and conducting the PazoQoL study in Switzerland, Roman Zagrosek, Compliance Solutions, GmbH, Stuttgart for his support of the digital part of PazoQoL and Katrin Linke, GWT-TUD GmbH, Medical Consulting, Dresden for project management.

Conflicts of Interest: The authors declare that they have no competing interest. The funders had no role in the design of the study; in the collection, analyses, or interpretation of data nor in the writing of the manuscript; or in the decision to publish the results.

References

1. Absolom, K.; Warrington, L.; Hudson, E.; Hewison, J.; Morris, C.; Holch, P.; Carter, R.; Gibson, A.; Holmes, M.; Clayton, B.; et al. Phase III Randomized Controlled Trial of eRAPID: eHealth Intervention During Chemotherapy. *J. Clin. Oncol.* **2021**, *39*, 734–747. [CrossRef] [PubMed]
2. Coens, C.; van der Graaf, W.T.; Blay, J.Y.; Chawla, S.P.; Judson, I.; Sanfilippo, R.; Manson, S.C.; Hodge, R.A.; Marreaud, S.; Prins, J.B.; et al. Health-related quality-of-life results from PALETTE: A randomized, double-blind, phase 3 trial of pazopanib versus placebo in patients with soft tissue sarcoma whose disease has progressed during or after prior chemotherapy-a European Organization for research and treatment of cancer soft tissue and bone sarcoma group global network study (EORTC 62072). *Cancer* **2015**, *121*, 2933–2941. [CrossRef] [PubMed]
3. Basch, E.; Stover, A.M.; Schrag, D.; Chung, A.; Jansen, J.; Henson, S.; Carr, P.; Ginos, B.; Deal, A.; Spears, P.A.; et al. Clinical Utility and User Perceptions of a Digital System for Electronic Patient-Reported Symptom Monitoring during Routine Cancer Care: Findings from the PRO-TECT Trial. *JCO Clin. Cancer Inform.* **2020**, *4*, 947–957. [CrossRef] [PubMed]
4. Gibbons, C.; Porter, I.; Goncalves-Bradley, D.; Stoilov, S.; Ricci-Cabello, I.; Tsangaris, E.; Gangannagaripalli, J.; Davey, A.; Gibbons, E.; Kotzena, A.; et al. Routine provision of feedback from patient-reported outcome measurements to healthcare providers and patients in clinical practice. *Cochrane Database Syst. Rev.* **2021**, CD011589. [CrossRef]
5. den Hollander, D.; Fiore, M.; Martin-Broto, J.; Kasper, B.; Casado Herraez, A.; Kulis, D.; Nixon, I.; Sodergren, S.C.; Eichler, M.; van Houdt, W.J.; et al. Incorporating the Patient Voice in Sarcoma Research: How Can We Assess Health-Related Quality of Life in This Heterogeneous Group of Patients? A Study Protocol. *Cancers* **2020**, *13*, 1. [CrossRef] [PubMed]
6. Meldahl, M.L.; Acaster, S.; Hayes, R.P. Exploration of oncologists' attitudes toward and perceived value of patient-reported outcomes. *Qual. Life Res.* **2013**, *22*, 725–731. [CrossRef] [PubMed]
7. Efficace, F.; Collins, G.S.; Cottone, F.; Giesinger, J.M.; Sommer, K.; Anota, A.; Schlussel, M.M.; Fazi, P.; Vignetti, M. Patient-Reported Outcomes as Independent Prognostic Factors for Survival in Oncology: Systematic Review and Meta-Analysis. *Value Health* **2021**, *24*, 250–267. [CrossRef] [PubMed]
8. Basch, E.; Deal, A.M.; Dueck, A.C.; Scher, H.I.; Kris, M.G.; Hudis, C.; Schrag, D. Overall Survival Results of a Trial Assessing Patient-Reported Outcomes for Symptom Monitoring during Routine Cancer Treatment. *JAMA* **2017**, *318*, 197–198. [CrossRef] [PubMed]
9. Abetz, L.; Coombs, J.H.; Keininger, D.L.; Earle, C.C.; Wade, C.; Bury-Maynard, D.; Copley-Merriman, K.; Hsu, M.A. Development of the cancer therapy satisfaction questionnaire: Item generation and content validity testing. *Value Health J. Int. Soc. Pharm. Outcomes Res.* **2005**, *8* (Suppl. 1), 41–53. [CrossRef] [PubMed]
10. Trask, P.C.; Tellefsen, C.; Espindle, D.; Getter, C.; Hsu, M.A. Psychometric validation of the cancer therapy satisfaction questionnaire. *Value Health* **2008**, *11*, 669–679. [CrossRef] [PubMed]
11. Dolan, P.; Gudex, C.; Kind, P.; Williams, A. Valuing health states: A comparison of methods. *J. Health Econ.* **1996**, *15*, 209–231. [CrossRef] [PubMed]
12. Valentí, V.; Ramos, J.; Pérez, C.; Capdevila, L.; Ruiz, I.; Tikhomirova, L.; Sánchez, M.; Juez, I.; Llobera, M.; Sopena, E.; et al. Increased survival time or better quality of life? Trade-off between benefits and adverse events in the systemic treatment of cancer. *Clin. Transl. Oncol.* **2020**, *22*, 935–942. [CrossRef] [PubMed]
13. Kozminski, M.A.; Neumann, P.J.; Nadler, E.S.; Jankovic, A.; Ubel, P.A. How long and how well: oncologists' attitudes toward the relative value of life-prolonging v. quality of life-enhancing treatments. *Med. Decis. Mak.* **2011**, *31*, 380–385. [CrossRef] [PubMed]
14. Aaronson, N.K.; Ahmedzai, S.; Bergman, B.; Bullinger, M.; Cull, A.; Duez, N.J.; Filiberti, A.; Flechtner, H.; Fleishman, S.B.; De Haes, J.C.J.M.; et al. The European organization for research and treatment of cancer QLQ-C30: A quality-of-life instrument for use in international clinical trials in oncology. *J. Natl. Cancer Inst.* **1993**, *85*, 365–376. [CrossRef] [PubMed]
15. Shiroiwa, T.; Hagiwara, Y.; Taira, N.; Kawahara, T.; Konomura, K.; Iwamoto, T.; Noto, S.; Fukuda, T.; Shimozuma, K. Randomized Controlled Trial of Paper-Based at a Hospital versus Continual Electronic Patient-Reported Outcomes at Home for Metastatic Cancer Patients: Does Electronic Measurement at Home Detect Patients' Health Status in Greater Detail? *Med. Decis. Mak.* **2022**, *42*, 60–67. [CrossRef] [PubMed]
16. Nixon, N.A.; Spackman, E.; Clement, F.; Verma, S.; Manns, B. Cost-effectiveness of symptom monitoring with patient-reported outcomes during routine cancer treatment. *J. Cancer Policy* **2018**, *15 Pt A*, 32–36. [CrossRef]
17. FDA. Guidance for Industry Patient-Reported Outcome Measures: Use in Medical Product Development to Support Labeling Claims. 2009. Available online: https://www.fda.gov/regulatory-information/search-fda-guidance-documents/patient-reported-outcome-measures-use-medical-product-development-support-labeling-claims (accessed on 12 February 2023).
18. European Medicines Agency. Committee for Medicinal Products for Human Use (CHMP) Appendix 2 to the Guideline on the Evaluation of Anticancer Medicinal Products in Man. The Use of Patient-Reported Outcome (PRO) Measures in Oncology Studies. 2016. Available online: https://www.ema.europa.eu/en/appendix-2-guideline-evaluation-anticancer-medicinal-products-man-use-patient-reported-outcome-pro (accessed on 12 February 2023).

Disclaimer/Publisher's Note: The statements, opinions and data contained in all publications are solely those of the individual author(s) and contributor(s) and not of MDPI and/or the editor(s). MDPI and/or the editor(s) disclaim responsibility for any injury to people or property resulting from any ideas, methods, instructions or products referred to in the content.

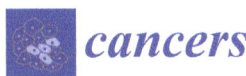

Review

Immunotherapy for Soft Tissue Sarcomas: Anti-PD1/PDL1 and Beyond

Mina Fazel [1,2], Armelle Dufresne [1], Hélène Vanacker [1,2], Waisse Waissi [1], Jean-Yves Blay [1,2] and Mehdi Brahmi [1,*]

[1] Centre Léon Bérard, 28 Rue Laënnec, 69008 Lyon, France
[2] Faculté de Médecine Lyon Est, Université Claude Bernard Lyon, 8 Avenue Rockefeller, 69008 Lyon, France
[*] Correspondence: mehdi.brahmi@lyon.unicancer.fr

Simple Summary: Although immunotherapy has revolutionized the standard of care of many cancers, its efficacy in soft tissue sarcomas has been disappointing so far. Nevertheless, some recent studies have reported meaningful activity in a few selected histotypes, especially alveolar soft part sarcoma (ASPS). Furthermore, emerging biomarkers, such as the presence of tertiary lymphoid structures, seem to be predictive of the efficacy of immune checkpoint inhibitors. Finally, innovative therapeutic agents (especially adoptive T-cell therapies) and the combination of immunotherapeutic agents with other therapies such as tyrosine kinase inhibitors represent promising prospects.

Abstract: Sarcomas gather a heterogeneous group of mesenchymal malignant tumors including more than 150 different subtypes. Most of them represent aggressive tumors with poor prognosis at the advanced stage, despite the better molecular characterization of these tumors and the development of molecular-driven therapeutic strategies. During the last decade, immunotherapy has been developed to treat advanced cancers, mainly thanks to immune checkpoint inhibitors (ICI) such as anti-PD1/PDL1 and later to adoptive immune cell therapies. In this review, we aim to summarize the state of the art of immunotherapy in soft tissue sarcomas (STS). Overall, the clinical trials of ICI that included a wide diversity of STS subtypes reported limited efficacy with some outlying responders. Both emerging biomarkers are of interest in selecting good candidates and in the development of combination therapies. Finally, the recent breakthroughs of innovative adoptive therapies in STS seem highly promising.

Keywords: soft tissue sarcomas; immunotherapy; immune checkpoint blockade; adoptive T-cell therapies

1. Introduction

Sarcomas gather a wide and heterogeneous group of rare malignant tumors of mesenchymal origins, representing less than 1% of all adult malignant tumors and 20% of childhood solid cancers [1–3]. They may occur on any site, at any age and are usually divided into soft tissue sarcomas (STS) and bone sarcomas. Furthermore, significant heterogeneity remains within these two subgroups, so that more than 150 distinct subtypes are described in the latest (fifth) WHO (World Health Organization) Classification of Soft Tissue and Bone Tumors [4]. Complete en-bloc R0 surgery is the cornerstone of the management of localized STS whereas the treatment of advanced STS remains challenging due to the rarity and the clinical and biological heterogeneity of these diseases [5]. Patients are treated with conventional chemotherapy (doxorubin, ifosfamide, etc.) or antiangiogenic tyrosine kinase inhibitors (TKI) (pazopanib), with a 3–6-month median progression free survival (PFS) and an 18-month median overall survival (OS) [6–8]. Therefore, advanced/metastatic STS represent a high unmet medical need.

Modern immunotherapy has been flourishing in the last decade, witnessing a significant expansion in the treatment of many solid and hematologic cancers [9]. Sarcomas

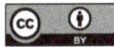

were first suggested as good candidates, due to an historical rationale. Indeed, the first immunotherapy was practiced in the 19th century by Coley [10], with the inoculation of erysipela samples directly into a sarcoma during surgery. He then observed tumor shrinkage, which is believed to be induced by the recruitment of immune cells. Nevertheless, early experiences with immunotherapy in trials recruiting unselected STS subtypes have been disappointing. Regardless, significant efficacy has been observed in a subset of patients and/or with genetically modified T cell-based adoptive immunotherapy approaches.

We conducted a literature review to describe the current approaches to immunotherapy in STS. Here, we discuss the current state of immunotherapy for STS, the ongoing clinical trials evaluating immune checkpoint inhibitors (ICI), alone or in combination, or adoptive cellular therapy and the investigations to identify predictive biomarkers.

2. Immune Checkpoint Inhibitors in STS: Therapeutic Options

2.1. ICI Trials (Mono or Dual Blockade)

During the last five years, a few clinical trials have been conducted to evaluate ICI in STS, targeting regulators of the immune response by blocking the PD1/PDL1 and CTLA4 axes. In the last decade, ICI have dramatically changed the vision of cancer management by emphasizing the importance of the immune system in cancer growth, contrasting with the previous, inefficient immunotherapy mostly based on the use of vaccines. Each step in T cell-mediated immunity is regulated by counterbalancing inhibitory signals, which are commonly overexpressed in tumor cells or in the tumoral microenvironment. Immune checkpoint receptors expressed by T cells or antigen-presenting cells, such as PD1/PDL1 and CTLA4, when combined to their ligand, induce immune tolerance. ICI are antibodies that target and prevent the inhibitory ligand–receptor interaction and can therefore activate the immune system [11] (Figure 1).

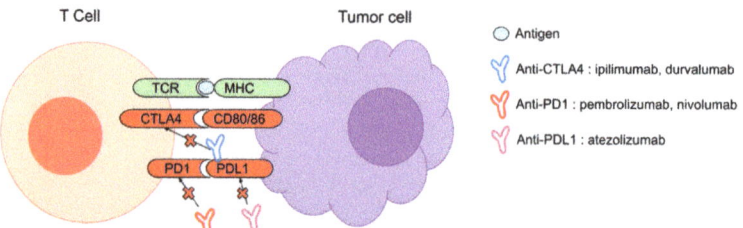

Figure 1. Mechanism of action of the most common ICI.

The results of these studies remain modest overall, in light of the fact that they include all patients with no preselection. The first study conducted by the MSKCC (Memorial Sloan Kettering Cancer Center) evaluated ipilimumab (anti-CTLA4) in patients with metastatic synovial sarcomas [12]. This study was closed prematurely due to the lack of both inclusion and efficacy, with only six patients enrolled and no objective response (OR). The PEMBROSARC trial, conducted by the French Sarcoma Group (FSG), was therefore the first completed phase II study to assess the efficacy of pembrolizumab (anti-PD1) combined with metronomic cyclophosphamide, to convey its immunomodulatory properties [13]. The results were disappointing, with a partial response (PR) of only 1/50. Despite the negative result, this study has fueled the first hypotheses concerning the mechanisms of immune evasion, in particular via macrophage infiltration and the activation of the IDO (indoleamine 2,3 dioxygenase) pathway. Shortly after, the American phase II study SARC028 tested pembrolizumab as a monotherapy on 80 patients, half of whom had STS and the other half of whom had bone sarcomas [14]. Seven out of 40 patients (18%) with STS had an OR, including 4/10 patients with undifferentiated pleomorphic sarcoma (UPS) and 2/10 patients with dedifferentiated liposarcoma (DD-LPS). Finally, the third pivotal phase II study was Alliance A091401, evaluating nivolumab (anti-PDL1) alone or with ipilimumab [15]. An OR was achieved in 5% (N = 2/38) of patients in the nivolumab group and in 16% (N = 6/38) of patients in the combination group, including patients with ASPS, angiosarcoma, UPS and DD-LPS. In addition, expansion cohorts have been developed to explore the activity of UPS and DD-LPS with response rates of around 23% and 10%, respectively [16]. Overall, these results suggest that immunotherapy might have a therapeutical impact on STS, especially in combination with other therapies, which highlights the need for the identification of a predictive biomarker.

Furthermore, immunotherapy seemed to cause meaningful clinical activity in some selected histological subtypes, especially ASPS, an ultra-rare subtype of STS [17,18]. A neoepitope arising from the ASPL::TFE3 fusion protein itself has been speculated to be immunogenic [19,20], even though the exact rationale for their increased sensitivity to immunotherapy remains unclear. As of today, more than 150 patients with ASPS have been treated in clinical trials evaluating anti-PD1/PDL1, with response rates ranging from 7.1% to 54.5% depending on the study [21,22]. The more recent study was a single-arm phase II study that evaluated atezolizumab in ASPS patients, showing an OR rate of 37.2% (16/43). Importantly, the median duration of the confirmed response was 16.5 months (range: 4.9–38.1 months). Although there is no clear predictive factor for treatment response, some hypotheses arise, such as the prior failure of TKI [23] or CD8+ infiltration and PD-L1 expression [21], but investigations need to be pursued, possibly through genomic and transcriptomic landscape evaluation. In light of these results, the Food and Drug Administration (FDA) recently approved atezolizumab for patients with unresectable or metastatic ASPS (9 December 2022). As for angiosarcomas, multiple case reports find a meaningful activity signal [24–27], which is partly explained by a mutational profile linked to DNA damage caused by UV exposure, as is the case of face and scalp cutaneous angiosarcomas [28]. An angiosarcoma cohort was extracted from the trial evaluating dual inhibition by anti-CTLA4 and anti-PD1 in rare tumors (DART) [29]. The ORR observed was 25% among the 16 studied patients. The 6-month PFS rate was 38%. A confirmed response was observed in 60% of patients (3/5) with primary cutaneous scalp or face tumors, supporting the theory about UV exposure. Otherwise, in a phase II trial, single-agent pembrolizumab caused significant and prolonged antitumor activity in a few selected rare sarcoma histotypes, mostly in ASPS (8 of 17 patients with an objective response), but also in chordoma and SMRT (SMARCA4 deleted/malignant rhabdoid tumor) [30].

All those data support ICI (mono or dual blockade) as efficient therapeutics only in patients with selected subtypes of STS. Nevertheless, we are still facing the limited efficacy of classical ICI in most STS trials, and those disappointing results are largely related to non-optimal patient selection. Furthermore, other strategies consist of combining ICI with other classical treatments.

2.2. Combination with Tyrosine Kinase Inhibitors

Several clinical trials have assessed the association of ICI with TKI, in particular targeting the VEGF pathway. In a phase II study combining the pan-VEGFR inhibitor axitinib with pembrolizumab, some remarkable responses or ORR were observed in 7 of 12 patients with ASPS (58%), but only two responses out of 21 (10%) among other STS patients (1 with epithelioid sarcoma and 1 with leiomyosarcoma) were observed [22]. Importantly, all patients with ASPS who had biopsy samples in this study expressed PD-L1 and most had high tumor lymphocyte infiltration scores, consistent with the so-called "inflamed phenotype" observed in melanoma and other cancers that respond to ICI. The median PFS was 12.4 months (95% CI 2.7–22.3) in ASPS patients, and the combination showed acceptable toxic effects, consistent with previous clinical trials of the drugs used as monotherapies. Another phase II study assessing the combination of sunitinib with nivolumab included 58 evaluable patients with STS. The objective response rate was 21%, mainly including patients with ASPS and angiosarcomas but also clear cell sarcomas, extraskeletal myxoid chondrosarcomas and synovial sarcomas. The PFS at 6 months was 48% and the 18-month overall survival proportion was 100% for those with an objective response [31]. Many additional studies are underway. Nevertheless, with the response rate remaining low in an unselected population, it remains crucial to identify biomarkers to help in therapeutic decisions. Furthermore, a trial comparing ICI alone versus ICI plus antiangiogenic therapy would be of interest.

2.3. Combination with Chemotherapy

Chemotherapy has been proposed to overcome resistance to immunotherapy in sarcomas, aiming at rewiring the immune-cold/immunosuppressive microenvironment. Clinical trials have tested agents that promote T-cells while downregulating Treg lymphocytes, immunosuppressive tumor-associated macrophages or immunosuppressive cytokines, thanks to a direct immune effect or immunogenic cancer cell death. As seen before, the PEMBROSARC study [13] aimed to evaluate the combination of metronomic cyclophosphamide, which has demonstrated the ability to suppress Treg lymphocytes and promote the development of T and NK lymphocytes, with pembrolizumab. Another strategy is based on the ability of anthracyclines to generate pro-inflammatory cytokines and damage-associated molecular patterns (DAMPs), activate the production of pro-inflammatory factor IFN1, deplete immunosuppressive cells and boost antigen presentation [32]. Based on this hypothesis, two phase II studies evaluated the combination of doxorubicin with pembrolizumab, in advanced or metastatic sarcomas. The OR rate was 19% in the first study, which included STS and osteosarcomas [33], and 36.7% in the second study, which included only STS [34]. The median PFS was 8.1 months (95% CI, 7.6–10.8) and 5.7 months (95% CI, 4.1–8.9), respectively, to put into perspective the 6.8-month median PFS with doxorubicin alone in a recent study [6]. Importantly, the heterogeneity between those two studies might be explained by the disparity between the two populations (in terms of histological subtypes). Moreover, some of the patients included could have been pre-treated with chemotherapy. In other cancers, immunotherapy alone or in combination with another therapy seems to be more efficient in the early course of the disease possibly due to increasing immune exhaustion over time and treatments. A typical example is small cell lung cancer [35], gastric [36] or triple-negative breast cancer [37], where first-line setting chemo-immunotherapy reached OS improvement whereas it failed in further lines of treatment. The relevance of bringing a chemo-immunotherapy combination to an earlier setting like the first-line treatment of the disease could be questioned. The rationale for the use of cytotoxic chemotherapy in combination with immunotherapy remains substantial and still need to be explored. Some innovative research approaches are ongoing, for example the use of different chemotherapies associated with a single or double blockade doxorubicin + ifosfamide (NCT04356872, NCT04606108), gemcitabine (NCT04577014, NCT03123276, NCT04535713), trabectedin (NCT03138161), eribulin (NCT03899805), etc.

2.4. Combination with Radiation Therapy

Radiation therapy is known to synergize with immunotherapy by inducing immune cell death. Indeed, it increases the level of calreticulin, ATP and HMGB1. By inducing these DAMPs, radiation may transform low-immunogenicity STS into so-called "hot" tumors, allowing better ICI efficacy. It is also believed to increase the presentation and diversity of tumor-specific antigens. Radiation-triggered immunogenic cell death releases tumor antigens, tumor cell DNA, cytokines and other danger signals [38]. For example, DNA double-strand breaks activate the pro-inflammatory cGAS–STING pathway [39]. Moreover, genetic damage caused by radiation increases the mutation load and leads to the generation and release of neoantigens, promoting the formation of antigen-presenting cells and thus activating T lymphocytes. The immunological microenvironment altered by irradiation also promotes tumor cell destruction. Changes in the endothelium of tumor blood vessels allow the enhanced migration of the immune cells to the tumor [40,41]. Based on the results of the SARC028 trial reporting encouraging results in UPS and DD-LPS, the SU2C–SARC032 trial aimed to evaluate perioperative pembrolizumab in 105 patients, with these two specific histological subtypes, who had had neoadjuvant radiotherapy [42]. To achieve the best synergies between ICI and radiotherapy, the sequence, dose and fractionation need to be optimized. Preclinical studies have shown that a high-dose per fraction is correlated with a better tumor immune response [43]. In addition to fractionation, one of the most crucial matters is the optimal timing of irradiation. Although there is a debate about sequential or concomitant ICI and radiotherapy, recent clinical data from a PACIFIC trial on non-small cell lung cancer showed survival benefits in the subgroup of patients receiving durvalumab within 14 days after irradiation. This could have been due to the recruitment of newly activated T cells that could destroy both tumors and distant metastases [44]. Although biological springs of the synergy between radiotherapy and immunotherapy still need to be explored, there is a strong rationale for adding ICI to irradiation in sarcoma settings.

Despite the diverse combinations, ICIs are still struggling to find their place in the therapeutic arsenal for the treatment of sarcomas, with variable ORR and PFS depending on the studies (Table 1), which reinforces the need to find effective biomarkers.

Table 1. Responses to checkpoint inhibitors and combinations in sarcomas.

Trial	Target	ICI	Combination Drug	ORR		Median PFS (Months) [95% CI]
PEMBROSARC Toulmonde et al. [12]	57 STS [1]	Pembrolizumab	Cyclophosphamide	2%		1.4 [1.2–1.4]
SARC028 Tawbi et al. [13]	40 BS [2] /40 STS [1]	Pembrolizumab	None	BS [2] STS [1]	5% 18%	2 [1.8–2.3] 4.5 [2–5.3]
SARC028 (expansion cohorts)	39 DDLPS [3] and 40 UPS [4]	Pembrolizumab	None	DDLPS [3] UPS [4]	10% 23%	2 [2–4] 3 [2–5]
Alliance A091401 D'Angelo et al. [14]	43 and 42 all sarcoma	Nivolumab +/− ipilimumab	None	Nivo Nivo + ipi	5% 16%	1.7 [1.4–4.3] 4.1 [2.6–4.7]
DART Wagner et al. [27]	16 AS [5]	Nivolumab + ipilimumab	None	25%		NA
Wilky et al. [21]	33 STS [1]	Pembrolizumab	Axitinib	25%		4.7 [3.0–9.4]
Martin-Broto et al. [29]	58 STS [1]	Nivolumab	Sunitinib	21%		5.6 [3.0–8.1]
Pollack et al. [31]	37 all sarcoma	Pembrolizumab	Doxorubicin	19%		8.1 [7.6–10.8]
Livingston et al. [32]	30 STS [1]	Pembrolizumab	Doxorubicin	36.7%		5.7 [4.1–8.9]
Somaiah et al.	57 all sarcoma	Durvalumab + tremelimumab	None	14.3%		4.5 [2.8–6.9]

[1] STS: soft tissue sarcoma; [2] BS: bone sarcoma; [3] DDLPS: dedifferenciated liposarcoma; [4] UPS: undifferentiated pleomorphic sarcoma; [5] AS: angiosarcoma.

3. Immune Checkpoint Inhibitors in STS: Challenge of Patient Selection and Stratification

As seen in the previous studies, the greatest challenge remains the improved selection of the patients most likely to benefit from immune therapy. Different hypotheses can be put forward, based on patients' tumor and/or pharmacological characteristics. Nevertheless, it is crucial to define objective biomarkers, which would allow the selection of the best candidates, as seen in other types of cancers with PDL1 and CPS scores, for example. To date, the investigations are still ongoing, as the biomarkers used to predict responses to ICI in other types of cancers do not seem to be as predictive in sarcomas.

3.1. PD1/PD-L1 Expression

PD1/PD-L1 is an efficient biomarker motivating ICI prescription in several cancers, based on results such as PDL1 staining, combined positive score (CPS) or tumor proportion score (TPS) [45]. In the case of STS, some studies suggest that elevated PD1/PD-L1 expression is associated with worse OS, while others suggest it is associated with favorable OS [46,47]. These controversial data might be explained by various confounding factors, such as the use of different antibody clones, different thresholds, the limitations of assays, and the disparity between the histological subtypes included, on top of sampling bias.

3.2. Tumor-Infiltrating Lymphocytes (TILs)

A biomarker more recently investigated in immunotherapy is the presence of TILs, which are white blood cells involved in innate and adaptive immunity, located in the tumor or in its stroma. As for PD-L1, the results of investigations remain conflicting, considering it either a positive or negative prognostic factor [48]. The genuine composition and role of these structures remain underexplored and can be different based on the tumor or the patient, either activating or suppressing immunosurveillance. Depending on the techniques used, some of the stromal TILs might be under-evaluated. It has been shown that patients with a greater population of CD8+- or PDL1-positive macrophages are better responders to pembrolizumab, compared to patients with a bigger proportion of immune regulation cells at the baseline. This was confirmed in sarcomas in a correlative analysis of SARC028, which established a correlation between the response to pembrolizumab and high densities of activated T cells (CD8+ CD3+ PD-1+) and an increased percentage of tumor-associated macrophages (TAM) expressing PD-L1 pre-treatment compared with non-responders [49].

3.3. Tumor Mutational Burden (TMB)/MicroSatellite Instability (MSI)

Tumor mutational burden (TMB) and microsatellite instability (MSI) are useful biomarkers in other cancer types, as the more mutated the tumor is, the more efficient the immunotherapy is expected to be. Unfortunately, sarcomas have a rather low TMB, with an average of 1.06 mutations/Mb, as reported in TCGA analysis [50]. Nevertheless, this TMB was heterogeneous with some tumors exhibiting a TMB of ≥ 10 mut/Mb, especially angiosarcomas (7.6%) and UPS (6.7%) [51]. Therefore, some particular histological subtypes may benefit from immunotherapy through a high TMB, such as STS caused by UV-associated mutations: face and scalp angiosarcomas and subcutaneous malignant peripheral nerve sheath tumors (MPSNT) [52]. The Angiosarcoma Project (ASCproject) is a research study that recently reported the results from a cohort of 47 angiosarcomas: 10 cases of the scalp and face had a median TMB of 20.7 mutations per megabase (Mb), and 37 cases of other localizations had a median TMB of 2.8 mutations per Mb [53]. Among the 10 angiosarcomas of the scalp and face, two had received ICI and showed remarkable and durable responses, while the three treated with anti-PD1 from the rest of the cohort did not benefit from it. These results are encouraging despite the very limited sample size. In other types of cancers, the identification of a MSI-high signature status directly allowed the use of pembrolizumab, implying the strength of this predictive factor. The small proportion of MSI in sarcomas (4/1893 sarcomas in the MSK cohort including 1 UPS, 2 uterine leiomyosarcomas and 1 leiomyosarcoma) seems too low to consider the use of this biomarker in routine practices [51].

3.4. Tertiary Lymphoid Structure (TLS)

More recent research has consisted of finding immune cell signatures by studying transcriptomic data, allowing us to identify immune cell signature clusters (low, moderated or high), named sarcoma immune classes (SIC). Petitprez and al. have recently demonstrated the correlation of immune cell signatures with responses to anti-PD1 therapy. Hence, patients in SIC-E class, which gathers a high immune activity signature sarcomas are more likely to have an objective response and a better PFS [54]. Some further analyses have demonstrated that class E was characterized by the presence of tertiary lymphoid structures (TLS) that contained T cells and more specifically DC LAMP+ dendritic cells and CD20+ B cells, which are the strongest prognostic factor even in the context of high or low CD8+ T cell and cytotoxic contents. TLS are organized aggregates of immune cells, not found under physiological conditions, but arising in the context of infection, auto immune diseases or, in this case, cancer. Their composition is very similar to that of secondary lymphoid organs, such as lymph nodes (Figure 2). This work discloses the potential of B-cell-rich TLS as a new to with which to select patients. Furthermore, an extended cohort of 48 TLS-positive STS patients out of 240 screened from the PEMBROSARC trial has emerged and resulted in an encouraging outcome. Indeed, among the 35 evaluable patients, the clinical benefit rate (CBR) was 63% (OR = 30%; SD = 33%), in comparison with the 2% OR when analyzing the whole population without prior selection. The median PFS and OS were 4.1 and 14.5 months, respectively [55]. Apart from the promising results of these two studies (Table 2), the CONGRATS study (NCT04095208), still recruiting, includes STS patients with a sarcoma enriched with TLS, evaluating treatment with nivolumab, anti-PDL1, which is associated with anti-LAG3, and relatlimab. The expression of LAG-3 in tumor immune cells has been observed in various tumors. It involves inhibiting a checkpoint on the surface of T cells by blocking lymphocyte activation gene 3. Preliminary data suggest that the dual blockade of LAG-3 and PD-1 has the potential to improve efficacy without substantially increasing toxicity compared to a PD-1 blockade alone. Another study (SPARTO and NCT05210413) evaluates the combination of spartalizumab (anti-PD1) and low-dose pazopanib in solid tumors including TLS-positive STS. Overall, further studies are needed to validate this biomarker, but it seems like another important step in the path of the optimized selection of patients.

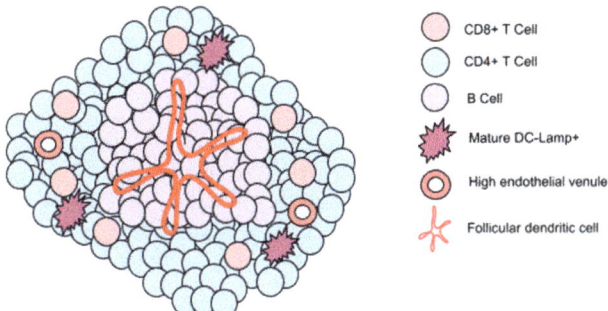

Figure 2. Composition of a tertiary lymphoid structure.

Table 2. Responses to checkpoint inhibitors in SIC-E and TLS$^+$ STS.

Trial	ICI	ORR	
SARC028 [14,54,56]	Pembrolizumab	Overall population (N = 47)	21.2%
		SIC-E Class (N = 10)	50% (with 1 CR)
PEMBROSARC [13,55]	Pembrolizumab	Unselected population (N = 50)	2%
		TLS$^+$ STS (N = 35)	30%

4. Adoptive Cellular Therapies: A New Opening Door in Sarcomas

As discussed before, one of the principles of immune evasion implies a lack of neoantigens or a defect in the antigen presentation and recognition pathway, preventing patients' immune systems from generating an adequate immune response to the invasion of the cancer. T lymphocyte activation requires an interaction between a T cell receptor (TCR) and the major histocompatibility complex (MHC). Thus, it is important to educate the host's immune system by exposing T cells to the tumor antigen for them to develop specific receptors and expand them to develop high-quality and high-avidity antigen-specific T-cell clones. Adoptive cellular therapy is a personalized treatment that involves the isolation of a patient's own immune cells, their ex vivo modification and expansion and their reinfusion, thus bypassing antigen presentation. Promising results have been attained in hematologic malignancies by using T cells transduced with vectors encoding TCRs recognizing HLA I-restricted antigens or with chimeric antigen receptors (CARs) recognizing cell surface proteins [57,58]. This cutting-edge technology requires investigations to find an antigen that is solely, or predominantly, expressed by tumor cells. The increased difficulty when it comes to sarcomas is due to their high heterogeneity, thus implying that there is a vast diversity of the selected antigens both in terms of histological subtypes but also within a single tumor.

4.1. Engineered T Cell Receptor Therapy

To redirect T cells against tumor cells, they can be engineered ex vivo to express cancer-antigen-specific T cell receptors (TCRs), generating products known as TCR-engineered T cells (TCR T). TCRs recognize HLA-presented peptides derived from the proteins of all cellular compartments, and this requires the presence of matched HLA allele subtypes in patients. As seen before, it is crucial to find a reliable neoantigen. Some cancer testis antigens (CTA), such as antigens with MAGE and NY-ESO expression in synovial sarcoma (SS) and myxoid LPS (MLPS), are exceptionally high in quantity and homogenous, ranging from 49% to 82%. While the normal function of the proteins remains elusive, NY-ESO-1 has been shown to interact with MAGE-C1 and may be important in tumor cell proliferation and tumor survival by the inhibition of p53 [59,60]. Afamitresgene autoleucel (afami-cel) and Letetresgene autoleucel (lete-cel) are two experimental therapies based on genetically engineered T cells. They consist of autologous CD4+ and CD8+ T cells that have been genetically modified to express a T-cell receptor (TCR) recognizing MAGE-A4 (afami-cel) or NY-ESO1 (lete-cel) bound to human leukocyte antigen A*02 (HLA-A*02) to induce anti-tumor responses in patients with SS and MLPS expressing those CTA. Afami-cel has been investigated in a phase I and a phase II trial dedicated to SS and MRCL MLPS (SPEARHEAD-1, NCT04044768) that is still recruiting. The preliminary results of the phase II trial was presented at the ASCO meeting in 2021 [61]. Among the 32 patients who received afami-cel at the data cut-off, 25 were evaluable for preliminary efficacy (23 with synovial sarcoma and 2 with MRCLPS). The investigator-assessed responses were for CR (2 patients), PR (8 patients), SD (11 patients) and PD (4 patients). Interestingly, 9 of the 10 responders had ongoing responses at the data cutoff. A pooled analysis from phase I of NCT03132922 and SPEARHEAD-1 gathered the data from 69 MAGE-A4+ patients and displayed 36.2% objective responses [62]. The efficacy and safety of lete-cel have also been previously evaluated in a phase I and a phase II clinical (NCT01343043 and NCT02992743). The preliminary efficacy results of phase I [63–65] reported impressive responses (50% and 40% objective responses for SS and MLPS, respectively, in patients who had received a high-dose lymphodepletion regimen, including 1 complete response). In addition, responses deepened over time and were durable; responses were ongoing in four patients (two with SS and two with MLPS). These preliminary data demonstrate that afami-cel and lete-cel are efficacious in heavily pre-treated patients (Table 3). Importantly, the safety profile has been favorable, with mainly a low-grade cytokine release syndrome ($\leq$Grade 2) and tolerable/reversible hematologic toxicities being directly correlated to lymphodepletive chemotherapy.

Table 3. Responses to TCR T cells in MAGE-A4[+] and NY-ESO [1] SS and MLPS: preliminary results.

Drug	Trial	Target	ORR [7]	Tolerance
Afami-cel	SPEARHEAD-1 NCT04044768	N = 32 28 MAGE-A4[+] SS + 4 MAGE-A4[+] MLPS	40% (2 CR [3], 8 PR [4], 11 SD [5], 4 PD [6])	59% CRS [8] with 95% ≤ Grade 2 and 0% ICANS [9]
Afami-cel	Pooled analyses from phase 1 NCT03132922 and SPEARHEAD-1 (NCT04044768)	N = 69	36.2%	Not applicable
Afami-cel	Pooled analyses from phase 1 NCT03132922 and SPEARHEAD-1 (NCT04044768)	59 MAGE-A4[+] SS [1]	40.7%	Not applicable
Afami-cel	Pooled analyses from phase 1 NCT03132922 and SPEARHEAD-1 (NCT04044768)	10 MAGE-A4[+] MLPS [2]	10.0%	Not applicable
Lete-cel	NCT0134043	N = 45 NY-ESO1[+] SS [1]	33% (15/45)	44% CRS [8] with 80% ≤ Grade 2
Lete-cel	NCT0134043	Cohort 1: high NY-ESO1 expression with cyclophosphamide + fludarabine lymphodepletion	50% (6/12) (1 CR [3], 5 PR [4], 5 SD [5], 1 PD [6])	44% CRS [8] with 80% ≤ Grade 2
Lete-cel	NCT0134043	Cohort 2: low NY-ESO1 expression with cyclophosphamide + fludarabine lymphodepletion	31% (4/13) (0 CR [3], 4 PR [4], 7 SD [5], 1 PD [6])	44% CRS [8] with 80% ≤ Grade 2
Lete-cel	NCT0134043	Cohort 3: high NY-ESO1 expression with cyclophosphamide only	20% (1/5) (0 CR [3], 1 PR [4], 3 SD [5], 0 PD [6])	44% CRS [8] with 80% ≤ Grade 2
Lete-cel	NCT0134043	Cohort 4: low NY-ESO1 expression with cyclophosphamide only	27% (4/15) (0 CR [3], 4 PR [4], 10 SD [5], 1 PD [6])	44% CRS [8] with 80% ≤ Grade 2
Lete-cel	NCT02992743	N = 20 NY-ESO1[+] MLPS [2]		80% CRS [8], with 75% ≤ Grade 2 and 0% ICANS [9]
Lete-cel	NCT02992743	Cohort 1: reduced-dose lymphodepletion	20% (2/10) (2 PR [4], 8 SD [5], 0 PD [6])	80% CRS [8], with 75% ≤ Grade 2 and 0% ICANS [9]
Lete-cel	NCT02992743	Cohort 2: standard-dose lymphodepletion	40% (4/10) (4 PR [4], 5 SD [5], 1 PD [6])	80% CRS [8], with 75% ≤ Grade 2 and 0% ICANS [9]

[1] SS: synovial sarcoma; [2] MLPS: myxoid liposarcoma; [3] CR: complete response; [4] PR: partial response; [5] SD: stable disease; [6] PD: progressive disease; [7] ORR: overall response rate; [8] CRS: cytokine release syndrome; [9] ICANS: immune effector cell-associated neurotoxicity syndrome.

4.2. CAR T Cell Therapy

Unlike TCRs, CAR T cells can target any cell surface protein, independently of HLA. One of the main obstacles to the use of this treatment is its limiting toxicity, caused via the release of cytokines caused by the stimulation of the immune system (systemic cytokine release syndrome). Thus, its position remains limited in the therapeutic arsenal of solid tumors, due to the difficulty of identifying a target that does not involve too-severe toxicities in the organs expressing this antigen. Some targets have been tested in sarcomas, including HER2, which is a ligand involved in the Ras/Raf/MEK/ERK1/2 pathway [66]. A phase I/II study studying HER2 CAR-T cell therapy included 19 patients with HER2+ sarcomas and found the OS to be 10.3 months, with an excellent safety profile. A preparation of this therapy with lymphodepleting chemotherapy seems to improve the results [67]. A following study included 10 patients with HER2+ sarcomas (including rhabdomyosarcoma and synovial sarcoma). The patient with rhabdomyosarcoma exhibited a complete response for 6 months [68]. Other targets are being investigated (EGFR (NCT03618381), PDGFRα and GD2 (NCT02107963, NCT04539366, NCT03721068, NCT03635632)) as well as another strategy combining this treatment with immune checkpoint inhibitors (NCT04995003) in order to increase its efficacy.

4.3. TIL Therapy

TIL therapy consists of extracting TILs from resected or biopsied human tumors, followed by ex vivo expansion away from the suppressive tumor microenvironment and reinfusion after lymphodepletive chemotherapy. TILs demonstrated the ability to target autologous tumor cells while saving MHC-compatible allogeneic tumor cells or normal autologous cells, in an early experimentation including ten sarcomas [69]. This was confirmed with their use in melanomas, displaying encouraging durable responses, with limited toxicity [70–72]. It has been shown that TILs derived from melanoma specifically target multiple antigens, thus standing out as an interesting treatment in the case of heterogeneous tumors, such as sarcomas [73]. Mullinax et al. confirmed that the feasibility of the treatment on sarcomas is of a degree required for clinical use [74]. A few clinical trials including sarcomas are ongoing, including a phase I (NCT04052334) and phase II (NCT03935893) trial. Sarcomas usually having poor lymphocytic infiltration, and some studies aim to assess the safety of combinations; for example, a study involving the use of LTX-315, an oncolytic peptide intended to increase TILs (NCT03725605) [75].

5. Conclusions

Immunotherapy with ICI has been reported to cause limited clinical activity in clinical trials. However, these trials included unselected populations of advanced STS patients. Nevertheless, a subset of patients showed remarkable and durable responses, after the failure of many traditional systemic treatments. Furthermore, recent research has restored hope in the possibility of sarcomas being treatable by immunotherapy [76]. One of the major challenges is to define the best candidates for these treatments by a better knowledge of each tumor's immune component's microenvironment and by the use of reliable biomarkers and response predictors, in order to optimize personalized medicine plans. The other great challenge is to expand the population that can benefit from them by overcoming immune evasion. Once these two obstacles have been overcome, immunotherapy could become one of the standard treatments for STS.

While the expression of PD-L1 has been reported with variable levels across studies and histotypes, this biomarker has not been found to be associated with the response to immunotherapy. Conversely, the presence of TLS in the primary tumor has been reported to be associated with a higher response rate, longer PFS and survival in both a retrospective study and a prospective study, across histological subtypes. Otherwise, ICI showed high clinical benefit rates in some selected STS histotypes; in particular, ASPS. Given the rarity of each sarcoma subtype, their heterogeneity and the small study sizes, other methodological approaches such as meta-analysis could be relevant. Finally, one of the most exciting approaches in sarcoma immunotherapy is the use of adoptive T cell therapies. By using overexpressed CTA MAGE-A4 and NY-ESO1, genetically modified T cells have been successfully developed to specifically target malignant cells in SS and MRCLS.

Other therapies aim to directly boost immunity by activating pro-inflammatory pathways. One of these involves an agonist of the IL2 pathway, NKTR-214, being combined with nivolumab to treat bone and STS (NCT03282344). Although significant and lasting responses were observed, the lack of a comparative arm is an important bias. Another phase II study is evaluating the addition of IFNy to pembrolizumab. Indeed, preliminary studies have shown that IFNy can activate the expression of MHC class I and therefore the infiltration of T lymphocytes [77]. These approaches seem promising in the activation of the primary immune response and the thwarting of the resistance mechanisms linked to the defect of innate immunity.

In conclusion, even if immunotherapy is not yet applied in the routine treatment of STS (excluding the recent FDA approval of atezolizumab for ASPS), there are promising perspectives based on the better selection of patients (in terms of histotypes and the presence of TLS), innovative therapeutic agents (especially adoptive T-cell therapies) and the combination of immunotherapeutic agents with other therapies.

Author Contributions: Conceptualization: M.F., A.D., H.V. and M.B.; writing—original draft preparation: M.F., A.D., H.V. and M.B.; writing—review and editing: M.F., A.D., H.V., W.W., J.-Y.B. and M.B.; supervision, M.B. All authors have read and agreed to the published version of the manuscript.

Funding: This research received no external funding.

Data Availability Statement: Not applicable.

Acknowledgments: We would like to thank the members of the multidisciplinary sarcoma tumor board of The Centre Léon Bérard for their assistance with the study.

Conflicts of Interest: The authors declare no conflict of interest.

References

1. Cormier, J.N.; Pollock, R.E. Soft Tissue Sarcomas. *CA Cancer J. Clin.* **2004**, *54*, 94–109. [CrossRef]
2. Siegel, R.L.; Miller, K.D.; Jemal, A. Cancer Statistics, 2018. *CA Cancer J. Clin.* **2018**, *68*, 7–30. [CrossRef] [PubMed]
3. de Pinieux, G.; Karanian, M.; Le Loarer, F.; Le Guellec, S.; Chabaud, S.; Terrier, P.; Bouvier, C.; Batistella, M.; Neuville, A.; Robin, Y.-M.; et al. Nationwide Incidence of Sarcomas and Connective Tissue Tumors of Intermediate Malignancy over Four Years Using an Expert Pathology Review Network. *PLoS ONE* **2021**, *16*, e0246958. [CrossRef] [PubMed]
4. WHO Classification of Tumours Editorial Board. *Soft Tissue and Bone Tumours*; WHO: Geneva, Switzerland, 2020; ISBN 978-92-832-4502-5.
5. Gronchi, A.; Miah, A.B.; Dei Tos, A.P.; Abecassis, N.; Bajpai, J.; Bauer, S.; Biagini, R.; Bielack, S.; Blay, J.Y.; Bolle, S.; et al. Soft Tissue and Visceral Sarcomas: ESMO-EURACAN-GENTURIS Clinical Practice Guidelines for Diagnosis, Treatment and Follow-Up☆. *Ann. Oncol. Off. J. Eur. Soc. Med. Oncol.* **2021**, *32*, 1348–1365. [CrossRef]
6. Tap, W.D.; Wagner, A.J.; Schöffski, P.; Martin-Broto, J.; Krarup-Hansen, A.; Ganjoo, K.N.; Yen, C.-C.; Abdul Razak, A.R.; Spira, A.; Kawai, A.; et al. Effect of Doxorubicin Plus Olaratumab vs Doxorubicin Plus Placebo on Survival in Patients with Advanced Soft Tissue Sarcomas: The ANNOUNCE Randomized Clinical Trial. *JAMA* **2020**, *323*, 1266–1276. [CrossRef]
7. van der Graaf, W.T.A.; Blay, J.-Y.; Chawla, S.P.; Kim, D.-W.; Bui-Nguyen, B.; Casali, P.G.; Schöffski, P.; Aglietta, M.; Staddon, A.P.; Beppu, Y.; et al. Pazopanib for Metastatic Soft-Tissue Sarcoma (PALETTE): A Randomised, Double-Blind, Placebo-Controlled Phase 3 Trial. *Lancet Lond. Engl.* **2012**, *379*, 1879–1886. [CrossRef]
8. Judson, I.; Verweij, J.; Gelderblom, H.; Hartmann, J.T.; Schöffski, P.; Blay, J.-Y.; Kerst, J.M.; Sufliarsky, J.; Whelan, J.; Hohenberger, P.; et al. Doxorubicin Alone versus Intensified Doxorubicin plus Ifosfamide for First-Line Treatment of Advanced or Metastatic Soft-Tissue Sarcoma: A Randomised Controlled Phase 3 Trial. *Lancet Oncol.* **2014**, *15*, 415–423. [CrossRef]
9. Couzin-Frankel, J. Breakthrough of the Year 2013. Cancer Immunotherapy. *Science* **2013**, *342*, 1432–1433. [CrossRef] [PubMed]
10. McCarthy, E.F. The Toxins of William B. Coley and the Treatment of Bone and Soft-Tissue Sarcomas. *Iowa Orthop. J.* **2006**, *26*, 154–158.
11. Pardoll, D.M. The Blockade of Immune Checkpoints in Cancer Immunotherapy. *Nat. Rev. Cancer* **2012**, *12*, 252–264. [CrossRef]
12. A Pilot Study of Anti-CTLA4 Antibody Ipilimumab in Patients with Synovial Sarcoma-PubMed. Available online: https://pubmed.ncbi.nlm.nih.gov/23554566/ (accessed on 1 March 2023).
13. Toulmonde, M.; Penel, N.; Adam, J.; Chevreau, C.; Blay, J.-Y.; Le Cesne, A.; Bompas, E.; Piperno-Neumann, S.; Cousin, S.; Grellety, T.; et al. Use of PD-1 Targeting, Macrophage Infiltration, and IDO Pathway Activation in Sarcomas: A Phase 2 Clinical Trial. *JAMA Oncol.* **2018**, *4*, 93–97. [CrossRef] [PubMed]
14. Tawbi, H.A.; Burgess, M.; Bolejack, V.; Van Tine, B.A.; Schuetze, S.M.; Hu, J.; D'Angelo, S.; Attia, S.; Riedel, R.F.; Priebat, D.A.; et al. Pembrolizumab in Advanced Soft-Tissue Sarcoma and Bone Sarcoma (SARC028): A Multicentre, Two-Cohort, Single-Arm, Open-Label, Phase 2 Trial. *Lancet Oncol.* **2017**, *18*, 1493–1501. [CrossRef] [PubMed]
15. D'Angelo, S.P.; Mahoney, M.R.; Van Tine, B.A.; Atkins, J.; Milhem, M.M.; Jahagirdar, B.N.; Antonescu, C.R.; Horvath, E.; Tap, W.D.; Schwartz, G.K.; et al. Nivolumab with or without Ipilimumab Treatment for Metastatic Sarcoma (Alliance A091401): Two Open-Label, Non-Comparative, Randomised, Phase 2 Trials. *Lancet Oncol.* **2018**, *19*, 416–426. [CrossRef] [PubMed]
16. Chen, J.L.; Mahoney, M.R.; George, S.; Antonescu, C.R.; Liebner, D.A.; Van Tine, B.A.; Milhem, M.M.; Tap, W.D.; Streicher, H.; Schwartz, G.K.; et al. A Multicenter Phase II Study of Nivolumab +/- Ipilimumab for Patients with Metastatic Sarcoma (Alliance A091401): Results of Expansion Cohorts. *J. Clin. Oncol.* **2020**, *38*, 11511. [CrossRef]
17. Stacchiotti, S.; Frezza, A.M.; Blay, J.-Y.; Baldini, E.H.; Bonvalot, S.; Bovée, J.V.M.G.; Callegaro, D.; Casali, P.G.; Chiang, R.C.-J.; Demetri, G.D.; et al. Ultra-Rare Sarcomas: A Consensus Paper from the Connective Tissue Oncology Society Community of Experts on the Incidence Threshold and the List of Entities. *Cancer* **2021**, *127*, 2934–2942. [CrossRef]
18. Brahmi, M.; Vanacker, H.; Dufresne, A. Novel Therapeutic Options for Alveolar Soft Part Sarcoma: Antiangiogenic Therapy, Immunotherapy and Beyond. *Curr. Opin. Oncol.* **2020**, *32*, 295–300. [CrossRef]

19. Lazar, A.J.F.; Das, P.; Tuvin, D.; Korchin, B.; Zhu, Q.; Jin, Z.; Warneke, C.L.; Zhang, P.S.; Hernandez, V.; Lopez-Terrada, D.; et al. Angiogenesis-Promoting Gene Patterns in Alveolar Soft Part Sarcoma. *Clin. Cancer Res. Off. J. Am. Assoc. Cancer Res.* **2007**, *13*, 7314–7321. [CrossRef]
20. Huan, C.; Kelly, M.L.; Steele, R.; Shapira, I.; Gottesman, S.R.S.; Roman, C.A.J. Transcription Factors TFE3 and TFEB Are Critical for CD40 Ligand Expression and Thymus-Dependent Humoral Immunity. *Nat. Immunol.* **2006**, *7*, 1082–1091. [CrossRef]
21. Naqash, A.R.; O'Sullivan Coyne, G.H.; Moore, N.; Sharon, E.; Takebe, N.; Fino, K.K.; Ferry Galow, K.V.; Hu, J.S.; Van Tine, D.A.; Burgess, M.A.; et al. Phase II Study of Atezolizumab in Advanced Alveolar Soft Part Sarcoma (ASPS). *J. Clin. Oncol.* **2021**, *39*, 11519. [CrossRef]
22. Wilky, B.A.; Trucco, M.M.; Subhawong, T.K.; Florou, V.; Park, W.; Kwon, D.; Wieder, E.D.; Kolonias, D.; Rosenberg, A.E.; Kerr, D.A.; et al. Axitinib plus Pembrolizumab in Patients with Advanced Sarcomas Including Alveolar Soft-Part Sarcoma: A Single-Centre, Single-Arm, Phase 2 Trial. *Lancet Oncol.* **2019**, *20*, 837–848. [CrossRef]
23. Shi, Y.; Cai, Q.; Jiang, Y.; Huang, G.; Bi, M.; Wang, B.; Zhou, Y.; Wang, G.; Ying, H.; Tao, Z.; et al. Activity and Safety of Geptanolimab (GB226) for Patients with Unresectable, Recurrent, or Metastatic Alveolar Soft Part Sarcoma: A Phase II, Single-Arm Study. *Clin. Cancer Res. Off. J. Am. Assoc. Cancer Res.* **2020**, *26*, 6445–6452. [CrossRef] [PubMed]
24. Florou, V.; Rosenberg, A.E.; Wieder, E.; Komanduri, K.V.; Kolonias, D.; Uduman, M.; Castle, J.C.; Buell, J.S.; Trent, J.C.; Wilky, B.A. Angiosarcoma Patients Treated with Immune Checkpoint Inhibitors: A Case Series of Seven Patients from a Single Institution. *J. Immunother. Cancer* **2019**, *7*, 213. [CrossRef] [PubMed]
25. Sindhu, S.; Gimber, L.H.; Cranmer, L.; McBride, A.; Kraft, A.S. Angiosarcoma Treated Successfully with Anti-PD-1 Therapy-a Case Report. *J. Immunother. Cancer* **2017**, *5*, 58. [CrossRef]
26. Xu, W.; Wang, K.; Gu, W.; Nie, X.; Zhang, H.; Tang, C.; Lin, L.; Liang, J. Case Report: Complete Remission with Anti−PD−1 and Anti−VEGF Combined Therapy of a Patient with Metastatic Primary Splenic Angiosarcoma. *Front. Oncol.* **2022**, *12*, 809068. [CrossRef] [PubMed]
27. Singh, G.; Haimes, B.; Klug, D. Immunotherapy and Chemotherapy for Cutaneous Angiosarcoma: A Systematic Review. *Int. J. Womens Dermatol.* **2019**, *5*, 201. [CrossRef]
28. Tomassen, T.; Weidema, M.E.; Hillebrandt-Roeffen, M.H.S.; van der Horst, C.; Desar, I.M.E.; Flucke, U.E.; Versleijen-Jonkers, Y.M.H.; PALGA group*. Analysis of PD-1, PD-L1, and T-Cell Infiltration in Angiosarcoma Pathogenetic Subgroups. *Immunol. Res.* **2022**, *70*, 256–268. [CrossRef] [PubMed]
29. Wagner, M.J.; Othus, M.; Patel, S.P.; Ryan, C.; Sangal, A.; Powers, B.; Budd, G.T.; Victor, A.I.; Hsueh, C.-T.; Chugh, R.; et al. Multicenter Phase II Trial (SWOG S1609, Cohort 51) of Ipilimumab and Nivolumab in Metastatic or Unresectable Angiosarcoma: A Substudy of Dual Anti-CTLA-4 and Anti-PD-1 Blockade in Rare Tumors (DART). *J. Immunother. Cancer* **2021**, *9*, e002990. [CrossRef] [PubMed]
30. Blay, J.-Y.; Penel, N.; Ray-Coquard, I.L.; Schott, R.; Saada-Bouzid, E.; Bertucci, F.; Chevreau, C.M.; Bompas, E.; Coquan, E.; Cousin, S.; et al. High Clinical Benefit Rates of Pembrolizumab in Very Rare Sarcoma Histotypes: First Results of the AcSé Pembrolizumab Study. *Ann. Oncol.* **2019**, *30*, v517. [CrossRef]
31. Martin-Broto, J.; Hindi, N.; Grignani, G.; Martinez-Trufero, J.; Redondo, A.; Valverde, C.; Stacchiotti, S.; Lopez-Pousa, A.; D'Ambrosio, L.; Gutierrez, A.; et al. Nivolumab and Sunitinib Combination in Advanced Soft Tissue Sarcomas: A Multicenter, Single-Arm, Phase Ib/II Trial. *J. Immunother. Cancer* **2020**, *8*, e001561. [CrossRef]
32. Galluzzi, L.; Humeau, J.; Buqué, A.; Zitvogel, L.; Kroemer, G. Immunostimulation with Chemotherapy in the Era of Immune Checkpoint Inhibitors. *Nat. Rev. Clin. Oncol.* **2020**, *17*, 725–741. [CrossRef]
33. Pollack, S.M.; Redman, M.W.; Baker, K.K.; Wagner, M.J.; Schroeder, B.A.; Loggers, E.T.; Trieselmann, K.; Copeland, V.C.; Zhang, S.; Black, G.; et al. Assessment of Doxorubicin and Pembrolizumab in Patients With Advanced Anthracycline-Naive Sarcoma: A Phase 1/2 Nonrandomized Clinical Trial. *JAMA Oncol.* **2020**, *6*, 1778–1782. [CrossRef]
34. Livingston, M.B.; Jagosky, M.H.; Robinson, M.M.; Ahrens, W.A.; Benbow, J.H.; Farhangfar, C.J.; Foureau, D.M.; Maxwell, D.M.; Baldrige, E.A.; Begic, X.; et al. Phase II Study of Pembrolizumab in Combination with Doxorubicin in Metastatic and Unresectable Soft-Tissue Sarcoma. *Clin. Cancer Res. Off. J. Am. Assoc. Cancer Res.* **2021**, *27*, 6424–6431. [CrossRef] [PubMed]
35. Goldman, J.W.; Dvorkin, M.; Chen, Y.; Reinmuth, N.; Hotta, K.; Trukhin, D.; Statsenko, G.; Hochmair, M.J.; Özgüroğlu, M.; Ji, J.H.; et al. Durvalumab, with or without Tremelimumab, plus Platinum-Etoposide versus Platinum-Etoposide Alone in First-Line Treatment of Extensive-Stage Small-Cell Lung Cancer (CASPIAN): Updated Results from a Randomised, Controlled, Open-Label, Phase 3 Trial. *Lancet Oncol.* **2021**, *22*, 51–65. [CrossRef] [PubMed]
36. Högner, A.; Moehler, M. Immunotherapy in Gastric Cancer. *Curr. Oncol.* **2022**, *29*, 1559–1574. [CrossRef] [PubMed]
37. Cortes, J.; Rugo, H.S.; Cescon, D.W.; Im, S.-A.; Yusof, M.M.; Gallardo, C.; Lipatov, O.; Barrios, C.H.; Perez-Garcia, J.; Iwata, H.; et al. Pembrolizumab plus Chemotherapy in Advanced Triple-Negative Breast Cancer. *N. Engl. J. Med.* **2022**, *387*, 217–226. [CrossRef]
38. Zhu, M.; Yang, M.; Zhang, J.; Yin, Y.; Fan, X.; Zhang, Y.; Qin, S.; Zhang, H.; Yu, F. Immunogenic Cell Death Induction by Ionizing Radiation. *Front. Immunol.* **2021**, *12*, 705361. [CrossRef]
39. STING-Dependent Cytosolic DNA Sensing Promotes Radiation-Induced Type I Interferon-Dependent Antitumor Immunity in Immunogenic Tumors-PubMed. Available online: https://pubmed.ncbi.nlm.nih.gov/25517616/ (accessed on 1 March 2023).
40. Hallahan, D.; Kuchibhotla, J.; Wyble, C. Cell Adhesion Molecules Mediate Radiation-Induced Leukocyte Adhesion to the Vascular Endothelium. *Cancer Res.* **1996**, *56*, 5150–5155.

41. Formenti, S.C.; Demaria, S. Combining Radiotherapy and Cancer Immunotherapy: A Paradigm Shift. *J. Natl. Cancer Inst.* **2013**, *105*, 256–265. [CrossRef]
42. Saif, A.; Verbus, E.A.; Sarvestani, A.L.; Teke, M.E.; Lambdin, J.; Hernandez, J.M.; Kirsch, D.G. A Randomized Trial of Pembrolizumab & Radiotherapy Versus Radiotherapy in High-Risk Soft Tissue Sarcoma of the Extremity (SU2C-SARC032). *Ann. Surg. Oncol.* **2023**, *30*, 683–685. [CrossRef]
43. Lugade, A.A.; Moran, J.P.; Gerber, S.A.; Rose, R.C.; Frelinger, J.G.; Lord, E.M. Local Radiation Therapy of B16 Melanoma Tumors Increases the Generation of Tumor Antigen-Specific Effector Cells That Traffic to the Tumor. *J. Immunol. Baltim. Md. 1950* **2005**, *174*, 7516–7523. [CrossRef]
44. Faivre-Finn, C.; Vicente, D.; Kurata, T.; Planchard, D.; Paz-Ares, L.; Vansteenkiste, J.F.; Spigel, D.R.; Garassino, M.C.; Reck, M.; Senan, S.; et al. Four-Year Survival with Durvalumab After Chemoradiotherapy in Stage III NSCLC-an Update from the PACIFIC Trial. *J. Thorac. Oncol. Off. Publ. Int. Assoc. Study Lung Cancer* **2021**, *16*, 860–867. [CrossRef] [PubMed]
45. Sajjadi, E.; Venetis, K.; Scatena, C.; Fusco, N. Biomarkers for Precision Immunotherapy in the Metastatic Setting: Hope or Reality? *Ecancermedicalscience* **2020**, *14*, 1150. [CrossRef]
46. Zheng, C.; You, W.; Wan, P.; Jiang, X.; Chen, J.; Zheng, Y.; Li, W.; Tan, J.; Zhang, S. Clinicopathological and Prognostic Significance of PD-L1 Expression in Sarcoma: A Systematic Review and Meta-Analysis. *Medicine* **2018**, *97*, e11004. [CrossRef]
47. Italiano, A.; Bellera, C.; D'Angelo, S. PD1/PD-L1 Targeting in Advanced Soft-Tissue Sarcomas: A Pooled Analysis of Phase II Trials. *J. Hematol. Oncol.* **2020**, *13*, 55. [CrossRef]
48. Zhu, M.M.T.; Shenasa, E.; Nielsen, T.O. Sarcomas: Immune Biomarker Expression and Checkpoint Inhibitor Trials. *Cancer Treat. Rev.* **2020**, *91*, 102115. [CrossRef] [PubMed]
49. Keung, E.Z.; Burgess, M.; Salazar, R.; Parra, E.R.; Rodrigues-Canales, J.; Bolejack, V.; Van Tine, B.A.; Schuetze, S.M.; Attia, S.; Riedel, R.F.; et al. Correlative Analyses of the SARC028 Trial Reveal an Association between Sarcoma-Associated Immune Infiltrate and Response to Pembrolizumab. *Clin. Cancer Res. Off. J. Am. Assoc. Cancer Res.* **2020**, *26*, 1258–1266. [CrossRef] [PubMed]
50. Cancer Genome Atlas Research Network. Electronic address: Elizabeth.demicco@sinaihealthsystem.ca; Cancer Genome Atlas Research Network Comprehensive and Integrated Genomic Characterization of Adult Soft Tissue Sarcomas. *Cell* **2017**, *171*, 950–965.e28. [CrossRef] [PubMed]
51. Clinical Sequencing of Soft Tissue and Bone Sarcomas Delineates Diverse Genomic Landscapes and Potential Therapeutic Targets | Nature Communications. Available online: https://www.nature.com/articles/s41467-022-30453-x (accessed on 1 March 2023).
52. Campbell, B.B.; Light, N.; Fabrizio, D.; Zatzman, M.; Fuligni, F.; de Borja, R.; Davidson, S.; Edwards, M.; Elvin, J.A.; Hodel, K.P.; et al. Comprehensive Analysis of Hypermutation in Human Cancer. *Cell* **2017**, *171*, 1042–1056.e10. [CrossRef]
53. Painter, C.A.; Jain, E.; Tomson, B.N.; Dunphy, M.; Stoddard, R.E.; Thomas, B.S.; Damon, A.L.; Shah, S.; Kim, D.; Gómez Tejeda Zañudo, J.; et al. The Angiosarcoma Project: Enabling Genomic and Clinical Discoveries in a Rare Cancer through Patient-Partnered Research. *Nat. Med.* **2020**, *26*, 181–187. [CrossRef] [PubMed]
54. Petitprez, F.; de Reyniès, A.; Keung, E.Z.; Chen, T.W.-W.; Sun, C.-M.; Calderaro, J.; Jeng, Y.-M.; Hsiao, L.-P.; Lacroix, L.; Bougoüin, A.; et al. B Cells Are Associated with Survival and Immunotherapy Response in Sarcoma. *Nature* **2020**, *577*, 556–560. [CrossRef]
55. Italiano, A.; Bessede, A.; Pulido, M.; Bompas, E.; Piperno-Neumann, S.; Chevreau, C.; Penel, N.; Bertucci, F.; Toulmonde, M.; Bellera, C.; et al. Pembrolizumab in Soft-Tissue Sarcomas with Tertiary Lymphoid Structures: A Phase 2 PEMBROSARC Trial Cohort. *Nat. Med.* **2022**, *28*, 1199–1206. [CrossRef] [PubMed]
56. Burgess, M.; Bolejack, V.; Schuetze, S.; Tine, B.; Attia, S.; Riedel, R.; Hu, J.; Davis, L.; Okuno, S.; Priebat, D.; et al. Clinical Activity of Pembrolizumab (P) in Undifferentiated Pleomorphic Sarcoma (UPS) and Dedifferentiated/Pleomorphic Liposarcoma (LPS): Final Results of SARC028 Expansion Cohorts. *J. Clin. Oncol.* **2019**, *37*, 11015. [CrossRef]
57. Zhao, L.; Cao, Y.J. Engineered T Cell Therapy for Cancer in the Clinic. *Front. Immunol.* **2019**, *10*, 2250. [CrossRef] [PubMed]
58. Huang, R.; Li, X.; He, Y.; Zhu, W.; Gao, L.; Liu, Y.; Gao, L.; Wen, Q.; Zhong, J.F.; Zhang, C.; et al. Recent Advances in CAR-T Cell Engineering. *J. Hematol. Oncol.* **2020**, *13*, 86. [CrossRef] [PubMed]
59. Ishihara, M.; Kageyama, S.; Miyahara, Y.; Ishikawa, T.; Ueda, S.; Soga, N.; Naota, H.; Mukai, K.; Harada, N.; Ikeda, H.; et al. MAGE-A4, NY-ESO-1 and SAGE MRNA Expression Rates and Co-Expression Relationships in Solid Tumours. *BMC Cancer* **2020**, *20*, 606. [CrossRef]
60. Kakimoto, T.; Matsumine, A.; Kageyama, S.; Asanuma, K.; Matsubara, T.; Nakamura, T.; Iino, T.; Ikeda, H.; Shiku, H.; Sudo, A. Immunohistochemical Expression and Clinicopathological Assessment of the Cancer Testis Antigens NY-ESO-1 and MAGE-A4 in High-Grade Soft-Tissue Sarcoma. *Oncol. Lett.* **2019**, *17*, 3937–3943. [CrossRef]
61. D'Angelo, S.P.; Van Tine, B.A.; Attia, S.; Blay, J.-Y.; Strauss, S.J.; Valverde Morales, C.M.; Abdul Razak, A.R.; Van Winkle, E.; Trivedi, T.; Biswas, S.; et al. SPEARHEAD-1: A Phase 2 Trial of Afamitresgene Autoleucel (Formerly ADP-A2M4) in Patients with Advanced Synovial Sarcoma or Myxoid/Round Cell Liposarcoma. *J. Clin. Oncol.* **2021**, *39*, 11504. [CrossRef]
62. D'Angelo, S.P.; Attia, S.; Blay, J.-Y.; Strauss, S.J.; Valverde Morales, C.M.; Abdul Razak, A.R.; Van Winkle, E.; Annareddy, T.; Sattigari, C.; Diamantopoulos, E.; et al. Identification of Response Stratification Factors from Pooled Efficacy Analyses of Afamitresgene Autoleucel ("Afami-Cel" [Formerly ADP-A2M4]) in Metastatic Synovial Sarcoma and Myxoid/Round Cell Liposarcoma Phase 1 and Phase 2 Trials. *J. Clin. Oncol.* **2022**, *40*, 11562. [CrossRef]

63. D'Angelo, S.; Demetri, G.; Tine, B.V.; Druta, M.; Glod, J.; Chow, W.; Pandya, N.; Hasan, A.; Chiou, V.; Tress, J.; et al. 298 Final Analysis of the Phase 1 Trial of NY-ESO-1-Specific T-Cell Receptor (TCR) T-Cell Therapy (Letetresgene Autoleucel; GSK3377794) in Patients with Advanced Synovial Sarcoma (SS). *J. Immunother. Cancer* **2020**, *8*, A325. [CrossRef]
64. D'Angelo, S.P.; Druta, M.; Van Tine, B.A.; Liebner, D.A.; Schuetze, S.; Nathenson, M.; Holmes, A.P.; D'Souza, J.; Kapoor, G.S.; Zajic, S.; et al. Primary Efficacy and Safety of Letetresgene Autoleucel (Lete-Cel; GSK3377794) Pilot Study in Patients with Advanced and Metastatic Myxoid/Round Cell Liposarcoma (MRCLS). *J. Clin. Oncol.* **2022**, *40*, 11500. [CrossRef]
65. D'Angelo, S.P.; Noujaim, J.C.; Thistlethwaite, F.; Abdul Razak, A.R.; Stacchiotti, S.; Chow, W.A.; Haanen, J.B.A.G.; Chalmers, A.W.; Robinson, S.I.; Van Tine, B.A.; et al. IGNYTE-ESO: A Master Protocol to Assess Safety and Activity of Letetresgene Autoleucel (Lete-Cel; GSK3377794) in HLA-A*02+ Patients with Synovial Sarcoma or Myxoid/Round Cell Liposarcoma (Substudies 1 and 2). *J. Clin. Oncol.* **2021**, *39*, TPS1158. [CrossRef]
66. Roskoski, R. The ErbB/HER Family of Protein-Tyrosine Kinases and Cancer. *Pharmacol. Res.* **2014**, *79*, 34–74. [CrossRef] [PubMed]
67. Ahmed, N.; Brawley, V.S.; Hegde, M.; Robertson, C.; Ghazi, A.; Gerken, C.; Liu, E.; Dakhova, O.; Ashoori, A.; Corder, A.; et al. Human Epidermal Growth Factor Receptor 2 (HER2) -Specific Chimeric Antigen Receptor-Modified T Cells for the Immunotherapy of HER2-Positive Sarcoma. *J. Clin. Oncol. Off. J. Am. Soc. Clin. Oncol.* **2015**, *33*, 1688–1696. [CrossRef] [PubMed]
68. Navai, S.A.; Derenzo, C.; Joseph, S.; Sanber, K.; Byrd, T.; Zhang, H.; Mata, M.; Gerken, C.; Shree, A.; Mathew, P.R.; et al. Abstract LB-147: Administration of HER2-CAR T Cells after Lymphodepletion Safely Improves T Cell Expansion and Induces Clinical Responses in Patients with Advanced Sarcomas. *Cancer Res.* **2019**, *79*, LB-147. [CrossRef]
69. Topalian, S.L.; Muul, L.M.; Solomon, D.; Rosenberg, S.A. Expansion of Human Tumor Infiltrating Lymphocytes for Use in Immunotherapy Trials. *J. Immunol. Methods* **1987**, *102*, 127–141. [CrossRef] [PubMed]
70. Besser, M.J.; Shapira-Frommer, R.; Itzhaki, O.; Treves, A.J.; Zippel, D.B.; Levy, D.; Kubi, A.; Shoshani, N.; Zikich, D.; Ohayon, Y.; et al. Adoptive Transfer of Tumor-Infiltrating Lymphocytes in Patients with Metastatic Melanoma: Intent-to-Treat Analysis and Efficacy after Failure to Prior Immunotherapies. *Clin. Cancer Res. Off. J. Am. Assoc. Cancer Res.* **2013**, *19*, 4792–4800. [CrossRef]
71. Rosenberg, S.A.; Yannelli, J.R.; Yang, J.C.; Topalian, S.L.; Schwartzentruber, D.J.; Weber, J.S.; Parkinson, D.R.; Seipp, C.A.; Einhorn, J.H.; White, D.E. Treatment of Patients with Metastatic Melanoma with Autologous Tumor-Infiltrating Lymphocytes and Interleukin 2. *J. Natl. Cancer Inst.* **1994**, *86*, 1159–1166. [CrossRef]
72. Yang, J.C. Toxicities Associated with Adoptive T-Cell Transfer for Cancer. *Cancer J. Sudbury Mass* **2015**, *21*, 506–509. [CrossRef]
73. Andersen, R.S.; Thrue, C.A.; Junker, N.; Lyngaa, R.; Donia, M.; Ellebæk, E.; Svane, I.M.; Schumacher, T.N.; Thor Straten, P.; Hadrup, S.R. Dissection of T-Cell Antigen Specificity in Human Melanoma. *Cancer Res.* **2012**, *72*, 1642–1650. [CrossRef] [PubMed]
74. Mullinax, J.E.; Hall, M.; Beatty, M.; Weber, A.M.; Sannasardo, Z.; Svrdlin, T.; Hensel, J.; Bui, M.; Richards, A.; Gonzalez, R.J.; et al. Expanded Tumor-Infiltrating Lymphocytes From Soft Tissue Sarcoma Have Tumor-Specific Function. *J. Immunother. Hagerstown Md. 1997* **2021**, *44*, 63–70. [CrossRef] [PubMed]
75. Nielsen, M.; Monberg, T.; Albieri, B.; Sundvold, V.; Rekdal, O.; Junker, N.; Svane, I.M. LTX-315 and Adoptive Cell Therapy Using Tumor-Infiltrating Lymphocytes in Patients with Metastatic Soft Tissue Sarcoma. *J. Clin. Oncol.* **2022**, *40*, 11567. [CrossRef]
76. Kerrison, W.G.J.; Lee, A.T.J.; Thway, K.; Jones, R.L.; Huang, P.H. Current Status and Future Directions of Immunotherapies in Soft Tissue Sarcomas. *Biomedicines* **2022**, *10*, 573. [CrossRef] [PubMed]
77. Zhang, S.; Kohli, K.; Black, R.G.; Yao, L.; Spadinger, S.M.; He, Q.; Pillarisetty, V.G.; Cranmer, L.D.; Van Tine, B.A.; Yee, C.; et al. Systemic Interferon-γ Increases MHC Class I Expression and T-Cell Infiltration in Cold Tumors: Results of a Phase 0 Clinical Trial. *Cancer Immunol. Res.* **2019**, *7*, 1237–1243. [CrossRef] [PubMed]

Disclaimer/Publisher's Note: The statements, opinions and data contained in all publications are solely those of the individual author(s) and contributor(s) and not of MDPI and/or the editor(s). MDPI and/or the editor(s) disclaim responsibility for any injury to people or property resulting from any ideas, methods, instructions or products referred to in the content.

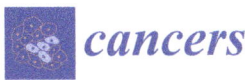

Article

Clinical Outcome of Low-Grade Myofibroblastic Sarcoma in Japan: A Multicenter Study from the Japanese Musculoskeletal Oncology Group

Munehisa Kito [1], Keisuke Ae [2], Masanori Okamoto [1,*], Makoto Endo [3], Kunihiro Ikuta [4], Akihiko Takeuchi [5], Naohiro Yasuda [6,7], Taketoshi Yasuda [8], Yoshinori Imura [9], Takeshi Morii [10], Kazutaka Kikuta [11], Teruya Kawamoto [12], Yutaka Nezu [13], Ichiro Baba [14], Shusa Ohshika [15], Takeshi Uehara [16], Takafumi Ueda [17], Jun Takahashi [1] and Hirotaka Kawano [18]

1. Department of Orthopaedic Surgery, Shinshu University School of Medicine, 3-1-1 Asahi, Matsumoto 390-8621, Japan
2. Department of Orthopaedic Surgery, Cancer Institute Hospital, Japanese Foundation for Cancer Research, 3-8-31 Ariake, Koto-ku, Tokyo 135-8550, Japan
3. Department of Orthopaedic Surgery, Graduate School of Medical Sciences, Kyushu University, 3-1-1 Maidashi, Higashi-ku, Fukuoka 812-8582, Japan
4. Department of Orthopaedic Surgery, Nagoya University Graduate School of Medicine, 65 Tsurumai, Showa-ku, Nagoya 466-8560, Japan
5. Department of Orthopaedic Surgery, Graduate School of Medical Sciences, Kanazawa University, 13-1 Takaramachi, Kanazawa 920-8641, Japan
6. Department of Orthopaedic Surgery, Osaka University Graduate School of Medicine, 2-2 Yamadaoka, Suita 565-0871, Japan
7. Department of Orthopaedic Surgery, National Hospital Organization Osaka National Hospital, 2-1-14 Houenzaka, Chuo-ku, Osaka 540-0006, Japan
8. Department of Orthopaedic Surgery, University of Toyama, 2630 Sugitani, Toyama 930-0194, Japan
9. Department of Orthopaedic Surgery, Osaka International Cancer Institute, 3-1-69 Otemae, Chuo-ku, Osaka 540-0008, Japan
10. Department of Orthopaedic Surgery, Kyorin University Faculty of Medicine, 6-20-2 Shinkawa, Tokyo 181-8621, Japan
11. Department of Musculoskeletal Oncology and Orthopaedic Surgery, Tochigi Cancer Center, 4-9-13 Yonan, Utsunomiya 320-0834, Japan
12. Department of Orthopaedic Surgery, Kobe University Graduate School of Medicine, 7-5-1 Kusunoki-cho, Chuo-ku, Kobe 650-0017, Japan
13. Department of Musculoskeletal Oncology and Rehabilitation, National Cancer Center Hospital, 5-1-1 Tsukigi, Chuo-ku, Tokyo 104-0045, Japan
14. Department of Orthopaedic Surgery, Osaka Medical and Pharmaceutical University, 2-7 Daigakumachi, Takatsuki 569-8686, Japan
15. Department of Orthopaedic Surgery, Hirosaki University Graduate School of Medicine, 5 Zaifu-cho, Hirosaki 036-8562, Japan
16. Department of Laboratory Medicine, Shinshu University School of Medicine, 3-1-1 Asahi, Matsumoto 390-8621, Japan
17. Department of Orthopaedic Surgery, Kodama Hospital, 1-3-2 Gotenyama, Takarazuka 665-0841, Japan
18. Department of Orthopaedic Surgery, Teikyo University School of Medicine, 2-11-1 Kaga, Itabashi-ku, Tokyo 173-0806, Japan
* Correspondence: ryouyuma@shinshu-u.ac.jp; Tel.: +81-263-37-2659

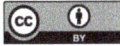

Simple Summary: Low-grade myofibroblastic sarcoma (LGMS) is one of the rarest sarcomas. We aimed to clarify the clinical outcomes of patients with LGMS. Twenty-two patients underwent surgical treatment for the primary tumor and two underwent radical radiotherapy (RT). The best overall response in the two patients who underwent radical RT was one complete response and one partial response. Local relapse-free survival was 91.3% at 2 years and 75.4% at 5 years. Relapsed tumors were treated with surgery in two cases and radical RT in three cases. None of the patients experienced a second local relapse. Disease-specific survival was 100% at 5 years. Wide excision is recommended due to its tendency to local relapse. However, RT was considered a viable option in unresectable cases or in cases where surgery may cause significant functional impairment.

Abstract: This retrospective multicenter study aimed to analyze the clinical features and prognosis of 24 patients diagnosed with LGMS between 2002 and 2019 in the Japanese sarcoma network. Twenty-two cases were surgically treated and two cases were treated with radical radiotherapy (RT). The pathological margin was R0 in 14 cases, R1 in 7 cases, and R2 in 1 case. The best overall response in the two patients who underwent radical RT was one complete response and one partial response. Local relapse occurred in 20.8% of patients. Local relapse-free survival (LRFS) was 91.3% at 2 years and 75.4% at 5 years. In univariate analysis, tumors of 5 cm or more were significantly more likely to cause local relapse ($p < 0.01$). In terms of the treatment of relapsed tumors, surgery was performed in two cases and radical RT was performed in three cases. None of the patients experienced a second local relapse. Disease-specific survival was 100% at 5 years. A wide excision aimed at the microscopically R0 margin is considered the standard treatment for LGMS. However, RT may be a viable option in unresectable cases or in cases where surgery is expected to cause significant functional impairment.

Keywords: low-grade myofibroblastic sarcoma; rare sarcoma; wide excision; radiotherapy; local relapse; prognosis

1. Introduction

Low-grade myofibroblastic sarcoma (LGMS) is a rare mesenchymal spindle cell neoplasm that exhibits fibromatosis-like features and differentiation of fibroblasts into myofibroblasts [1]. The disease was first described by Mentzel et al. in 1998 and classified as a novel disease in the World Health Organization (WHO) classification of tumors of soft tissue and bone in 2002 [2]. It is known to occur frequently in the subcutaneous and deep soft tissues of the head, neck, and extremities with a diffusely infiltrative growth pattern and a tendency to cause local relapse. However, because it is a low-grade malignant tumor, distant metastasis is rare. Four small retrospective observational studies [1,3–5], two analytical studies using the Surveillance, Epidemiology, and End Results (SEER) database [6,7], and multiple case reports [8–22] have been reported to date. Because the local relapse rate is higher with simple excision than with wide excision, wide excision is generally the recommended treatment method. In terms of adjuvant radiotherapy (RT)/chemotherapy, Mentzel et al. [1] and Montgomery et al. [3] reported that local relapse was not observed in patients who underwent excision and adjuvant RT; however, Xu et al. [7] recommended against the routine use of adjuvant RT/chemotherapy due to the limited effects on survival. There are few reports on radical RT in unresectable cases. Distant metastasis is rare, but the treatment strategy for distant metastasis remains controversial. Regarding survival rates, an analysis of the SEER database by Chan et al. [6] showed an 80% survival at 3 years and 76.3% at 5 years, while Xu et al. [7] reported a 93% survival at 1 year, 79% at 5 years, and 76% at 10 years. However, due to the rarity of LGMS, many aspects of the disease remain unknown, such as the survival rate. There is presently no consensus regarding the optimal treatment strategy for LGMS. The purpose of this study is to investigate treatment of LGMS cases at facilities that are members of the Japanese Musculoskeletal Oncology Group (JMOG) and to clarify the clinical outcome for LGMS.

2. Materials and Methods

2.1. Study Design and Evaluation

From 2002, when LGMS was included in the WHO classification, to 2019, patients diagnosed and treated for LGMS at 14 JMOG tertiary referral centers for musculoskeletal tumors were included in this research. This study was a retrospective, multicenter study that was approved by the institutional review board at each institution and conducted in accordance with the Declaration of Helsinki. The following clinical information was collected: age, sex, initial presentation (primary or relapse), primary site of occurrence, localization, maximum tumor diameter, treatment method for the primary tumor, complications associated with treatment, presence of local relapse, presence of distant metastases, treatment methods for local relapse/distant metastases, and oncological outcome at final follow-up. Information on the pathological margins was collected from those who underwent surgery. The pathological margins were assessed by residual (R) tumor classification [23], with R0 corresponding to no residual tumor, R1 to microscopic residual tumor, and R2 to macroscopic residual tumor. In patients who underwent RT/chemotherapy, evaluation of the response to the treatment was determined according to the RECIST guideline [24], and local relapse was defined as tumor regrowth from the time of the best overall response. The following histopathological information was collected: mitotic count, tumor necrosis, and immunohistochemical study (α-SMA, desmin, calponin, h-caldesmon, CD34, β-catenin, S-100, CK AE/AE3, and Ki-67). The mitotic count and tumor necrosis were assessed using the National Cancer Institute and French Federation of Cancer Centers Sarcoma Group (FNCLCC) grading system [25]. The pathological diagnosis was performed by experienced pathologists specializing in bone and soft-tissue tumors at each facility.

2.2. Statistical Analysis

The local relapse-free survival (LRFS) and disease-specific survival (DSS) were calculated using the Kaplan–Meier method. To identify factors associated with LRFS, univariate analysis was performed using the log-rank test. A p-value of 0.05 or less was considered statistically significant. IBM SPSS Statistics (version 28) was used for data analysis.

3. Results

3.1. Patient Characteristics

Ten males and fourteen females were included in this study. Detailed patient characteristics are shown in Table 1. The mean age was 45.7 years (11–83 years), and the condition of the sarcoma at the initial visit was primary in 23 cases and relapse in 1 case. None of the patients had distant metastases. The primary tumor sites were 10 cases in the trunk (buttock, 3 cases; back, 3 cases; chest wall, 1 case; abdominal wall, 1 case; axilla, 1 case; groin, 1 case), 5 cases in the head and neck (neck, 3 cases; vocal cord, 1 case; tongue, 1 case), 6 cases in the lower extremity (thigh, 3 cases; lower leg, 2 cases; foot, 1 case), and 3 cases in the upper extremity (upper arms, 2 cases; forearm, 1 case). In terms of localization, 13 cases were deep-seated, and 11 cases were superficial. The mean maximum tumor diameter was 4.7 cm (1–14 cm), with 15 cases < 5 cm and 9 cases $\geq$ 5 cm. The mean follow-up period (from the date of intervention to last follow-up) was 79 months (4–181 months).

3.2. Pathological Features

Histologically, spindle cells with mild atypia had proliferated while forming complex and irregular fascicles, thus indicating infiltration into the surrounding tissues (Figure 1a,b). The mitotic count score was one in all cases. There were no cases with tumor necrosis. The results of the immunohistochemical study were as follows: α-SMA, 24 positive and 0 negative; desmin, 3 positive, 20 negative, and 1 untested; calponin, 7 positive, 1 negative, and 16 untested; h-caldesmon: 0 positive, 12 negative, and 12 untested; CD34, 3 positive, 17 negative, and 4 untested; β-catenin, 0 positive, 11 negative, and 13 untested; S-100, 2 positive, 19 negative, and 3 untested; CK AE/AE3, 1 positive, 12 negative and 11 untested; and Ki-67, mean 9.7% (20 cases, 2–40%). A-SMA, a marker for unstriated muscle cells and myofibroblasts, was positive in all cases. As for other muscle markers, desmin was negative in 20 out of 23 cases, calponin was positive in 7 out of 8 cases, and h-caldesmon was negative in all 12 cases (Figure 1c–f).

Table 1. Patient characteristics.

No.	Age (y)	Sex	Initial Presentation	Primary Site	Localization	Maximum Diameter (cm)	F/U Periods (m)
1	46	F	Primary	Back	Deep	2.5	113
2	58	F	Primary	Neck	Deep	3.5	101
3	48	M	Primary	Abdominal wall	Superficial	1	104
4	64	M	Primary	Vocal cords	Deep	1.4	34
5	30	F	Primary	LE (ankle)	Superficial	1.6	83
6	67	M	Primary	Chest wall	Deep	3	161
7	11	M	Primary	UE (upper arm)	Superficial	2.8	96
8	19	F	Primary	LE (thigh)	Superficial	3.7	94
9	12	M	Primary	LE (foot)	Superficial	2.8	118
10	36	M	Primary	Back	Deep	6.1	46
11	79	F	Primary	UE (forearm)	Superficial	4	50
12	27	F	Relapse	UE (upper arm)	Superficial	2.5	32
13	19	F	Primary	Groin	Superficial	3	55
14	68	M	Primary	Buttock	Deep	6.2	38
15	74	F	Primary	LE (lower leg)	Deep	9.5	54
16	33	M	Primary	LE (thigh)	Deep	2.8	73
17	26	F	Primary	Axilla	Deep	7	181
18	86	F	Primary	LE (thigh)	Deep	10	88
19	76	F	Primary	Buttock	Superficial	6.2	4
20	83	F	Primary	Buttock	Superficial	5.4	58
21	38	F	Primary	Tongue	Superficial	1.5	93
22	47	M	Primary	Back	Deep	4	11
23	28	M	Primary	Neck	Deep	14	121
24	22	F	Primary	Neck	Deep	7.2	75

LE: lower extremities, UE: upper extremities, F/U: follow-up.

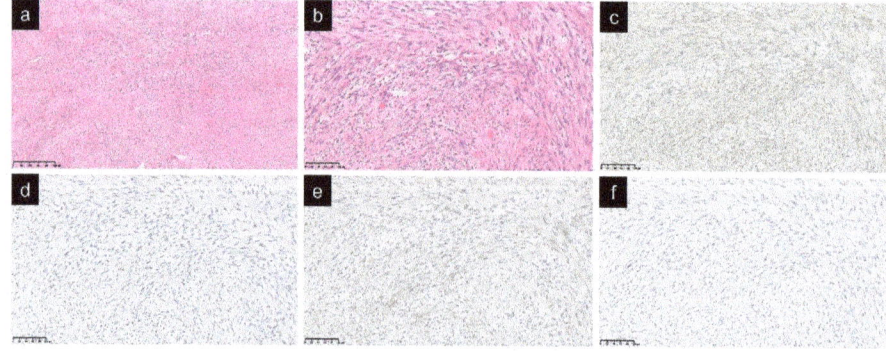

Figure 1. Spindle cells with mild atypia were observed with irregular fascicles. Hematoxylin and eosin staining: magnification ×50 (**a**); magnification ×200 (**b**). In an immunochemical study of muscle markers, α-SMA was positive (**c**), desmin was negative (**d**), calponin was positive (**e**), and h-caldesmon was negative (**f**); ((**c**–**f**) magnification ×200).

3.3. Treatment and Outcome of Initial Tumor

Details are shown in Table 2. Twenty-two cases underwent surgical treatment. The surgical method was wide excision in 17 cases, marginal excision in 4 cases, and intralesional excision in 1 case. One case of intralesional excision of a tumor arising from the subcutaneous tissue was performed under local anesthesia; however, this was an unplanned excision that left gross residual tumor tissues due to adhesion to muscles. The pathological margin was R0 in 14 cases, R1 in 7 cases, and R2 in 1 case. Although the indication for adjuvant RT was determined by each institution, four patients received postoperative adjuvant RT, of which three cases had an R1 pathological margin (No. 10, 11, and 18) and one case had an R0 margin in close proximity to a tumor (No. 15). Two cases (No. 23 and 24) were determined to be difficult to undergo surgical treatment and underwent radical RT (intensity-modulated radiation therapy: IMRT). The best overall response after RT was one case of complete response (Figure 2) and one case of partial response.

Table 2. Treatment and outcome of initial tumor.

No.	Treatment	Margin Status	Local Relapse	Metastases	Outcome
1	Wide excision	R0	-	-	CDF
2	Wide excision	R0	-	-	CDF
3	Intralesional excision	R2	-	-	AWD
4	Wide excision	R0	-	-	CDF
5	Marginal excision	R1	-	-	CDF
6	Wide excision	R0	+	-	NED
7	Wide excision	R0	-	-	CDF
8	Wide excision	R0	-	-	CDF
9	Wide excision	R0	-	-	CDF
10	Marginal excision + adjuvant RT (50 Gy)	R1	-	-	CDF
11	Wide excision + adjuvant RT (48 Gy)	R1	-	-	CDF
12	Wide excision	R1	-	-	NED
13	Wide excision	R0	-	-	CDF
14	Wide excision	R0	-	-	CDF
15	Wide excision + adjuvant RT (60 Gy)	R0	+	-	AWD
16	Wide excision	R0	-	-	CDF
17	Marginal excision	R1	+	-	NED
18	Wide excision + adjuvant RT (66 Gy)	R1	-	-	CDF
19	Wide excision	R0	-	-	CDF
20	Marginal excision	R1	+	+	AWD
21	Wide excision	R0	-	-	CDF
22	Wide excision	R0	-	-	CDF
23	IMRT (60 Gy)	No surgery	-	-	CDF
24	IMRT (60 Gy)	No surgery	+	-	AWD

IMRT: intensity-modulated radiation therapy, CDF: completely disease-free, NED: no evidence of disease, AWD: alive with disease, DOD: dead of disease.

Local relapse occurred in 20.8% of cases (5 cases: No. 6, 15, 17, 20, 24). The mean time to local relapse was 27 months (6–36 months). The LRFS was 91.3% at 2 years and 75.4% at 5 years (Figure 3).

In univariate analysis, the only factor associated with the LRFS was the maximum tumor diameter, and tumors with a diameter of 5 cm or more were significantly more likely to exhibit local relapse ($p < 0.01$) (Table 3).

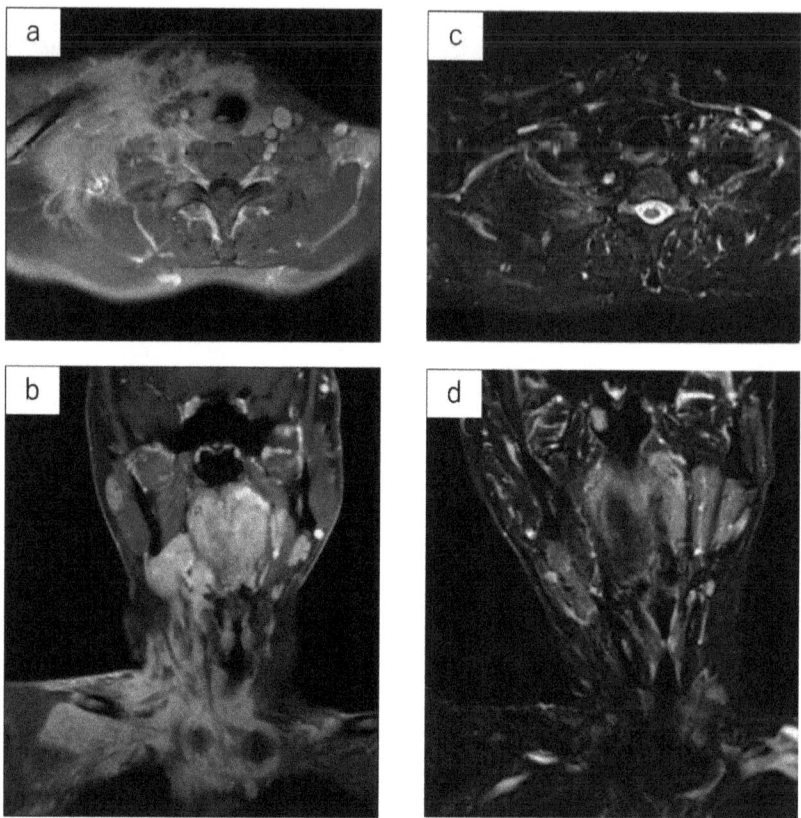

Figure 2. LGMS arising from the neck of a 29-year-old male. Contrast-enhanced MRI prior to irradiation. Signal changes are observed across a large area of the neck (**a**,**b**). MRI STIR image at 10.1 years after irradiation (IMRT: 60 Gy). The tumor has completely subsided (**c**,**d**).

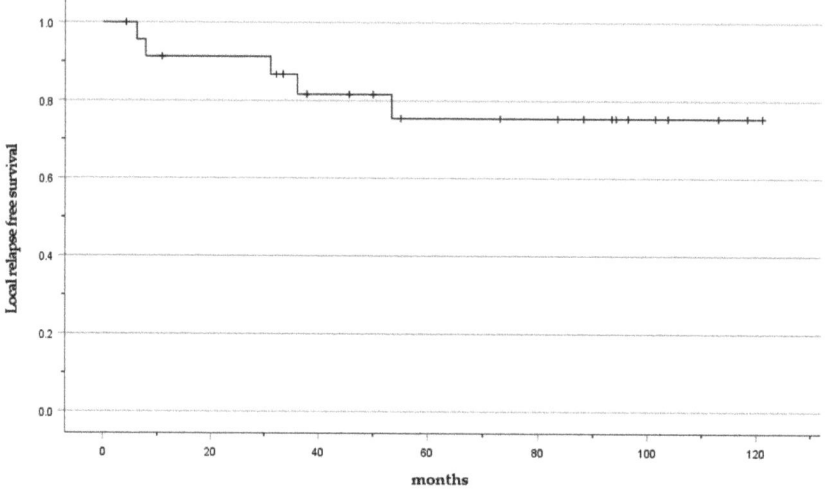

Figure 3. Kaplan–Meier curve presenting the LRFS.

Table 3. Risk factors for local relapse.

Variables	n	5-Year Survival (%)	p-Value
Age (years)			
45>	12	83.3	0.52
45≤	12	63.4	
Sex			
male	10	83.3	0.25
female	14	68.4	
Primary site			
trunk	10	57.1	0.68
head and neck	5	80	
LE	6	83.3	
UE	3	100	
Localization			
deep	13	63.5	0.19
superficial	11	88.9	
Maximum diameter (cm)			
5>	15	90.9	<0.01
5≤	9	50.0	
Treatment			
surgery	18	79	0.58
Surgery + adjuvant RT	4	75	
RT	2	50	
Surgical methods (only surgical cases)			
wide excision	17	84.4	0.16
marginal + intra excision	5	60.0	
Margin status (only surgical cases)			
R0	14	82.1	0.49
R1 + R2	8	72.9	
Ki-67 (%)			
10>	12	71.4	0.78
10≤	12	79.5	

LE: lower extremities, UE: upper extremities.

3.4. Treatment and Outcome of Relapsed Tumor

Details on the treatment and outcomes for relapsed tumors are shown in Table 4. Two cases underwent surgical treatment. Radical RT was performed on three patients for whom surgical treatment was determined to be difficult. Case No. 24 underwent radical RT during the initial treatment. Although the evaluation of the response was determined to be a partial response, there was tumor relapse outside the irradiated field and re-irradiation was, subsequently, performed. The type of radiation was X-ray in two cases and carbon ion in one case. None of the patients experienced a second local relapse at a mean of 79 months (22–175 months) after retreatment. A case arising from the axilla treated with carbon ion RT (No. 17) had grade 3 neuropathy according to the Common Terminology Criteria for Adverse Events version 5.0 (CTCAE). No adverse events occurred in the re-irradiated case (No. 24) at 43 months after re-irradiation.

3.5. Distant Metastases and Disease-Specific Survival

Distant metastases occurred in 4.2% of cases (one case: No. 20). The time to distant metastases was 36 months. The metastatic organs were the lungs and lymph nodes. The patient is currently undergoing routine follow-up without treatment, but is still alive at 22 months from the diagnosis of metastasis. The DSS was 100% at 5 years. The oncological outcome was completely disease-free in 17 cases, no evidence of disease in 3 cases, and alive with disease in 4 cases.

Table 4. Treatment for local tumor relapse.

No. (Refer to Table 1)	Time to Local Relapse (m)	Treatment	Margin Status	Best Overall Response	Re-Local Relapse	F/U Periods after Treatment (m)
6	53	Surgery	R0	N/A	-	108
15	8	RT (60 Gy)	No surgery	PR	-	46
17	6	Carbon ion RT (70.4 Gy)	No surgery	SD	-	175
20	36	Surgery	R0	N/A	-	22
24	31	IMRT (60 Gy)	No surgery	PR	-	43

IMRT: intensity-modulated radiation therapy, N/A: not available, PR: partial response, SD: stable disease, F/U: follow-up.

4. Discussion

LGMS was first reported by Mentzel et al. in a case series of 18 cases in 1998. Histologically, the sarcoma shows a diffusely infiltrative growth pattern and is composed of spindle-shaped tumor cells arranged in fascicles. In immunohistochemical studies of muscle markers, α-SMA can be positive in most cases, but desmin can be both positive and negative [2,26]. In addition, calponin can often be positive, but h-caldesmon is negative. This is important for its differentiation from leiomyosarcoma (which is positive for both calponin and h-caldesmon) [27]. CK/CD34/S100 is often negative. In this study, α-SMA was positive in all cases, and desmin was almost always negative. In terms of calponin and h-caldesmon, approximately half of the cases were tested, but most of them were shown to be calponin-positive and h-caldesmon-negative. The results of the immunohistochemical study were considered consistent with past reports. Mentzel et al. [1] also reported that tumor cells showed moderate nuclear atypia and the mitotic cell count was 1 to 6 figures per 10 HPF in most cases; however, no tumor necrosis was observed. Montgomery et al. [3] reported 15 cases of which 5 cases were histological grade 2 (the presence of necrosis (up to 15%) and 6 or more mitotic figures per 10 HPF). Meng et al. [4] reported 20 cases that included 6 grade 2 cases. Using the SEER database, Xu et al. [7] reported that 22.9% of cases were histologically grade 2 or 3, according to the FNCLCC grading system. These reports included non-low-grade myofibroblastic sarcomas, which might affect the survival analysis. In this study population, the mitosis count score was one for all cases, and there were no cases with tumor necrosis; thus, we believe this study contains the true number of LGMS cases.

Local relapse of LGMS has been reported to range from 13.3% to 44.4% [1,3–5]. The local relapse rate is especially prominent in simple excisions and accounts for up to 28.6–100% of cases. In this study, the local relapse rate was 20%. Despite 14 patients achieving R0 margins, local relapse occurred in 2 patients (14.2%). Fujiwara et al. [28] reported a 100% local control in low-grade soft-tissue sarcoma with excision margins of ≥2 mm. LGMS is, thus, believed to be a tumor with a high relapse rate among low-grade sarcomas. Although dependent on the site of occurrence, a wide excision with the preservation of as much normal tissue as possible is desirable for local treatment, rather than a simple R0 excision. Only the tumor size was shown to be statistically associated with local relapse in this study. Because local relapse of soft-tissue sarcoma is reported to be less common when the tumor diameter is less than 5 cm [29], we believe that our results are acceptable.

The use of adjuvant RT/chemotherapy for LGMS remains debatable, considering that previous reports have only included a limited number of cases. Mentzel et al. [1] reported that two patients who underwent excision and RT showed no local relapse, and Montgomery et al. [3] also reported two patients who underwent excision and RT without local relapse. Meng et al. [4] reported local relapse in one of two patients who underwent excision and RT, while local relapse occurred in three of four patients with excision and chemotherapy. Khosla et al. [14] reported no local relapse for 14 months after partial excision and RT for LGMS arising from the larynx. Peng et al. [10] reported that excision and chemotherapy for LGMS arising from the pancreas had remained continuously disease-free for 5 years. A report by Xu et al. [7] using the SEER database stated that RT and chemotherapy should not be routinely performed when a negative margin can be secured, due to the limited improvement in survival rates. In this study, postoperative RT was performed in one case with R1 marginal excision, two cases with R1 wide excision, and one case with R0 wide excision of a tumor in close proximity to the stump. Local control was obtained in 75% of cases (three cases). Therefore, it is necessary to consider more cases in a future study; however, in patients with positive excision margins, adjuvant RT may be considered. Although the recommendation of adjuvant chemotherapy may be outside the scope of this study, due to the lack of applicable patients in this study, further collection of data is warranted for a future study, considering the scarcity of previous reports on this subject matter.

Presently, there are almost no reports on the results of radical RT. Xu et al. [7] reported three patients who underwent RT without surgical treatment, but did not provide detailed outcomes. Zoltán et al. [9] performed 66 Gy radical RT for local relapse of LGMS of the tongue and reported good local control at 50 months after irradiation. On the other hand, Yu et al. [30] reported that 66 Gy of radical RT was performed on LGMS of the mandibular canal, but the tumor again increased in size 6 months later. Oral intake subsequently became impossible, leading to death from disease. In this study, radical RT (radiation dose: 60 Gy, four cases; 70.4 Gy, one case) was performed in two cases of unresectable primary tumors and three cases of relapsed tumors. In one patient who underwent irradiation of a primary tumor, re-irradiation was performed due to a local relapse that occurred outside the irradiated field. Local control was achieved 43 months after re-irradiation. In other cases, good local control was obtained after one irradiation. Although we cannot make a definitive statement due to the small number of cases, RT may be a useful treatment option in unresectable cases or in cases where surgery results in significant functional impairment due to the potential radiosensitivity of LGMS. However, one case relapsed outside of the area of irradiation. Considering that LGMS shows a growth pattern that infiltrates the surrounding tissue, close attention must be paid in setting the area for irradiation. Since the tumor is surrounded by important tissues in head and neck lesions, the use of an intensity modulated technique to reduce irradiation to normal tissues and to reduce adverse events [31], and the use of carbon ion beams and proton beams to obtain good local control with fewer adverse events [32–34], may be necessary in these cases. In this study, distant metastases occurred in 4.2% of patients, which was comparable to previous reports (0–9.1%) [1,3,5]. However, there is no consensus on the optimal treatment strategy following the occurrence of metastases. Because cases with metastasis in this study did not undergo post-metastatic treatment, a recommendation for treatment is outside the scope of this study.

Table 5 compares the local relapse and distant metastases rates, according to the local treatment used in previous reports and this study.

Table 5. Summary of local relapse and distant metastases of LGMS in previous reports and this study.

Authors, Year of Publication	n	Local Relapse					Distant Metastases
		Simple Excision	Wide Excision	Excision + RT	Excision + Chemotherapy	Radical RT	
Mentzel et al., 1998 [1]	11	28.6% (2/7)	0% (0/1)	0% (0/3)	N/A	N/A	9.1% (1/11)
Montgomery et al., 2001 [3]	13	66.7% (6/9)	50% (1/2)	0% (0/2)	N/A	N/A	7.7% (1/13)
Meng et al., 2007 [4]	14	12.5% (1/8)		50% (1/2)	75% (3/4)	N/A	0% (0/14)
Kim et al., 2021 [5]	15	100% (2/2)	0% (0/13)	N/A	N/A	N/A	0% (0/15)
This study	24	50% (2/4)	7.1% (1/14)	25% (1/4)	N/A	50% (1/2)	4.2% (1/24)

RT: radiotherapy, N/A: not available.

In terms of DSS, Chan et al. [6] reported 80% at 3 years and 76.3% at 5 years, and Xu et al. [7] reported 93% at 1 year, 85% at 3 years, 79% at 5 years, and 76% at 10 years. These reports are analytical studies using the SEER database. In the report by Xu et al., 22.9% of cases were histological grade 2 or 3, and 8.3% had distant metastases at initial presentation. Non-low-grade myofibroblastic sarcoma was included in their study, as evidenced by their database search term "third-edition ICD-O (ICD-O-3) histological code 8825/3: Myofibroblastoma, malignant." In this study, DSS was 100% at 5 years, showing characteristics consistent with a low-grade tumor. Cases with a low mitotic count and no tumor necrosis were collected in this study, and we believe that the prognosis of LGMS was accurately evaluated.

There were notable limitations to this research. Firstly, this was a retrospective asymmetric observational study with a small number of patients, and the possibility of selection bias in the patients and treatments cannot be ruled out. Moreover, the sample size was too small for statistical analysis. Therefore, it is possible that the prognosis and optimal treatment cannot be accurately determined. Secondly, the examination for confirming the diagnosis was inconsistent due to the lack of a central pathology review. This carries the potential risk of diagnostic problems. However, since pathologists for tertiary referral centers for musculoskeletal tumor performed the diagnosis, we expect that most cases were correctly diagnosed. A future prospective study may warrant a larger sample size.

5. Conclusions

Although a wide excision aiming at the R0 margin is considered the standard treatment for LGMS, RT may provide some degree of response and may be a viable option in unresectable cases, or in cases where surgery is expected to cause significant functional impairment.

Author Contributions: Conceptualization, M.K., M.O. and K.A.; methodology, M.K. and K.A.; software, M.K.; validation, M.K., M.O. and K.A.; formal analysis, M.K.; investigation, M.K., M.E., K.I., A.T., N.Y., T.Y., Y.I., T.M., K.K., T.K., Y.N., I.B., S.O. and T.U. (Takeshi Uehara); resources, M.K., M.E., K.I., A.T., N.Y., T.Y., Y.I., T.M., K.K., T.K., Y.N., I.B., S.O. and T.U. (Takeshi Uehara); data curation, M.K.; writing—original draft preparation, M.K.; writing—review and editing, K.A.; visualization, M.K.; supervision, J.T., T.U. (Takafumi Ueda) and H.K.; project administration, M.K., M.O., K.A. and H.K.; funding acquisition, M.K. All authors have read and agreed to the published version of the manuscript.

Funding: This research was supported by the Japan Orthopaedic and Traumatology Foundation (Grant No.476). The funders had no role in the study design, data collection, analysis, manuscript writing, or submitting the manuscript for publication.

Institutional Review Board Statement: This study was conducted according to the guidelines of the Declaration of Helsinki and approved by the Institutional Review Board of Shinshu University (No. 4795, 13 July 2020).

Informed Consent Statement: Informed consent was obtained from all subjects involved in the study.

Data Availability Statement: No new data were created or analyzed in this study. Data sharing is not applicable to this article.

Acknowledgments: We conducted a questionnaire survey for all JMOG member facilities in carrying out this research. We would like to express our gratitude to all members and secretaries of JMOG for their contribution.

Conflicts of Interest: The authors declare no conflict of interest.

References

1. Mentzel, T.; Dry, S.; Katenkamp, D.; Fletcher, C.D. Low-grade myofibroblastic sarcoma: Analysis of 18 cases in the spectrum of myofibroblastic tumors. *Am. J. Surg. Pathol.* **1998**, *22*, 1228–1238. [CrossRef] [PubMed]
2. Fletcher, C.D.M. World Health Organization; International Agency for Research on Cancer. In *WHO Classification of Tumours of Soft Tissue and Bone*, 4th ed.; IARC Press: Lyon, France, 2013.

3. Montgomery, E.; Goldblum, J.R.; Fisher, C. Myofibrosarcoma: A clinicopathologic study. *Am. J. Surg. Pathol.* **2001**, *25*, 219–228. [CrossRef]
4. Meng, G.Z.; Zhang, H.Y.; Bu, H.; Zhang, X.L.; Pang, Z.G.; Ke, Q.; Liu, X.; Yang, G. Myofibroblastic sarcomas: A clinicopathological study of 20 cases. *Chin. Med. J.* **2007**, *120*, 363–369. [CrossRef]
5. Kim, J.H.; Choi, W.; Cho, H.S.; Lee, K.S.; Park, J.K.; Kim, B.K. Surgical treatment and long-term outcomes of low-grade myofibroblastic sarcoma: A single-center case series of 15 patients. *World J. Surg. Oncol.* **2021**, *19*, 339. [CrossRef] [PubMed]
6. Chan, J.Y.; Gooi, Z.; Wong, E.W.; Ng, S.K.; Tong, M.C.; Vlantis, A.C. Low-grade myofibroblastic sarcoma: A population-based study. *Laryngoscope* **2017**, *127*, 116–121. [CrossRef] [PubMed]
7. Xu, Y.; Xu, G.; Wang, X.; Mao, M.; Wu, H.; Baklaushev, V.P.; Chekhonin, V.P.; Peltzer, K.; Wang, G.; Zhang, C. Is there a role for chemotherapy and radiation in the treatment of patients with low-grade myofibroblastic sarcoma? *Clin. Transl. Oncol.* **2021**, *23*, 344–352. [CrossRef]
8. Yonezawa, H.; Yamamoto, N.; Hayashi, K.; Takeuchi, A.; Miwa, S.; Igarashi, K.; Langit, M.B.; Kimura, H.; Shimozaki, S.; Kato, T.; et al. Low-grade myofibroblastic sarcoma of the levator scapulae muscle: A case report and literature review. *BMC Musculoskelet. Disord.* **2020**, *21*, 836. [CrossRef]
9. Takácsi-Nagy, Z.; Muraközy, G.; Pogány, P.; Fodor, J.; Orosz, Z. Myofibroblastic sarcoma of the base of tongue. Case report and review of the literature. *Strahlenther. Onkol.* **2009**, *185*, 198–201. [CrossRef] [PubMed]
10. Peng, L.; Tu, Y.; Li, Y.; Xiao, W. Low-grade myofibroblastic sarcoma of the pancreas: A case report and literature review. *J. Cancer Res. Ther.* **2018**, *14* (Suppl. 3), S796–S799. [PubMed]
11. Morii, T.; Mochizuki, K.; Sano, H.; Fujino, T.; Harasawa, A.; Satomi, K. Occult myofibroblastic sarcoma detected on FDG-PET performed for cancer screening. *Ann. Nucl. Med.* **2008**, *22*, 811–815. [CrossRef]
12. Saito, T.; Mitomi, H.; Kurisaki, A.; Torigoe, T.; Takagi, T.; Suehara, Y.; Okubo, T.; Kaneko, K.; Yao, T. Low-grade myofibroblastic sarcoma of the distal femur. *Int. J. Surg. Case Rep.* **2013**, *4*, 195–199. [CrossRef] [PubMed]
13. Arora, R.; Gupta, R.; Sharma, A.; Dinda, A.K. A rare case of low-grade myofibroblastic sarcoma of the femur in a 38-year-old woman: A case report. *J. Med. Case Rep.* **2010**, *4*, 121. [CrossRef] [PubMed]
14. Khosla, D.; Yadav, B.S.; Kumar, R.; Ghoshal, S.; Vaiphei, K.; Verma, R.; Sharma, S.C. Low-grade myofibroblastic sarcoma of the larynx: A rare entity with review of literature. *J. Cancer Res. Ther.* **2013**, *9*, 284–286. [PubMed]
15. Murakami, Y.; Tsubamoto, H.; Hao, H.; Nishimoto, S.; Shibahara, H. Long-term disease-free survival after radical local excision of low-grade myofibroblastic sarcoma of the vulva. *Gynecol. Oncol. Case Rep.* **2013**, *5*, 34–36. [CrossRef]
16. Humphries, W.E., 3rd; Satyan, K.B.; Relyea, K.; Kim, E.S.; Adesina, A.M.; Chintagumpala, M.; Jea, A. Low-grade myofibroblastic sarcoma of the sacrum. *J. Neurosurg. Pediatr.* **2010**, *6*, 286–290. [CrossRef] [PubMed]
17. Han, S.R.; Yee, G.T. Low Grade Myofibroblastic Sarcoma Occurred in the Scalp. *J. Korean Neurosurg. Soc.* **2015**, *58*, 385–388. [CrossRef]
18. Qiu, J.Y.; Liu, P.; Shi, C.; Han, B. Low-grade myofibroblastic sarcomas of the maxilla. *Oncol. Lett.* **2015**, *9*, 619–625. [CrossRef]
19. Miyazawa, M.; Naritaka, Y.; Miyaki, A.; Asaka, S.; Isohata, N.; Yamaguchi, K.; Murayama, M.; Shimakawa, T.; Katsube, T.; Ogawa, K.; et al. A low-grade myofibroblastic sarcoma in the abdominal cavity. *Anticancer Res.* **2011**, *31*, 2989–2994.
20. Katalinic, D.; Santek, F. Giant low-grade primary myofibroblastic sarcoma of the posterior chest wall. *World J. Surg. Oncol.* **2017**, *15*, 96. [CrossRef]
21. Yamada, T.; Yoshimura, T.; Kitamura, N.; Sasabe, E.; Ohno, S.; Yamamoto, T. Low-grade myofibroblastic sarcoma of the palate. *Int. J. Oral Sci.* **2012**, *4*, 170–173. [CrossRef]
22. Kuo, Y.R.; Yang, C.K.; Chen, A.; Ramachandran, S.; Lin, S.D. Low-Grade Myofibroblastic Sarcoma Arising From Keloid Scar on the Chest Wall After Thoracic Surgery. *Ann. Thorac. Surg.* **2020**, *110*, e469–e471. [CrossRef]
23. Wittekind, C.; Compton, C.C.; Greene, F.L.; Sobin, L.H. TNM residual tumor classification revisited. *Cancer* **2002**, *94*, 2511–2516. [CrossRef]
24. Eisenhauer, E.A.; Therasse, P.; Bogaerts, J.; Schwartz, L.H.; Sargent, D.; Ford, R.; Dancey, J.; Arbuck, S.; Gwyther, S.; Mooney, M.; et al. New response evaluation criteria in solid tumours: Revised RECIST guideline (version 1.1). *Eur. J. Cancer* **2009**, *45*, 228–247. [CrossRef] [PubMed]
25. Guillou, L.; Coindre, J.M.; Bonichon, F.; Nguyen, B.B.; Terrier, P.; Collin, F.; Vilain, M.O.; Mandard, A.M.; Le Doussal, V.; Leroux, A.; et al. Comparative study of the National Cancer Institute and French Federation of Cancer Centers Sarcoma Group grading systems in a population of 410 adult patients with soft tissue sarcoma. *J. Clin. Oncol.* **1997**, *15*, 35. [CrossRef] [PubMed]
26. Fisher, C. Myofibrosarcoma. *Virchows Arch.* **2004**, *445*, 215–223. [CrossRef] [PubMed]
27. Watanabe, K.; Kusakabe, T.; Hoshi, N.; Saito, A.; Suzuki, T. h-Caldesmon in leiomyosarcoma and tumors with smooth muscle cell-like differentiation: Its specific expression in the smooth muscle cell tumor. *Hum. Pathol.* **1999**, *30*, 392–396. [CrossRef]
28. Fujiwara, T.; Kaneuchi, Y.; Tsuda, Y.; Stevenson, J.; Parry, M.; Jeys, L. Low-grade soft-tissue sarcomas: What is an adequate margin for local disease control? *Surg. Oncol.* **2020**, *35*, 303–308. [CrossRef]
29. Maki, R.G.; Moraco, N.; Antonescu, C.R.; Hameed, M.; Pinkhasik, A.; Singer, S.; Brennan, M.F. Toward better soft tissue sarcoma staging: Building on american joint committee on cancer staging systems versions 6 and 7. *Ann. Surg. Oncol.* **2013**, *20*, 3377–3383. [CrossRef]
30. Yu, Y.; Xiao, J.; Wang, L.; Yang, G. Low-Grade Myofibroblastic Sarcoma in the Mandibular Canal: A Case Report. *J. Oral Maxillofac. Surg.* **2016**, *74*, e1501–e1505. [CrossRef]

31. Yang, J.; Gao, J.; Qiu, X.; Hu, J.; Hu, W.; Wu, X.; Zhang, C.; Ji, T.; Kong, L.; Lu, J.J. Intensity-Modulated Proton and Carbon-Ion Radiation Therapy in the Management of Head and Neck Sarcomas. *Cancer Med.* **2019**, *8*, 4574–4586. [CrossRef]
32. Allignet, B.; Sunyach, M.P.; Geets, X.; Waissi, W. Is there a place for definitive radiotherapy in the treatment of unresectable soft-tissue sarcoma? A systematic review. *Acta Oncol.* **2022**, *61*, 720–729. [CrossRef] [PubMed]
33. Jingu, K.; Tsujii, H.; Mizoe, J.E.; Hasegawa, A.; Bessho, H.; Takagi, R.; Morikawa, T.; Tonogi, M.; Tsuji, H.; Kamada, T.; et al. Carbon ion radiation therapy improves the prognosis of unresectable adult bone and soft-tissue sarcoma of the head and neck. *Int. J. Radiat. Oncol. Biol. Phys.* **2012**, *82*, 2125–2131. [CrossRef] [PubMed]
34. Musha, A.; Kubo, N.; Kawamura, H.; Okano, N.; Sato, H.; Okada, K.; Osu, N.; Yumisaki, H.; Adachi, A.; Takayasu, Y.; et al. Carbon-ion Radiotherapy for Inoperable Head and Neck Bone and Soft-tissue Sarcoma: Prospective Observational Study. *Anticancer Res.* **2022**, *42*, 1439–1446. [CrossRef] [PubMed]

Disclaimer/Publisher's Note: The statements, opinions and data contained in all publications are solely those of the individual author(s) and contributor(s) and not of MDPI and/or the editor(s). MDPI and/or the editor(s) disclaim responsibility for any injury to people or property resulting from any ideas, methods, instructions or products referred to in the content.

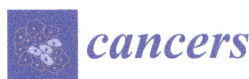

Communication

Preoperative Dose-Escalated Intensity-Modulated Radiotherapy (IMRT) and Intraoperative Radiation Therapy (IORT) in Patients with Retroperitoneal Soft-Tissue Sarcoma: Final Results of a Clinical Phase I/II Trial

Katharina Seidensaal [1,2,3,4,*], Matthias Dostal [1,2], Andreas Kudak [1,2], Cornelia Jaekel [1], Eva Meixner [1,2,3,4], Jakob Liermann [1,2,3], Fabian Weykamp [1,2,3], Philipp Hoegen [1,2,3], Gunhild Mechtersheimer [5], Franziska Willis [6], Martin Schneider [6] and Jürgen Debus [1,2,3,4,7,8]

[1] Department of Radiation Oncology, Heidelberg University Hospital, 69120 Heidelberg, Germany
[2] Heidelberg Institute of Radiation Oncology (HIRO), 69120 Heidelberg, Germany
[3] National Center for Tumor Diseases (NCT), 69120 Heidelberg, Germany
[4] Heidelberg Ion-Beam Therapy Center (HIT), Department of Radiation Oncology, Heidelberg University Hospital, 69120 Heidelberg, Germany
[5] Institute of Pathology, University of Heidelberg, 69120 Heidelberg, Germany
[6] Department of General, Visceral and Transplantation Surgery, University Hospital Heidelberg, 69120 Heidelberg, Germany
[7] Clinical Cooperation Unit Radiation Oncology, German Cancer Research Center (DKFZ), 69120 Heidelberg, Germany
[8] German Cancer Consortium (DKTK), Partner Site Heidelberg, 69120 Heidelberg, Germany
* Correspondence: katharina.seidensaal@med.uni-heidelberg.de

Citation: Seidensaal, K.; Dostal, M.; Kudak, A.; Jaekel, C.; Meixner, E.; Liermann, J.; Weykamp, F.; Hoegen, P.; Mechtersheimer, G.; Willis, F.; et al. Preoperative Dose-Escalated Intensity-Modulated Radiotherapy (IMRT) and Intraoperative Radiation Therapy (IORT) in Patients with Retroperitoneal Soft-Tissue Sarcoma: Final Results of a Clinical Phase I/II Trial. *Cancers* **2023**, *15*, 2747. https://doi.org/10.3390/cancers15102747

Academic Editors: Shinji Miwa, Po-Kuei Wu and Hiroyuki Tsuchiya

Received: 27 March 2023
Revised: 6 May 2023
Accepted: 7 May 2023
Published: 13 May 2023

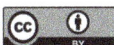

Copyright: © 2023 by the authors. Licensee MDPI, Basel, Switzerland. This article is an open access article distributed under the terms and conditions of the Creative Commons Attribution (CC BY) license (https://creativecommons.org/licenses/by/4.0/).

Simple Summary: Retroperitoneal sarcomas represent a very rare entity. The most common pattern of recurrence and cause of death is local recurrence, and the rates of locoregional recurrences are high even at high-volume centers. In contrast to soft-tissue sarcomas of the extremities, the role of radiotherapy in retroperitoneal sarcoma is not fully established. The aim of the study was to report the results of a prospective single-center trial for preoperative dose-escalated intensity-modulated radiotherapy with an intraoperative boost in patients with retroperitoneal sarcoma after all surviving patients had achieved a follow-up of at least 60 months. The primary endpoint of a 5-year local control of 70% was not met; the local control of the cohort was 59.6%. In those patients who received a dose > 50 Gy and the intraoperative boost, the local control was promising at 64.8%.

Abstract: Background: To report the final results of a prospective, one-armed, single-center phase I/II trial (NCT01566123). Methods: Between 2007 and 2017, 37 patients with primary or recurrent (N = 6) retroperitoneal sarcomas were enrolled. Treatment included preoperative IMRT of 45–50 Gy with a simultaneous integrated boost of 50–56 Gy, surgery and IORT. The primary endpoint was local control (LC) at 5 years. The most common histology was dedifferentiated liposarcoma (51%), followed by leiomyosarcoma (24%) and well-differentiated liposarcoma (14%). The majority of lesions were high-grade (FNCLCC G1: 30%, G2: 38%, G3: 27%, two missing). Five patients were excluded from LC analysis per protocol. Results: The minimum follow-up of the survivors was 62 months (median: 109; maximum 162). IORT was performed for 27 patients. Thirty-five patients underwent gross total resection; the pathological resection margin was mostly R+ (80%) and, less often, R0 (20%). We observed 10 local recurrences. The 5-year LC of the whole cohort was 59.6%. Eleven patients received a dose > 50 Gy plus IORT boost; LC was 64.8%; the difference, however, was not significant ($p = 0.588$). Of 37 patients, 15 were alive and 22 deceased at the time of final analysis. The 5-year OS was 59.5% (68.8% per protocol). Conclusions: The primary endpoint of a 5-year LC of 70% was not met. This might be explained by the inclusion of recurrent disease and the high rate of G3 lesions and leiomyosarcoma, which have been shown to profit less from radiotherapy. Stratification by grading and histology should be considered for future studies.

Keywords: retroperitoneal sarcoma; radiotherapy; IORT; intraoperative radiotherapy; dose-escalated radiotherapy; simultaneous integrated boost

1. Introduction

Retroperitoneal sarcomas (RPSs) constitute 15% of all soft-tissue sarcomas [1]. High-grade tumors are the most common; the spectrum of histological diagnoses is broad and ranges from lipo- and leiomyosarcoma to less common diagnoses [2,3]. In contrast to extremity soft-tissue sarcomas, local control (LC) is the central issue in the treatment of retroperitoneal sarcomas. Local recurrences are quite common and represent the leading cause of death. RPSs remain asymptomatic without specific symptoms for a long time; thus, many patients are diagnosed with large tumors of 16–21 cm median tumor size [2]. The primary treatment for initial and recurrent disease is surgery; however, incomplete resection with microscopic positive margins occurs in up to 65% of cases due to the immense size these tumors commonly achieve and the complex anatomy of the retroperitoneum [4]. Compartmental resection of organs adjacent to the tumor is the current surgical technique and has increased LC [5]. Although many undergo several consecutive multivisceral resections, the outcomes of retroperitoneal sarcomas are substantially less satisfactory compared to soft-tissue sarcomas at other sites. As known from extremity soft-tissue sarcoma, preoperative radiotherapy has the potential to increase LC; however, the available data are still limited, and further insight is needed. The only prospective trial published so far is the EORTC STRASS trial. The results did not support a broad use of radiotherapy in RPS and were contradictory to many other publications [1]. In an additional analysis, the results from STRASS have been pooled in a propensity-score-matched analysis with patients treated outside the trial (STREXIT). A benefit of additional radiotherapy was shown especially for patients with well-differentiated liposarcoma (WDLS) and dedifferentiated liposarcoma G1 and G2 [6,7]. The anatomy of the retroperitoneum complicates not only surgery but also radiotherapy; clinical target volume (CTV) margins known from extremity soft-tissue sarcomas cannot be adopted due to the necessary limitations to the adjacent organs at risk, mainly the bowel. Previous analyses have demonstrated that recurrence commonly occurs at the posterior margin of the tumor. Therefore, a simultaneous integrated boost (SIB) was tested on this high-risk margin with photon IMRT and protons before, with promising results, although with only a comparably short follow-up [8]. Intraoperative radiation therapy (IORT) has additional potential to increase the dose to the high-risk margin as identified during the resection. Herein, we present the final results of a phase I/II feasibility trial which combined a photon IMRT with a SIB plus an IORT boost. All of the surviving trial participants have achieved a minimum follow-up period of 60 months.

2. Methods

Retro-WTS was designed as a prospective single-center one-armed phase I/II study. The study design, as well as an unplanned interim analysis, have been published elsewhere [9,10]. In short, patients with histologically confirmed, primary or locally recurrent soft-tissue sarcoma of the retroperitoneal space judged to be at least marginally resectable were enrolled. Absence of primary metastases, tumor size of 5 cm or more were additional inclusion criteria. Exclusion criteria included desmoid tumors, gastrointestinal stroma tumors (GISTs), prior irradiation to the abdominal region, inflammatory bowel disease and incomplete staging. Immobilization was performed with individual body masks or vacuum mattresses. Planning was performed either with contrast-enhanced CT or MRI. Patients were treated with IMRT. The attempted dose was 45–50 Gy prescribed to the planning target volume (PTV) with a SIB of 50–56 Gy to the gross target volume (GTV) in 25 fractions. For target volume delineation, a 1.5 cm margin was added to the GTV to receive the CTV. CTV margins were reduced to respect the non-infiltrated adjacent organs at risk and anatomical borders. Surgery was scheduled approximately six weeks after the end of radiotherapy. Before surgery, re-evaluation with an abdominal CT or MRI was performed. An intraoperative radiation boost was dedicated to the whole tumor bed or the high-risk region for positive resection margins, which was defined by the surgeon together with the radiation oncologist. The patients received no pre- or postoperative chemotherapy. Regular follow-up visits including abdominal CT or MRI were performed every three months for the first two years, and every six months up to the end of the study follow-up interval of five years.

The primary objective of the trial was the LC rate after five years. The calculated sample size was 37 patients to detect an improvement in the 5-year LC rate from 50% to 70% with a statistical power of 80%. Data should be analyzed by the per protocol population and full-set population. Secondary endpoints included distant control (DC) and overall survival (OS). LC was defined as absence from abdominal recurrence. Data of those without recurrence were censored at the time of the last local MRI or CT. DC was defined as absence from distant metastases; data of those without distant progression were censored at the time of last thoracic CT. Timeframes were calculated from beginning of radiotherapy; survival analysis was performed by the Kaplan–Meier method. Data on acute toxicity and perioperative morbidity were published in an unplanned interim analysis [9].

The survival data of those lost to follow-up or those who were not followed with repetitive imaging after five years were updated by information from the German Cancer registry and the resident's registration offices.

The study was approved by the Ethics Committee of Heidelberg University. Written informed consent was obtained from each patient prior to study entry.

3. Results

Between 2007 and 2017, a total of 37 patients with primary or recurrent (N = 6) retroperitoneal sarcomas were enrolled. The median age of the patients was 61.5 years (range 36–76 years); the gender distribution was homogeneous (male 49%, female 51%). The most common histology was dedifferentiated liposarcoma (51%), followed by leiomyosarcoma (24%) and well-differentiated liposarcoma (14%). The majority of lesions were high-grade (FNCLCC G1: 30%, G2: 38%, G3: 27%, two missing; Table 1); grading was determined at the time of the initial biopsy.

Table 1. Patient characteristics.

		N	Range or Percent
		N = 37	
Age (median, range)		61	(36–76)
Gender			
	Male	18	49
	Female	19	51
Primary vs. recurrence			
	Primary	31	84
	Recurrent	6	16
Histology			
	Liposarcoma	26	70
	Leiomyosarcoma	9	24
	SFT	1	3
	NOS	1	3
Grading (FNCLCC)			
	G1	11	30

Table 1. Cont.

		N	Range or Percent
	G2	14	38
	G3	10	27
	Missing	2	5
Survival			
	Deceased	22	59
	Alive	15	41

Of the 37 patients enrolled in the trial, 34 finished the neoadjuvant therapy per protocol. Percutaneous RT was performed as step-and-shoot IMRT in most cases (N = 32) and as helical IMRT in four cases. In total, four patients did not receive a SIB. The most common fractionation was 45 Gy in 25 fractions with a SIB up to 50 Gy (35%), followed by 45 Gy in 25 fractions with a SIB up to 54 Gy or 55 Gy (18% and 18%, Table 2). Gross total resection was performed in 35 cases. Two patients did not receive surgery; in one case, infiltration of the mesentery root was confirmed with intraoperative frozen sample analysis, and in the second case, inoperability was stated during surgery. On final pathology, the resection margin was mainly microscopic margin-positive R1 (N = 24, 69%). In one case, gross residual disease remained (R2, 3%). In two cases, the presence of residual tumor could not be assessed (RX, 6%), and in one case, the resection was described as marginal (3%). Seven patients received a microscopic margin-negative R0 resection (20%).

Table 2. Treatment characteristics.

			N	Range or Percent
Neoadjuvant IMRT			N = 37	
	Completed		34	91
	Terminated prematurely		2	6
	Upfront surgery		1	3
Percutaneous RT technique			N = 36	
	Step-and-shoot IMRT		32	89
	Helical IMRT		4	11
Percutaneous RT				
Total dose for the main plan, boost and the number of fractions **			N = 34	
	SIB	Fx.		
45	50	25	12	35
45	54	25	6	18
50	55	25	6	18
41.4	46	23	1	3
45	50.4	25	1	3
45	55	25	1	3
50	-	25	3	9
50.4	-	28	2	6
55	-	25	1	3
45	-	25	1	3

Table 2. *Cont.*

		N	Range or Percent
Surgery		N = 37	
	Gross total	35	94
	Not performed	2	6
Resection margin		N = 35	
	R1	24	69
	R0	7	20
	RX	2	6
	R2	1	3
	Marginal	1	3
IORT		N = 36 *	
	Yes	27	75
	No	9	25
IORT total dose		N = 27	
	12 Gy	20	74
	15 Gy	4	15
	10 Gy	2	7
	20 Gy	1	4
IORT energy		N = 27	
	8 MeV	16	60
	6 MeV	9	33
	12 MeV	2	7
IORT cones (cm)			
Squircle (horseshoe-shaped)		N = 13	48
	6 × 7	2	
	7 × 8	2	
	10 × 10	1	
	10 × 11	2	
	10 × 13	4	
Straight round (diameter)		N = 5	19
	5	2	
	6	1	
	7	1	
	8	1	
Beveled round (diameter), angle up to 30%		N = 9	33
	5	1	
	6	2	
	7	1	
	8	4	
	9	1	

* one patient did not receive surgery after confirmation of infiltration of the mesentery root. He received IORT.
** preliminary cessation of RT excluded.

The IORT boost was performed in 75% of patients. The main reason for omission of IORT was the intraoperative difficulty in identifying a coverable high-risk region, as well as the fact that irradiating the whole tumor bed was not feasible due to its sheer size. One patient did not receive surgery due to the aforementioned infiltration of the mesentery root, but an IORT boost was applied. The most common IORT dose was 12 Gy (74%) prescribed to the 90% isodose, the most common energy applied was 8 MeV (60%).

The median follow-up of the survivors for OS was 109 months (range: 62–162 months). Of the 37 patients, 15 were alive and 22 deceased at the time of final analysis. Two patients died due to postoperative complications in the prolonged postoperative period, and one patient died 91 months after the beginning of RT and 10 months after his last follow-up presentation, at the age of 75, due to unknown reasons. The 5-year OS of the whole cohort was 59.5%. The 5-year OS of those treated per protocol accumulated to 68.8%.

Five patients were excluded from LC analysis per protocol. Of those, two patients had a preliminary termination of radiotherapy due to progression after 13 and 23 fractions, two patients did not receive surgery and one received upfront surgery without preoperative radiotherapy, as the tumor was rapidly progressing on planning CT.

The median follow-up for LC of those without local progression was defined as the timeframe from the beginning of radiotherapy until the last abdominal MRI, or, in exceptional cases, CT. The median FU time for LC was 60.5 months (range: 4–154 months). In total, 10 patients had local progression during the observation interval, while 22 did not progress. Of ten patients, five progressed within two years and an additional five within five years. The 3-year LC was 70% and the 5-year LC was 59.6% (Figure 1). Of five patients treated per protocol for recurrent disease, three developed local progression, one developed distant progression and one developed local and distant progression.

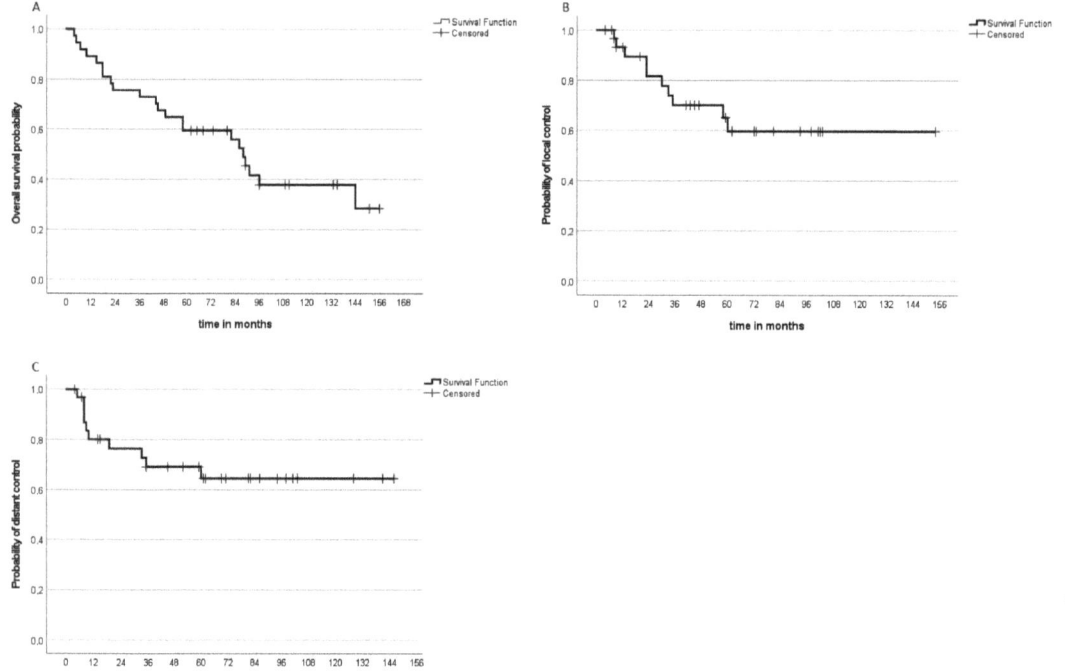

Figure 1. Kaplan–Meier analysis displays the probability of (**A**) overall survival, (**B**) local control and (**C**) distant control.

Eleven patients received a total dose above 50.4 Gy plus IORT boost. The LC was 64.8%; however, the difference was not significant ($p = 0.588$). We did not identify factors influencing LC or OS on univariate analysis; only the comparison of recurrent vs. primary tumors showed a clear trend towards a higher LC probability for primary tumors ($p = 0.006$).

Of the 32 patients treated per protocol, 10 developed distant progression (4 pulmonary, 2 bone, 2 pulmonary and hepatic, 1 hepatic, 1 bone and soft tissue). Of eight leiomyosarcoma patients, five developed distant progression. The 5-year DC of those treated per protocol was 64.6%. On univariate analysis, the histology leiomyosarcoma was correlated with distant progression ($p = 0.005$).

4. Discussion

The role of preoperative radiotherapy in addition to surgery has been controversial for many years, and several contradicting retrospective studies have been published so far [11–15]. At present, only one prospective phase III trial for retroperitoneal sarcoma investigating this issue has completed patient recruitment. In the STRASS trial, 266 patients were enrolled and randomly assigned to surgery or preoperative radiotherapy of 50.4 Gy in 28 fractions followed by surgery. The results have been published preliminarily after a median follow-up of 43 months. The trial was powered for an increase of 20% in abdominal-recurrence-free survival (ARFS) at five years, which was not reached. The scientifically invalidated composite endpoint received much criticism after the full publication of the paper in Lancet Oncology in 2020. The data monitoring committee of the trial recommended performing additional analyses and modifying the endpoint. Thus, progression on preoperative imaging and becoming medically unfit where excluded from the primary endpoint in the second sensitivity analysis for those patients who had a subsequent macroscopic complete resection. It was demonstrated that the liposarcoma group had an increased 3-year ARFS of 75.5% after treatment with radiotherapy and surgery compared to 65.2% after surgery alone. As the trial was not powered to evaluate specific subtypes, the authors concluded that preoperative radiotherapy should not be considered the standard of care for retroperitoneal sarcomas [6]. The results of the STRASS trial were translated into quite contradictory clinical approaches. While some institutions decided not to offer preoperative radiotherapy to patients with retroperitoneal sarcomas outside of clinical trials, others have implemented a broader use of radiotherapy for patients with retroperitoneal well-differentiated liposarcoma. Valuable information on the topic was provided by the STREXIT results, published in 2022 by Callegaro et al. Additional 831 patients treated by the institutions participating in the STRASS trial were included in the analysis. A 1:1 propensity score matching was performed for 202 patients and the cohorts from STRASS and STREXIT were investigated in a pooled analysis. ARFS was defined as R2 resection, abdominal recurrence or death. Administration of radiotherapy was associated with an improved ARFS in patients with liposarcoma, especially in well-differentiated liposarcoma and G1–G2 dedifferentiated liposarcoma, while patients with leiomyosarcoma or G3 dedifferentiated liposarcoma did not benefit from radiotherapy [7]. The biological heterogeneity of retroperitoneal sarcomas and the different clinical behaviors clearly indicate a histology-tailored approach and management strategy. The next-generation STRASS 2 trial evaluates neoadjuvant chemotherapy in leiomyosarcoma and high-risk liposarcoma.

The results of the present trial did not reach the primary endpoint of an LC of 70% at five years. The 3-year ARFS in the aforementioned second sensitivity analysis of those who received preoperative radiotherapy and surgery in the STRASS trial was 71.3%. Our trial shows that relapse also occurs later than at three years; thus, an observational period of five years should be considered for further trials. The STRASS data will be published with a longer follow-up after five years, which will show whether the results achieved here are comparable to the results of bigger cohorts. The rate of microscopically complete R0 resections was 20%, but the role of R0 resection in RPS is controversial. Resection margins have been shown to be a strong prognostic factor for, at least, LC [4]. On the other hand, due to the retroperitoneal location with a close anatomical relationship to the spine and large blood vessels and the average tumor size of 15–30 cm, no large safety margins can be maintained during the resection. The evaluation of R1 resections in retroperitoneal sarcomas differs significantly from soft-tissue sarcomas of the extremities and trunk, and postoperative histopathological examination of the resection margins is less reliable [16]. In several publications, a distinction is only made between a macroscopically complete (R0/R1) and incomplete (R2) resection [3,6,17].

The survival rates at 3 years were lower, with 73% compared to the 84% of the STRASS trial [6], which might be also explained by the inclusion of recurrent tumors and the longer follow-up.

Prospective comparative data for the application of an IORT boost are, so far, not available. Nonetheless, IORT is considered to be well tolerated and a reasonable option to achieve dose escalation and improve LC, with a low risk of wound healing disorders or gastrointestinal toxicity [4,18–20]. Additional care should be taken to limit dose to the ureters and reduce the risk of ureter stenosis. The single prospective NCI trial identified neuropathy as a possible risk of IORT of the retroperitoneal space. Here, patients were randomized to postoperative high-dose RT (50 to 55 Gy) or IORT (20 Gy) in combination with postoperative percutaneous radiation therapy of 35 to 40 Gy [21].

Performing preoperative radiotherapy with a SIB above 50.4 Gy plus IORT boost was not possible or reasonable for several patients, but we observed increased rates of LC for those who received the combination of both. Applying a boost to the high-risk GTV (a smaller volume than the whole GTV, which constituted the SIB volume in this trial) is one additional option of dose escalation. The high-risk GTV generally includes the posterolateral abdominal wall, posterior retroperitoneal musculature, ipsilateral pre- and paravertebral space, major vessels or organs that will remain in situ after surgery [22]. This approach of neoadjuvant intensity-modulated proton therapy was investigated in a phase I pilot study (n = 11). The average-risk CTV received a dose of 50.4 Gy in 28 fractions and a SIB was performed to the high-risk CTV with 60.2 GyRBE, 61.6 GyRBE or 63 GyRBE. Beside one case of hydronephrosis, the treatment was tolerated well [8]. Further results of the phase 2 arm of the trial are eagerly awaited. In a plan comparison of 3D conformal proton therapy (3D CPT), intensity-modulated proton therapy (IMPT) and intensity-modulated photon therapy, 3D CPT and IMPT achieved lower organ-at-risk doses and IMPT achieved the closest conformity [23].

The standard neoadjuvant RT regimen is delivered in 25–28 fractions, but there is a growing interest in more condensed hypofractionated treatment approaches minimizing patient burden and psychological stress. Several ongoing trials are investigating different fractionation concepts for extremity and trunk soft-tissue sarcomas [24–26]. Particle therapy provides an improved dose distribution with a high dose conformity and reduction in dose to healthy tissue [27]. In analogy to our extremity soft-tissue sarcoma trial, we are currently investigating a hypofractionated particle treatment with carbon ions or protons with 13 fractions of 3 GyRBE single doses in a single-center, randomized, prospective phase II pilot trial for retroperitoneal sarcoma, combining the benefits of reduced organ-at-risk doses of protons or carbon ion with hypofractionation [28,29].

5. Conclusions

The data of a prospective phase II trial are presented. The strength of the cohort is the long follow-up in the prospective setting. The main limitation of the trial is the small sample size. The primary endpoint of a 5-year LC of 70% was not met. This might be explained by the inclusion of recurrent disease and the high rate of G3 lesions and leiomyosarcoma, which have been shown to profit less from radiotherapy in the time since the beginning of the trial. Stratification by grading and histology should be considered for future studies.

Author Contributions: Conceptualization, J.D., K.S. and M.S.; methodology, K.S.; software, M.D. and A.K.; formal analysis, K.S. and E.M.; investigation, F.W. (Fabian Weykamp), J.L., P.H., G.M., F.W. (Franziska Willis) and M.S.; resources, J.D.; data curation, K.S.; writing—original draft preparation, K.S.; writing—review and editing, F.W. (Fabian Weykamp), F.W. (Franziska Willis), J.L. and P.H.; supervision, C.J. and J.D.; project administration, C.J. All authors have read and agreed to the published version of the manuscript.

Funding: J.L. is funded by the Physician-Scientist Program of Heidelberg University, Faculty of Medicine.

Institutional Review Board Statement: The study was conducted in accordance with the Declaration of Helsinki and approved by the Ethics Committee of Medical Faculty at the University of Heidelberg.

Informed Consent Statement: Informed consent was obtained from all subjects involved in the study.

Data Availability Statement: The raw data supporting the conclusions of this article will be made available by the authors, without undue reservation.

Acknowledgments: We appreciate the contribution of Stefanie Arnold, who digitalized the case report forms.

Conflicts of Interest: The authors declare no conflict of interest.

References

1. Nussbaum, D.P.; Rushing, C.N.; Lane, W.O.; Cardona, D.M.; Kirsch, D.G.; Peterson, B.L.; Blazer, D.G., 3rd. Preoperative or postoperative radiotherapy versus surgery alone for retroperitoneal sarcoma: A case-control, propensity score-matched analysis of a nationwide clinical oncology database. *Lancet Oncol.* **2016**, *17*, 966–975. [CrossRef] [PubMed]
2. Raut, C.P.; Miceli, R.; Strauss, D.C.; Swallow, C.J.; Hohenberger, P.; van Coevorden, F.; Rutkowski, P.; Fiore, M.; Callegaro, D.; Casali, P.G.; et al. External validation of a multi-institutional retroperitoneal sarcoma nomogram. *Cancer* **2016**, *122*, 1417–1424. [CrossRef] [PubMed]
3. Gronchi, A.; Strauss, D.C.; Miceli, R.; Bonvalot, S.; Swallow, C.J.; Hohenberger, P.; Van Coevorden, F.; Rutkowski, P.; Callegaro, D.; Hayes, A.J.; et al. Variability in Patterns of Recurrence After Resection of Primary Retroperitoneal Sarcoma (RPS): A Report on 1007 Patients From the Multi-institutional Collaborative RPS Working Group. *Ann. Surg.* **2016**, *263*, 1002–1009. [CrossRef] [PubMed]
4. Roeder, F.; Alldinger, I.; Uhl, M.; Saleh-Ebrahimi, L.; Schimmack, S.; Mechtersheimer, G.; Büchler, M.W.; Debus, J.; Krempien, R.; Ulrich, A. Intraoperative Electron Radiation Therapy in Retroperitoneal Sarcoma. *Int. J. Radiat. Oncol. Biol. Phys.* **2018**, *100*, 516–527. [CrossRef]
5. Swallow, C.J.; Strauss, D.C.; Bonvalot, S.; Rutkowski, P.; Desai, A.; Gladdy, R.A.; Gonzalez, R.; Gyorki, D.E.; Fairweather, M.; van Houdt, W.J.; et al. Management of Primary Retroperitoneal Sarcoma (RPS) in the Adult: An Updated Consensus Approach from the Transatlantic Australasian RPS Working Group. *Ann. Surg. Oncol.* **2021**, *28*, 7873–7888. [CrossRef]
6. Bonvalot, S.; Gronchi, A.; Le Péchoux, C.; Swallow, C.J.; Strauss, D.; Meeus, P.; van Coevorden, F.; Stoldt, S.; Stoeckle, E.; Rutkowski, P.; et al. Preoperative radiotherapy plus surgery versus surgery alone for patients with primary retroperitoneal sarcoma (EORTC-62092: STRASS): A multicentre, open-label, randomised, phase 3 trial. *Lancet Oncol.* **2020**, *21*, 1366–1377. [CrossRef]
7. Callegaro, D.; Raut, C.P.; Ajayi, T.; Strauss, D.; Bonvalot, S.; Ng, D.; Stoeckle, E.; Fairweather, M.; Rutkowski, P.; van Houdt, W.J.; et al. Preoperative Radiotherapy in Patients With Primary Retroperitoneal Sarcoma: EORTC-62092 Trial (STRASS) Versus Off-trial (STREXIT) Results. *Ann. Surg.* **2022**, *2022*, 10–97. [CrossRef]
8. DeLaney, T.F.; Chen, Y.-L.; Baldini, E.H.; Wang, D.; Adams, J.; Hickey, S.B.; Yeap, B.Y.; Hahn, S.M.; De Amorim Bernstein, K.; Nielsen, G.P.; et al. Phase 1 trial of preoperative image guided intensity modulated proton radiation therapy with simultaneously integrated boost to the high risk margin for retroperitoneal sarcomas. *Adv. Radiat. Oncol.* **2017**, *2*, 85–93. [CrossRef]
9. Roeder, F.; Ulrich, A.; Habl, G.; Uhl, M.; Saleh-Ebrahimi, L.; Huber, P.E.; Schulz-Ertner, D.; Nikoghosyan, A.V.; Alldinger, I.; Krempien, R.; et al. Clinical phase I/II trial to investigate preoperative dose-escalated intensity-modulated radiation therapy (IMRT) and intraoperative radiation therapy (IORT) in patients with retroperitoneal soft tissue sarcoma: Interim analysis. *BMC Cancer* **2014**, *14*, 617. [CrossRef]
10. Roeder, F.; Schulz-Ertner, D.; Nikoghosyan, A.V.; Huber, P.E.; Edler, L.; Habl, G.; Krempien, R.; Oertel, S.; Saleh-Ebrahimi, L.; Hensley, F.W.; et al. A clinical phase I/II trial to investigate preoperative dose-escalated intensity-modulated radiation therapy (IMRT) and intraoperative radiation therapy (IORT) in patients with retroperitoneal soft tissue sarcoma. *BMC Cancer* **2012**, *12*, 287. [CrossRef]
11. Bonvalot, S.; Rivoire, M.; Castaing, M.; Stoeckle, E.; Le Cesne, A.; Blay, J.Y.; Laplanche, A. Primary retroperitoneal sarcomas: A multivariate analysis of surgical factors associated with local control. *J. Clin. Oncol. Off. J. Am. Soc. Clin. Oncol.* **2009**, *27*, 31–37. [CrossRef] [PubMed]

12. Le Péchoux, C.; Musat, E.; Baey, C.; Al Mokhles, H.; Terrier, P.; Domont, J.; Le Cesne, A.; Laplanche, A.; Bonvalot, S. Should adjuvant radiotherapy be administered in addition to front-line aggressive surgery (FAS) in patients with primary retroperitoneal sarcoma? *Ann. Oncol. Off. J. Eur. Soc. Med. Oncol.* **2013**, *24*, 832–837. [CrossRef]
13. Kelly, K.J.; Yoon, S.S.; Kuk, D.; Qin, L.X.; Dukleska, K.; Chang, K.K.; Chen, Y.L.; Delaney, T.F.; Brennan, M.F.; Singer, S. Comparison of Perioperative Radiation Therapy and Surgery Versus Surgery Alone in 204 Patients With Primary Retroperitoneal Sarcoma: A Retrospective 2-Institution Study. *Ann. Surg.* **2015**, *262*, 156–162. [CrossRef] [PubMed]
14. Gronchi, A.; Lo Vullo, S.; Fiore, M.; Mussi, C.; Stacchiotti, S.; Collini, P.; Lozza, L.; Pennacchioli, E.; Mariani, L.; Casali, P.G. Aggressive surgical policies in a retrospectively reviewed single-institution case series of retroperitoneal soft tissue sarcoma patients. *J. Clin. Oncol. Off. J. Am. Soc. Clin. Oncol.* **2009**, *27*, 24–30. [CrossRef] [PubMed]
15. Gronchi, A.; Miceli, R.; Colombo, C.; Stacchiotti, S.; Collini, P.; Mariani, L.; Sangalli, C.; Radaelli, S.; Sanfilippo, R.; Fiore, M.; et al. Frontline extended surgery is associated with improved survival in retroperitoneal low- to intermediate-grade soft tissue sarcomas. *Ann. Oncol. Off. J. Eur. Soc. Med. Oncol.* **2012**, *23*, 1067–1073. [CrossRef]
16. Kirane, A.; Crago, A.M. The importance of surgical margins in retroperitoneal sarcoma. *J. Surg. Oncol.* **2016**, *113*, 270–276. [CrossRef]
17. Toulmonde, M.; Le Cesne, A.; Mendiboure, J.; Blay, J.Y.; Piperno-Neumann, S.; Chevreau, C.; Delcambre, C.; Penel, N.; Terrier, P.; Ranchère-Vince, D.; et al. Long-term recurrence of soft tissue sarcomas: Prognostic factors and implications for prolonged follow-up. *Cancer* **2014**, *120*, 3003–3006. [CrossRef]
18. Petersen, I.A.; Haddock, M.G.; Donohue, J.H.; Nagorney, D.M.; Grill, J.P.; Sargent, D.J.; Gunderson, L.L. Use of intraoperative electron beam radiotherapy in the management of retroperitoneal soft tissue sarcomas. *Int. J. Radiat. Oncol. Biol. Phys.* **2002**, *52*, 469–475. [CrossRef]
19. Krempien, R.; Roeder, F.; Oertel, S.; Weitz, J.; Hensley, F.W.; Timke, C.; Funk, A.; Lindel, K.; Harms, W.; Buchler, M.W.; et al. Intraoperative electron-beam therapy for primary and recurrent retroperitoneal soft-tissue sarcoma. *Int. J. Radiat. Oncol. Biol. Phys.* **2006**, *65*, 773–779. [CrossRef]
20. Roeder, F.; Morillo, V.; Saleh-Ebrahimi, L.; Calvo, F.A.; Poortmans, P.; Ferrer Albiach, C. Intraoperative radiation therapy (IORT) for soft tissue sarcoma—ESTRO IORT Task Force/ACROP recommendations. *Radiother. Oncol.* **2020**, *150*, 293–302. [CrossRef]
21. Sindelar, W.F.; Kinsella, T.J.; Chen, P.W.; DeLaney, T.F.; Tepper, J.E.; Rosenberg, S.A.; Glatstein, E. Intraoperative Radiotherapy in Retroperitoneal Sarcomas: Final Results of a Prospective, Randomized, Clinical Trial. *Arch. Surg.* **1993**, *128*, 402–410. [CrossRef] [PubMed]
22. Baldini, E.H.; Bosch, W.; Kane, J.M., 3rd; Abrams, R.A.; Salerno, K.E.; Deville, C.; Raut, C.P.; Petersen, I.A.; Chen, Y.L.; Mullen, J.T.; et al. Retroperitoneal sarcoma (RPS) high risk gross tumor volume boost (HR GTV boost) contour delineation agreement among NRG sarcoma radiation and surgical oncologists. *Ann. Surg. Oncol.* **2015**, *22*, 2846–2852. [CrossRef]
23. Chung, C.; Trofimov, A.; Adams, J.; Kung, J.; Kirsch, D.G.; Yoon, S.; Doppke, K.; Bortfeld, T.; Delaney, T.F. Comparison of 3D Conformal Proton Therapy, Intensity-Modulated Proton Therapy, and Intensity-Modulated Photon Therapy for Retroperitoneal Sarcoma. *Sarcoma* **2022**, *2022*, 5540615. [CrossRef] [PubMed]
24. Koseła-Paterczyk, H.; Szacht, M.; Morysiński, T.; Ługowska, I.; Dziewirski, W.; Falkowski, S.; Zdzienicki, M.; Pieńkowski, A.; Szamotulska, K.; Świtaj, T.; et al. Preoperative hypofractionated radiotherapy in the treatment of localized soft tissue sarcomas. *Eur. J. Surg. Oncol.* **2014**, *40*, 1641–1647. [CrossRef] [PubMed]
25. Pennington, J.D.; Eilber, F.C.; Eilber, F.R.; Singh, A.S.; Reed, J.P.; Chmielowski, B.; Eckardt, J.J.; Bukata, S.V.; Bernthal, N.M.; Federman, N.; et al. Long-term Outcomes With Ifosfamide-based Hypofractionated Preoperative Chemoradiotherapy for Extremity Soft Tissue Sarcomas. *Am. J. Clin. Oncol.* **2018**, *41*, 1154–1161. [CrossRef]
26. Valle, L.F.; Bernthal, N.; Eilber, F.C.; Shabason, J.E.; Bedi, M.; Kalbasi, A. Evaluating Thresholds to Adopt Hypofractionated Preoperative Radiotherapy as Standard of Care in Sarcoma. *Sarcoma* **2021**, *2021*, 3735874. [CrossRef] [PubMed]
27. Santos, A.; Penfold, S.; Gorayski, P.; Le, H. The Role of Hypofractionation in Proton Therapy. *Cancers* **2022**, *14*, 2271. [CrossRef]
28. Brügemann, D.; Lehner, B.; Kieser, M.; Krisam, J.; Hommertgen, A.; Jaekel, C.; Harrabi, S.B.; Herfarth, K.; Mechtesheimer, G.; Sedlaczek, O.; et al. Neoadjuvant irradiation of extremity soft tissue sarcoma with ions (Extrem-ion): Study protocol for a randomized phase II pilot trial. *BMC Cancer* **2022**, *22*, 538. [CrossRef] [PubMed]
29. Seidensaal, K.; Kieser, M.; Hommertgen, A.; Jaekel, C.; Harrabi, S.B.; Herfarth, K.; Mechtesheimer, G.; Lehner, B.; Schneider, M.; Nienhueser, H.; et al. Neoadjuvant irradiation of retroperitoneal soft tissue sarcoma with ions (Retro-Ion): Study protocol for a randomized phase II pilot trial. *Trials* **2021**, *22*, 134. [CrossRef]

Disclaimer/Publisher's Note: The statements, opinions and data contained in all publications are solely those of the individual author(s) and contributor(s) and not of MDPI and/or the editor(s). MDPI and/or the editor(s) disclaim responsibility for any injury to people or property resulting from any ideas, methods, instructions or products referred to in the content.

MDPI
St. Alban-Anlage 66
4052 Basel
Switzerland
www.mdpi.com

MDPI Books Editorial Office
E-mail: books@mdpi.com
www.mdpi.com/books

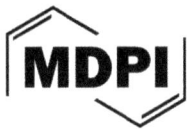

Disclaimer/Publisher's Note: The statements, opinions and data contained in all publications are solely those of the individual author(s) and contributor(s) and not of MDPI and/or the editor(s). MDPI and/or the editor(s) disclaim responsibility for any injury to people or property resulting from any ideas, methods, instructions or products referred to in the content.

www.ingramcontent.com/pod-product-compliance
Lightning Source LLC
LaVergne TN
LVHW070444100526
838202LV00014B/1665